Nov' 84

EMERGING DIMENSIONS
OF SEXOLOGY

Sexual Medicine, Volume 2
HAROLD I. LIEF, M.D., SERIES EDITOR

OTHER VOLUMES IN THE SERIES

Lief and Hoch: **International Research in Sexology, 1984**
Selected Papers from the Fifth World Congress

EMERGING DIMENSIONS OF SEXOLOGY

Selected Papers from the Proceedings of the Sixth World Congress of Sexology

Edited by

R. Taylor Segraves, M.D., Ph.D.
and Erwin J. Haeberle, Ph.D., Ed.D.

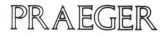

PRAEGER SPECIAL STUDIES • PRAEGER SCIENTIFIC

New York • Philadelphia • Eastbourne, UK
Toronto • Hong Kong • Tokyo • Sydney

Library of Congress Cataloging in Publication Data

World congress of Sexology (6th : 1983 : Washington, D.C.)
    Emerging dimensions of sexology.

    (Sexual Medicine ; v. 2)
    Includes bibliographies and index.
    1. Sexual disorders—Congresses. 2. Sex—Congresses.
I. Segraves, R. Taylor, 1941- . II. Haeberle, Erwin J.
III. Title. IV. Series. (DNLM: 1. Sex—Congresses.
2. Sex disorders—Therapy—Congresses. W1 SE99F v.2 /
HQ 21)
RC556.W67   1983   616.6'9   83-26890
ISBN 0-03-064006-7 (alk. paper)

Published in 1984 by Praeger Publishers
CBS Educational and Professional Publishers
a Division of CBS, Inc.
521 Fifth Avenue, New York, New York 10175, U.S.A.

456789 052 987654321
Printed in the United States of America
on acid-free paper

Foreword

The pioneers in sex research and education—Magnus Hirschfeld in Germany, and Alfred Kinsey, William Masters, Virginia Johnson, and Mary Calderone in the United States, for example—have been on the receiving end of abuse and vilification as if, through investigating and explaining our sexual natures, they were perverted purveyors of smut. Sigmund Freud was not excluded from this prejudice. When Freud's theories were being propounded at a medical society meeting in Hamburg in 1910, a distinguished medical professor banged his fist on the table and shouted, "This is not a topic for discussion at a scientific meeting; it is a matter for the police" [1]. In 1900, for similar reasons, the editor of the *Journal of the American Medical Association* refused to publish a paper by Denslow Lewis, a distinguished Chicago gynecologist, entitled "The Gynecologic Consideration of the Sexual Act." Eighty years later, the *JAMA* acknowledged the original error in judgment and published it as a "Delayed Communication" [2].

The world congresses of sexology are but one indication that the attitudes of the public, certainly of the professional public, have become far more accepting. It seems strange to have had to justify for at least a century that our sexual nature was a legitimate subject for scientific investigation and scrutiny. Yet it is only now that the field of sexology (sexual matters cannot be restricted to one particular discipline or area of inquiry, hence the term "sexology," implying its broad base in medicine and the behavioral sciences as well as the arts and humanities, including law) is gaining recognition as a discipline in its own right.

The papers from the 6th World Congress of Sexology (the first in the United States) form the content of this volume. They have been admirably edited by R. Taylor Segraves and Erwin J. Haeberle, who indicate in their introduction the accelerating body of knowledge that gives us hope that with the passage of time the mysteries and intricacies of the sexual aspects of our personalities may become ever more comprehensible. I welcome this volume to the series on "Sexual Medicine" of which I am general editor.

—Harold I. Lief, M.D.
Philadelphia, Pennsylvania
December 1983

NOTES

1. Jones, E. *The Life and Work of Sigmund Freud,* Volume 2. New York: Basic Books, 1955, 109.

2. Lewis, D. The Gynecologic Consideration of the Sexual Act, *Journal of the American Medical Association,* 1983, 250:222.

Preface

This publication consists of representative papers from the proceedings of the Sixth World Congress in Sexology held in Washington, D.C., May 22–27, 1983. The congress was sponsored by the World Association for Sexology and organized by the United States Consortium for Sexology. The United States Consortium for Sexology is made up of representatives from sexological organizations in the United States who are members of the World Association for Sexology. These sponsoring organizations include the Akron Sex Forum, the American Association of Sex Educators, Counselors and Therapists (AASECT), the Institute for Advanced Study of Human Sexuality, the Sex Information and Education Council of the United States (SIECUS), the Society for Sex Therapy and Research (SSTAR), and The Association of Sexologists (TAOS).

The selection of papers in this volume was organized to permit a wide sampling of researchers working in areas of significance to the future of sex research. Similarly, the titles of papers included in this volume indicate the co-editors' conviction that the advancement of knowledge in human sexuality requires a multidisciplinary and multinational collaborative effort. We regret that space limitations did not allow inclusion of all presentations at the World Congress.

Acknowledgements

Special acknowledgements are due to various individuals who made the Sixth World Congress of Sexology possible. Without their active participation, this congress could not have occurred. These individuals and their roles in the congress are listed below.

World Association for Sexology

President: Gilbert Tordjman, M.D.   France
Secretary-General: Fernando J. Bianco, M.D.   Venezuela
Vice-President: Zwi Hoch, M.D.   Israel

Sixth World Congress—Honorary Presidents

Mary S. Calderone, M.D., M.P.H.   New York
Harold Lief, M.D.   Philadelphia
Wardell Pomeroy, Ph.D.   San Francisco

Contents

List of Contributors

Pierre Alarie, M.D.
  Groupe de Recherche Clinique, Université du Quebec à
  Montréal, Montréal, Canada

Bernard Apfelbaum, Ph.D.
  Berkeley Sex Therapy Group, Oakland, California

John Bancroft, M.D.
  MRC Reproductive Biology Unit, Edinburgh, Scotland

G. F. Baraghini, M.D.
  Department of Endocrinology and Physiology, University
  of Modena, Modena, Italy

Edouard Beltrami, M.D., F.R.C.P.
  Groupe de Recherche Clinique, Université du Quebec à
  Montréal, Montréal, Canada

Charles Blake, M.D.
  University of Nebraska Medical Center, 602 South 45th
  Street, Omaha, Nebraska

Ernest Borneman, Ph.D.
  A-4612 Scharten, Austria

F. Borruto, M.D.
  Institute of Clinical Obstetrics and Gynecology,
  University of Verona, Verona, Italy

Deryck Calderwood, Ph.D.
  Director, Human Sexuality Program, New York
  University, New York, New York

Gabriella Bravi Cantoni, M.D.
  Department of Psychiatry, University of Brescia,
  Brescia, Italy

C. Carani, M.D.
  Department of Endocrinology and Physiology, University
  of Modena, Modena, Italy

M. F. Celani, M.D.
Department of Endocrinology and Physiology, University
of Modena, Modena, Italy

Sven Daelemans, Ph.D.
Institute for Family and Sexuality Research, Catholic
University of Leuven, Groot Park 3, B-3042, Lovenjoel,
Belgium

Marian E. Dunn, Ph.D.
Center for Human Sexuality, SUNY, Downstate Medical
Center, Brooklyn, New York

Wolf Eicher, M.D.
Faculty of Medicine, University of Mannheim,
Diakonissenkrankenhaus, Mannheim, Germany

Charles Fisher, M.D., Ph.D.
Department of Psychiatry, Mount Sinai School of
Medicine, New York, New York

Joseph Gartner, M.D.
University of Nebraska Medical Center, 602 South 45th
Street, Omaha, Nebraska

Kenneth D. George, Ph.D.
Human Sexuality Program, University of Pennsylvania,
Philadelphia, Pennsylvania

Octavio Giraldo-Neira, Ph.D.
Department of Psychology, Universidad del Valle,
Apartado Aereo 25360, Cali, Colombia

Andrew Glover, Ph.D.
Department of Psychiatry, Mt. Sinai School of Medicine,
New York, New York

Juliette Goldman, Ph.D.
La Trobe University, Bundoora 3083, Melbourne,
Australia

Ronald Goldman, Ph.D.
La Trobe University, Bundoora 3083, Melbourne,
Australia

Bernard Goldstein, Ph.D.
Human Sexuality Studies Program, San Francisco State
University, 1600 Holloway Avenue, San Francisco,
California

Benjamin Graber, M.D.
    University of Nebraska Medical Center, 602 South 45th
    Street, Omaha, Nebraska

N. Grafeille, M.D.
    Hospital Saint-André, 1 rue Jean Burquet, 33075
    Bordeaux-Cedex

Erwin J. Haeberle, Ph.D., Ed.D.
    Institute for Advanced Study of Human Sexuality,
    1523 Franklin Street, San Francisco, California

J. C. Joutard, M.D.
    Centre Psychotherapique Departemental, BP 12–84140,
    Montfavet

Simi Kelley-Linton
    Coalition of Sexuality and Disability, New York,
    New York

Aziz Ahmed Khattab, M.D.
    Department of Clinical Pathology, Ain Shams University
    Medical School, Cairo, Egypt

E. W. Klimowsky, Ph.D.
    Tel-Aviv, Israel

Dennis J. Krauss, M.D.
    VA Medical Center, 800 Irving Avenue, Syracuse,
    New York

Wolfgang Kröhn, M.D.
    Sexualmedizinische Forschungs-und Beratungsstelle,
    Universität Kiel, Hospitalstrasse 17/19, 2300 Kiel,
    West Germany

Hans Lehfeldt, M.D.
    26 East 93rd Street, New York, New York

Joseph Josy Levy, Ph.D.
    Head, Department of Sexology, Université du Québec à
    Montréal, Montréal, Canada

Bengt Lundström, M.D., Ph.D.
    St. Jörgen's Hospital, S-422 03 Hisings Backa, Sweden

Maureen Luyens, Ph.D.
    Institute for Family and Sexuality Research, Catholic
    University of Leuven, Lovenjoel, Belgium

Francesca Maggiorano, Ph.D.
  I Cattedra di Psicologia Fisiologica, Universita di Roma,
  Rome, Italy

Fausto Manara, M.D.
  Department of Psychiatry, University of Brescia,
  Brescia, Italy

Augustinus Marlinata, M.D.
  School of Medicine, Airlangga University, Surabaya,
  Indonesia

P. Marrama, M.D.
  Department of Endocrinology and Physiology, University
  of Modena, Modena, Italy

Shinobu Miyahara, M.D., M.P.H.
  Department of Maternal and Child Health, Faculty of
  Medicine, University of Tokyo, Tokyo, Japan

John Money, Ph.D.
  Department of Psychiatry, John Hopkins University,
  Baltimore, Maryland

V. Montamini, M.D.
  Department of Endocrinology and Physiology, University
  of Modena, Modena, Italy

Herman Musaph, M.D., F.R.C.
  Professor of Medical Sexology, University of Utrecht,
  Utrecht, Netherlands

Sharon G. Nathan, Ph.D., M.P.H.
  Department of Psychiatry, Cornell University Medical
  College, New York, New York

Piet Nijs, M.D.
  Department of Obstetrics/Gynecology, University
  Hospital, Lueven, Belgium

Giuseppe Pascale, Ph.D.
  I Cattedra dr Psicologia Fisiologica, Universita di Roma,
  Rome, Italy

R. M. Pederzini, M.D.
  Department of Psychiatry, University of Parma, Parma,
  Italy

Michael A. Perelman, Ph.D.
  Department of Psychiatry, New York Hospital—Cornell
  Medical Center, New York, New York

Wardell B. Pomeroy, Ph.D.
  Academic Dean, Institute for Advanced Study of Human
  Sexuality, San Francisco, California

Michael Quadland, Ph.D.
  Department of Psychiatry, Mt. Sinai School of Medicine,
  New York, New York

June Machover Reinisch, Ph.D.
  Director, Kinsey Institute for Research in Sex, Gender,
  and Reproduction, Indiana University, Bloomington,
  Indiana

Harilyn Rousso, ACSW
  Disabilities Unlimited Counseling Services, New York,
  New York

A. Ruffie, M.D.
  Université De Bordeaux II, 146 Rue Leo Saignat, 33076
  Bordeaux-Cedex

Raul C. Schiavi, M.D.
  Department of Psychiatry, Mount Sinai School of
  Medicine, New York, New York

John Schipke, M.D.
  Department of Psychiatry, University of Chicago,
  Chicago, Illinois

Kathleen Blindt Segraves, M.A.
  Department of Psychiatry, University of Chicago,
  Chicago, Illinois

Chiara Simonelli, Ph.D.
  I Cattedra di Psicologia Fisiologica, Universita di Roma,
  Rome, Italy

Gilbert Tordjman, M.D.
  Paris 21 Brd Brune 75014, Paris, France

A. Tridenti, M.D.
  Department of Psychiatry, University of Parma, Parma,
  Italy

Alfons Vansteenwegen, Ph.D.
Institute for Family and Sexuality Research, Catholic
University of Leuven, Groot Park 3 B-3042, Lovenjoel,
Belgium

G. Vecchietti, M.D.
Institute of Clinical Obstetrics and Gynecology,
University of Verona, Verona, Italy

Riccardo Venturini, Ph.D.
I Cattedra di Psicologia Fisiologica, Universita di Roma,
Rome, Italy

Alan J. Wabrek, M.D.
Hartford Hospital, Hartford, Connecticut

Gorm Wagner, M.D.
Panum Institute, University of Copenhagen, Copenhagen,
Denmark

John Wålinder, M.D., Ph.D.
Linköping University, Department of Psychiatry, S-581
85 Linköping, Sweden

Reinhard Wille, M.D.
Sexualmedizinische Forschungs-und Beratungsstelle,
Hospitalstrasse 17/19, Universität Kiel, 2300 Kiel,
West Germany

James E. Wilson, Pharm, D.
University of Nebraska Medical Center, 602 South 45th
Street, Omaha, Nebraska

D. Zini, M.D.
Department of Endocrinology and Physiology, University
of Modena, Modena, Italy

Committees and Sponsors

ORGANIZING COMMITTEE

Richard Bennett, M.D., Ph.D. (Akron)
Oliver Bjorksten, M.D. (Charleston)
Michael Carrera, Ed.D. (New York)
Robert Dickes, M.D. (New York)
Lewis Durham, Mth, Ed.D. (San Francisco)
Thomas Gertz, MHS (Akron)
William Granzig, M.D. (Washington, D.C.)
Loretta Haroian, Ph.D. (Fresno)
Mickey Apter-Marsh, Ph.D. (Oakland)
Robert McIvenna, MDIV, Ph.D. (San Francisco)
Alan Wabrek, M.D. (Hartford)
Ann Welbourne, RN, Ph.D. (Stony Brook)
Shirley Zussman, Ed.D. (New York)

INTERNATIONAL SCIENTIFIC COMMITTEE

Co-Chairmen

Erwin J. Haeberle, Ph.D., Ed.D. (San Francisco)
R. Taylor Segraves, M.D., Ph.D. (Chicago)

Members

Georges Abraham, M.D., Ph.D. (Geneva, Switzerland)
Sally Binford, Ph.D. (Paia, Hawaii)
Ernest Borneman, Ph.D. (Scharten, Austria)
Vern Bullough, Ph.D. (Buffalo)
Michael Carrera, Ed.D. (New York)
Dudley Chapman, D.O. (North Madison, Ohio)
Larry Constantine, LCSW (Acton, MA)
Susan Daniels, Ph.D. (New Orleans)
Clive Davis, Ph.D. (Syracuse)
John De Cecco, Ph.D. (San Francisco)
Milton Diamond, Ph.D. (Honolulu)
Wolf Eicher, M.D. (Munich, Germany)
Anke Erhardt, Ph.D. (New York)

Albert Ellis, Ph.D. (New York)
H. J. Eysenck, Ph.D. (London, England)
Robert Francoeur, Ph.D. (Rockaway, NJ)
Jos Frenken, Ph.D. (Zeist, Netherlands)
John Gagnon, Ph.D. (Stony Brook)
Paul Gebhard, Ph.D. (Bloomington)
Robert Gemme, Ph.D. (Montreal, Canada)
Harvey Gochros, DSW (Honolulu)
Richard Green, M.D. (Stony Brook)
William Hartman, Ph.D. (Long Beach)
Preben Hertoft, M.D. (Copenhagen, Denmark)
Evelyn Hooker, Ph.D. (Santa Monica)
Kazimierz Imielinski, M.D. (Warsaw, Poland)
James Jones, Ph.D. (Houston)
Thomas Jones, M.D. (Chicago)
Phyllis Katz (Boulder)
Lester Kirkendall, Ph.D. (Portland)
Robert Kolodny, M.D. (St. Louis)
Carol Lassen, Ph.D. (Denver)
Steven Levine, M.D. (Cleveland)
Brian McNaught (Brookline, MA)
David McWhirter, M.D. (San Diego)
Heino Meyer-Bahlburg, M.D. (New York)
Howard Moltz, Ph.D. (Chicago)
Herman Musaph, M.D. (Utrecht, Netherlands)
Piet Nijs, M.D. (Leuven, Belgium)
Willy Pasini, M.D. (Geneva, Switzerland)
Jan Raboch, DSc (Prague, Czechoslovakia)
James Ramey, Ph.D. (New York)
Ira Reiss, Ph.D. (Minneapolis)
Leah Schaefer, Ed.D. (New York)
Raul Schiavi, M.D. (New York)
Harry Schoenberg, M.D. (Chicago)
Dorothy Strauss, Ph.D. (Brooklyn)
Gilbert Tordjman, M.D. (Paris, France)
Pierre Vallay, M.D. (Paris, France)
Gerald Valle, M.D. (Paris, France)
Gorm Wagner, M.D. (Copenhagen, Denmark)
Maj-Briht Bergström-Walan, Ph.D. (Stockholm, Sweden)
Paul Walker, Ph.D. (San Francisco)
Peter Webb, M.A. (London, England)
James Weinrich, Ph.D. (Baltimore)
Reinhard Wille, M.D. (Kiel, Germany)
Mildred Hope Witkin, Ph.D. (New York)

INTRODUCTION

Sex Therapy and Research: Current Status

R. T. Segraves and E. J. Haeberle

The Proceedings of the Sixth World Congress of Sexology document that sexology is beginning to evolve as a respectable field of scientific inquiry. One can clearly see the rudiments of a growing data base and the striving for an acceptable methodology within this multidisciplinary field. As Gagnon [1] has emphasized, the history of scientific sex research is difficult to separate completely from the social context of sexual ideologies. It is only in the last century that serious investigators have begun to study sexual behavior. Cultural attitudes have influenced the scientific community, and with a few notable exceptions, only recently have highly qualified and established investigators entered the field of sexology. As Yolles [2] points out, similar situations existed in the early investigations of drug and alcohol abuse and even in psychotherapy research. It is comparatively recently that serious investigators and clinicians could specialize in this area of inquiry without compromising their professional careers or losing the respect of colleagues. Contemporary investigators, of course, owe a tremendous debt to the courageous and pioneering work of the pioneers who began to establish human sexuality as a legitimate area of inquiry. All of us in the field owe a tremendous debt to pioneers such as Iwan Bloch, Sigmund Freud, Magnus Hirschfeld, Havelock Ellis, Alfred C. Kinsey, and William Masters. The recent interest of biomedical investigators in sexology may be, in part, the result of the legitimization of sexology by the addition of courses in human sexuality to the standard medical school curriculum [3,4].

1

The readers of this text, of course, do not need to be reminded how important it is for the investigation of human sexuality to come out of the closet. Serious investigators can now begin to dare choose sexology as a legitimate area of specialization without necessarily compromising their careers. The implicit philosophy of the scientific community has always been that the merit of any academic or scientific pursuit should be assessed by the academic rigor or scientific methodology utilized and not by the social acceptability of the object of study.

It is ironic that a byproduct of past social taboos against the investigation of human sexuality may be the current close association between clinical research and practice. So much basic information concerning human sexuality is lacking that academic clinicians are doing basic research in order to gain knowledge related to their practices. This model of combined clinical practice and research, of course, was set by Masters and Johnson and is currently exemplified by John Bancroft, Raul Schiavi, and many others. The importance of basic research being done by practitioners cannot be overemphasized. In other areas, such as psychotherapy research, clinical research has had minimal influence on practitioners [5,6]. This dichotomy between clinical research and practice means that practitioners, the appropriate consumers of psychotherapy research, have felt that much of psychotherapy research has been irrelevant to the practice of psychotherapy. We hope that such a schism will not occur in our burgeoning field.

RECENT GAINS IN KNOWLEDGE

Clinician-practitioners are beginning to build a data base concerning the prevalence and natural history of sexual disorders in the general population [7,8]. Epidemiological studies have indicated that sexual dysfunction is quite common in the general population (approximately 50 percent in some studies). Similarly, sexual problems have been found to occur with a high frequency in the medical population [9]. This is especially true of disorders such as multiple sclerosis [10], renal failure [11], and diabetes mellitus [12]. Similarly, the pharmacological side-effects of many drugs, including hypotensive agents, on sexual functioning is beginning to be appreciated [13]. Clinicians will not be surprised to learn that approximately one-half of physician referrals to sex therapists are not completed [14] and that recent research has indicated that the spontaneous remission rates of some sexual disorders is quite low [15].

The last decade has witnessed a growth in practical research related to the treatment of sexual disorders. Efforts have begun to isolate both patient [16] and treatment variables [17] which are related to clinical outcome. Controlled outcome studies have indicated that behavioral sex therapy is effective for some disorders such as anorgasmia [18] and not for other disorders such as erectile problems [19]. Other research has indicated that a high relapse rate may be common in some sexual disorders after successful treatment [20]. In this research, one sees the beginning of an effort to specify which subgroups of patients will respond to standard treatment approaches. Such knowledge will, of course, lead to clinical innovation.

One of the most exciting new areas of sex research concerns the biological factors involved in sexual desire and behavior. Most of these advances have been in the understanding of erectile function. A considerable technology including nocturnal penile tumescence studies, pudendal nerve conduction studies, investigation of pelvic and penile blood flow, and complex endocrinological investigations have become standard procedures in many sexual dysfunction centers [21]. Again, clinicians aware of the limited state of current knowledge have conducted basic investigations concerning the neurologic and vascular mechanisms involved in the human sexual response cycle.

An exciting byproduct of biological diagnostic evaluation has been the realization that it is often impossible to dichotomize the etiology of sexual complaints as either organic or psychogenic. In many cases, appropriate clinical management requires that sexual function be considered as resulting from a complicated interplay of biological and psychological factors. Sexual function clearly interfaces with numerous biological, psychological, and sociological influences. This realization emphasizes the necessity of sexology being truly a multidisciplinary field.

NEED FOR FUTURE RESEARCH

In spite of significant advances in the field, the potential for future advances in our understanding of human sexuality is almost limitless. Male sexual function has been investigated far more than female sexual function and behavior. Realizing this, it is sobering to realize that cerebral structures mediating sexual arousal and erection are virtually uninvestigated in the human [22]. It is unclear whether penile erection is mediated by peripheral acetylcholine pathways or whether adrenergic fibers [23] play a significant role. The vascular mechanisms involved are unclear. The role of venous constriction in erection is unclear [24], and the previously accepted fact of penile "polsters" redistributing blood flow to produce erections has been questioned [25]. These findings assume clinical significance when one begins to evaluate patients for the etiology of their complaints. The lack of reliable information concerning the physiology of the human sexual response severely hampers the delineation of causative factors in sexual dysfunction.

OVERVIEW OF TEXT

A representative selection of papers from the proceedings of the Sixth World Congress are organized into eight major sections. The first section concerns the history of the sexology movement, and the second section deals with the investigation of childhood sexuality. The next few sections concern treatment and include sections on diagnostic evaluation, psychotherapy, surgical and medical interventions. The seventh section has been named "transcultural" and includes papers reflective of sexuality in specific cultures. The last section is included for papers which do not logically fit any of the previous headings.

NOTES

1. Gagnon, J. H. Sex research and social change. *Archives of Sexual Behavior,* 1975, 4:111–41.

2. Yolles, S. F. Opening address. *Archives of Sexual Behavior,* 1975, 4:323–28.

3. Calderone, M. S. "Historical perspectives on the human sexuality movement: Hindsights, insights, foresights." In: N. Rosenzweig, and F. P. Pearsall (eds.) *Sex Education for the Health Professional: A curriculum guide,* 7–21. New York: Grune and Stratton, 1978.

4. Lief, H. I. "Sex education in medicine: Retrospect and prospect." In: N. Rosenzweig, and F. P. Pearsall (eds.) *Sex Education for the Health Professional: A curriculum guide,* 23–361. New York: Grune and Stratton, 1978.

5. Stupp, H. Psychotherapy research and practice: An overview. In: S. L. Garfield, and A. E. Bergin (eds.) *Handbook of Psychotherapy and Behavior Change: An empirical analysis,* 3–22. New York: John Wiley & Sons, 1978.

6. Segraves, R. T. *Marital Therapy: A Combined Psychodynamic-behavioral Model*. New York: Plenum Press, 1982.

7. Frank, E., C. Anderson, and D. Rubinstein. Frequency of sexual dysfunction in normal couples. *New England Journal of Medicine,* 1978, 229:111–15.

8. Nettelbladt, P., and N. Uddenberg. Sexual dysfunction and sexual satisfaction in 58 married Swedish men. *Journal of Psychosomatic Research,* 1979, 23:141–47.

9. Slag, M. F., J. E. Morley, M. K. Elson, D. L. Trence, C. J. Nelson, A. E. Nelson, W. B., Kinlaw, H. S. Beyer, F. G. Nuttall, and R. B. Shafer. Impotence in medical clinic outpatients. *Journal of the American Medical Association,* 1983, 249:1736–40.

10. Lilius, H., E. Valtonen, and J. Wilkstrom. Sexual problems in patients suffering from multiple sclerosis. *Journal of Chronic Diseases,* 1976, 29: 643–47.

11. Abram, H. S., L. R. Hester, and W. F. Sheridan. Sexual functioning in patients with chronic renal failure. *Journal of Nervous and Mental Diseases,* 1975, 160:220–26.

12. Karacan, I., P. J. Salis, J. C. Ware, B. Dervent, R. L. Williams, F. B. Scott, S. L. Attia, and L. E. Beutler. Nocturnal penile tumescence and diagnosis in diabetic impotence. *American Journal of Psychiatry,* 1978, 135:191–97.

13. Segraves, R. T. Pharmacological agents causing sexual dysfunction. *Journal of Sex and Marital Therapy,* 1973, 3:157:76.

14. Segraves, R. T., H. W. Schoenberg, C. K. Zarins, P. Camic, and J. Knopf. Characteristics of erectile dysfunction as a function of medical care system entry point. *Psychosomatic Medicine,* 1981, 43:227–34.

15. Segraves, R. T., J. Knopf, and P. Camic. Spontaneous remission in erectile impotence. *Behavior Research and Therapy,* 1982, 20:89–91.

16. Cooper, A. J. Disorders of sexual potency in the male: A clinical and statistical study of some factors related to short-term prognosis. *British Journal of Psychiatry,* 1969, 115:709–19.

17. LoPiccolo, J. "Effects of variation in format on sex therapy outcome." Read at annual meeting of Society for Sex Therapy and Research, Charleston, SC, May, 1982.

18. Riley, A. J. and E. J. Riley. A controlled study to evaluate directed masturbation in the management of primary orgasmic failure in women. *British Journal of Psychiatry,* 1978, 133:404–09.

19. Ansari, J. Impotence prognosis (a controlled study). *British Journal of Psychiatry,* 1978, 128:194–98.

20. Levine, S. B. and D. Agle. The effectiveness of sex therapy for chronic secondary psychological impotence. *Journal Sex and Marital Therapy,* 1978, 4:235–38.

21. Segraves, R. T. and H. W. Schoenberg. Evaluation of the etiology of erectile failure. In: R. T. Segraves, and H. W. Schoenberg (eds.) *Erectile Impotence.* New York: Plenum Press, 1983.

22. Leiter, E. Causes of erectile dysfunction. *Sexuality and Disability,* 1981, 4:80–85.

23. Benson, G. S., J. A. McConnell, L. I. Lipschultz, J. N. Corriene, and J. Wood. Neuromorphology and neuropharmacology of the human penis. *Journal of Clinical Investigation,* 1980, 65:506–13.

24. Krane, R. J. and M. B. Siroky. Neurophysiology of erection. *Urologic Clinics of North America,* 1981, 8:91–102.

25. Benson, G. S., J. A. McConnell, and W. A. Schmitt. Penile polsters: Functional structures or atherosclerosis changes? *Journal of Urology,* 1981, 125, 800–03.

PART I

History of Sexology

Most American investigators are aware of the early research efforts of Alfred C. Kinsey and colleagues and of the later contributions of William Masters and Virginia Johnson. These two investigative teams clearly influenced sex therapy and research in the United States, legitimizing this area of inquiry. However, few investigators are aware of the earlier contributions to sexology. Erwin J. Haeberle details the early German efforts in the field of human sexology and, in particular, documents the importance of early sexologists such as Iwan Bloch, Magnus Hirschfeld, and Harry Benjamin. Dr. Haeberle reveals previously undisclosed letters by Hirschfeld. His contribution is complemented by that of Hans Lehfeldt on the history of International Sexological congresses before and after World War II. Dr. Lehfeldt's contribution details the history of the birth control clinics in Europe and North America.

Early sexologists faced considerable opposition to their work. The climate of anti-eroticism is captured in the manuscript from John Money. Social taboos against masturbation were extreme and masturbation was held to contribute to hereditarily transmitted genetic defects. The last article in this section is a speculative one by E. W. Klimowsky on the changing sex roles in history. He postulates that the current blending of sex roles can be traced to a fierce struggle between these roles in earlier times.

1

Sexology: Conception, Birth, and Growth of a Science

E. J. Haeberle

Our present congress marks a double anniversary: 75 years ago—in 1908—the first *Journal for Sexology* was published in Berlin, and in 1913—70 years ago—the first *Society for Sexology* was founded, also in Berlin. Indeed, there is a third historical date worth commemorating today, a date that gives all of us cause for somber reflection: exactly 50 years ago, in May 1933, the first *Institute for Sexology* was destroyed by the Nazis in Berlin. This event signaled the end of sexology in Europe, because soon thereafter, Fascism extended its power over the entire continent. The sexological pioneers, most of them German and Austrian Jews, had to flee into exile; their books and journals were burned, their societies dissolved, their well-established international congresses were discontinued, and thus their accomplishments were eventually forgotten. In short, a whole promising young science fell victim to the holocaust.

Even now many sexologists are unaware of the rich and respectable past which has been stolen from them, and they realize even less why and how this theft occurred. Thus, they neither understand the scientific logic which led to the establishment of sexology as a science, nor the social and political forces that oppose this logic, and that have always tried to destroy sexology. These forces still exist. They succeeded once before, and they are again gathering strength. We can defeat them only if we reclaim our lost heritage and thereby anchor ourselves in the general scientific tradition of which our endeavor is a legitimate and integral part.

At our previous congress in Jerusalem, I had the opportunity to summarize the Jewish contribution to the development of sexology and thus to provide a rough outline of its first decades, which, as already mentioned, were dominated by Jewish scientists [1]. I will not repeat this outline here. Instead, I would now like to flesh it out with some human detail and, at the same time, attempt to put our science in a wider historical context. This alternating focus on the microcosm and macrocosm of its pioneering phase may help us understand the dialectics of sexology itself. Indeed, this "micro-macro method" will perhaps reveal some parallels to our present situation and allow us to sense the true significance of our work. Fortunately, since our last meeting in Israel, we have seen several hopeful developments. Indeed, I now have the great pleasure of acknowledging the contributions of three German and Austrian government agencies to our congress. The Institute for Foreign Cultural Relations in Stuttgart and the Austrian Institute in New York have enabled us to display a selection of documents in a historical exhibition on the birth of sexology. The Senator for Science and Research in Berlin has financed the printing of an illustrated brochure for our congress participants. As we take this pictorial and textual evidence home with us, we can provide our friends and colleagues with the first handy reference to our honorable lost tradition.

Special credit is also due to the Kinsey Institute in Bloomington, Indiana, which, for the last two years, has been supporting research in this area and has provided the basis for the more recent specific German and Austrian efforts. Thus, through his legacy, Alfred C. Kinsey, the first great American sexologist, has provided the link to our European past. His enormous collection of original German and Austrian material, which was not fully appreciated or even widely known at the time, now allows us to find our roots. In short, more than 25 years after his death, Kinsey proves once again that he was the "compleat sexologist," a man who cared about the history not only of sex, but also of sex research. In his spirit, let us therefore reflect on the conception, birth, and growth of our science.

Let us also, right from the start, emphasize that this science is of a somewhat complex, unstable, and elusive character. In dialectical fashion, it looks—now alternately, now simultaneously—at both the natural and cultural aspects of human life. In a never-ending process it combines and recombines elements of both the natural and cultural sciences and, in so doing, it is constantly forced to shift ground. In short, it possesses neither a fixed method nor a fixed object of its own. Indeed, concepts like "sexuality," "homosexuality," "sex drive," "sexual behavior," "sexual response," and so on, which today represent the objects of sexology, are new. Even the expressions themselves did not exist before the 19th century. They are the products of a particular historical development, which is still in progress, and in which we ourselves are playing a still largely unconscious role.

Still, many of the actual phenomena which now concern us in a new way have long been studied by various methods in many cultures. After all, men and women everywhere have always reproduced, they have always experienced love, desire, and sensual pleasure, and they have always tried to gain some practical and theoretical control over these experiences. Thus, there have long been two distinct, if related, approaches to our present theme, and these can be called the erotological and the sexological.

Erotology—the practical study of lovemaking or *ars amatoria*—is the older of these two approaches, reaching back into a religious past. Originally, it involved a personal initiation over a lengthy period, a carefully cultivated sense of the mystery of life, and an attitude of devotion. The early great Hindu love manuals still convey much of this spirit, which is now so sadly lacking in our own civilization. Yet recent American and European movements have turned to older Eastern philosophies in search of erotic fulfillment, proving that this spirit is still alive and may even grow again.

Sexology, on the other hand—the theoretical study of sex or *scientia sexualis*—has always come more easily to the Western mind, at least since the days of classical Greece. Its aim has always been objective understanding, and although our specific modern concept for this effort was still lacking, ancient philosophers and physicians already tried to make objective and systematic observations of love and reproduction. In this sense, men like Hippocrates and Aristotle can be claimed as legitimate forefathers of sexology.

Continued by the great medieval Islamic scholars, their tradition of impersonal, dispassionate research was finally adopted in the new European medical schools and universities and led to another great flowering in the Renaissance. The genius of Leonardo da Vinci left enough evidence of this new, unflinching, and penetrating view in his notebooks and therefore has rightly been called—among other things—the first modern sexologist [2].

Later researchers like Fallopio, Bartholinus, and de Graaf increased our understanding of our sexual anatomy, and the 18th and 19th centuries then began to describe, list, and classify all possible forms of human sexual behavior. The fact that these classifications were often prejudiced by an unsound medical ideology does not invalidate their scientific intent. Indeed, the inherent objective tendency of science finally exposed the bias and led to the founding of sexology in our present, more specific sense. Its pioneers—Iwan Bloch, Albert Moll, Magnus Hirschfeld, and Max Marcuse—are properly honored on this double anniversary. Following their lead, other scientists all over the world have pursued sexological studies and have produced impressive results. Indeed, in the next few days this very congress will again increase our objective understanding of sex.

As we proceed with our work, however, it behooves us to see the example of our pioneers not only as an inspiration, but also as a challenge. Just as the ancient erotological tradition has been debased and its spiritual dimension ignored in countless cheap "marriage manuals" and "gourmet guides to lovemaking," so our sexological classics—the two great studies by Kinsey, for example—are always in danger of being exploited in ever-new pseudo-scientific surveys or so-called "sex reports," which are eagerly sensationalized by the mass media, but which in the end only undermine the credibility of our work.

However, as our pioneers knew, this credibility must be earned the hard way—through persistent honest effort, constant self-criticism, and painstaking impartial observation. For the sexologist, scientific objectivity is not merely an ideal, it is the very justification for his existence. It is the only basis from which he can hope to reach his ultimate goal: a better life for himself and his fellow human beings. For even as he tries to preserve his neutrality in order to be useful at all, he can never remove himself from the world. In our Western civilization, his science presents one of the many indispensable correctives which, fortunately, have developed together with the excesses, with negative social trends and destructive political power. Sexology can be, and has been, ignored and destroyed, but if allowed to grow, it will work as one of the positive forces which keep society in some functioning balance.

This has been true of sexology from the moment of its conception. When, in 1906, Iwan Bloch proposed a science of sex and named it *Sexualwissenschaft* or sexology, he saw it as a necessary first step on the way to meaningful sexual reform which led to the concept of a special science as the best means of achieving it. Beginning with the rise of the middle classes and the industrial revolution, and accelerating in the 19th century, human sexuality had more and more turned into a problem. Malthus' dismal calculations about growing populations and dwindling food supplies [3], the repeatedly frustrated efforts of the neo-Malthusians to promote birth control as a way to escape disaster, the fear of "degeneracy" promoted by French psychiatrists from Morel to Charcot [4], a corresponding "eugenics" movement, led by the Englishman Galton [5], in Russia and Austria, Kaan's and Krafft-Ebing's disturbing descriptions of "sexual psychopathy" [6]—these and many other new concerns increasingly focused public attention on "sex" as a worrisome subject. At the same time, Western societies experienced rapid economic growth and modernization in many areas of life, yet irrational sexual attitudes and antiquated sex laws persisted. For this reason alone, a unified scientific effort to deal with sex became all but inevitable. Sex was on everyone's mind, not as erotic pleasure, but as an oppressive, dark, unsettling force, as a potential threat demanding attention.

In the 1920s, when sexology was already firmly established, Hans Kunz, in a contribution to the *Zeitschrift für Sexualwissenschaft*, reflected on the earlier anxious situation and concluded:

> It was mostly the enormous importance of sexuality in life that played . . . the decisive role in the creation of the term sexology (*Sexualwissenschaft*) by Iwan Bloch. This is in contrast to other disciplines where the affective element played a more subordinate, unconscious . . . role. The fact that we do not have a special science of "smell" or "hunger" is not due to logical insight—the justification would be the same as that for sexology—but is due alone to that affective element [7].

The strong feelings that gave sexuality its "enormous importance in life" had not arisen accidentally. In many ways they were symptoms of a deep frustration. Bloch himself was impatient with the lack of progress in solving the problem of prostitution. When he began to edit his *Comprehensive Handbook of Sexology* (1912) [8], he therefore wrote the first volume himself on this very subject. For him, prostitution was the key problem of sexology, because it combined the biological and cultural aspects of sex in the most dramatic and obvious fashion. Thus, only a new interdisciplinary approach combining the natural and cultural sciences, indeed only a new science—sexology—could hope to do justice to it. In turn, and by the same token, only the proper scientific understanding could lead to a lasting solution. A solution was clearly necessary, however, since in Berlin alone there were about 60,000 prostitutes, of whom only 10 percent were registered and regularly examined by the health agencies.

As a dermatologist, Bloch was further interested in the problem of venereal diseases. He himself had written a widely acclaimed study on *The Origin of Syphilis* (2 vols. 1901 and 1910) [9], and saw with satisfaction how other German scientists from Albert Neisser to August von Wasserman, Paul Ehrlich, and Alfred Blaschko achieved the first significant victories in the fight against syphilis and gonorrhea. In the final analysis, of course, the control of venereal diseases was also tied to solving the problem of prostitution.

Prostitution was related as well to the discrimination against unmarried mothers, because as despised "fallen women" many of them found no other way to survive. At the time, access to contraception was still greatly restricted, and every twelfth child in Germany was born "illegitimate"—about 180,000 every year. As a rule, these children were given up for adoption or raised in foster homes. This allowed some of the working mothers to cling to their jobs. Female teachers, for example, were expected to be celibate. Not only could they never "disgrace themselves"—they even had to leave their position upon marriage. Within marriage, on the other hand, they did not enjoy equal rights with their husbands, but rather became dependents. Moreover, women in general were second-class citizens, powerless to bring about change, since they did not have the right to vote. Obviously, all of this cried out for reform.

Bloch soon found himself educated on this whole cluster of issues by Helene Stöcker, one of the great figures in the German women's movement. As a co-founder and president of the German Association for the Protection of Mothers (Deutscher Bund für Mutterschutz und Sexualreform, founded in 1905), she fought for the rights of unmarried mothers and children, all "women's rights over their own bodies," and new sexual ethics based on full sexual equality. As a tireless organizer, writer, and editor, she helped countless women, but also made many enemies. Especially her demand for legalized abortion disturbed more conservative feminists and split the movement in Germany. Sickened by the mindless brutality of the First World War, she increasingly turned to pacifism, had to flee Nazi Germany, and finally came to the United States, where she died, alone and forgotten, in 1943. Even today, many politically active women have never heard of her—a great pity, because she was one of the most important feminists of our century. Her dramatic life would certainly make for a highly educational television series.

Another co-founder of Helene Stöcker's organization was the young Max Marcuse, although he eventually turned away from her after taking over her first journal *Mutterschutz* (Protection of Mothers). However, as already mentioned, her friendship with Iwan Bloch remained strong, as did that with Magnus Hirschfeld. She not only collaborated and consulted with both of them, but also joined Hirschfeld's World League for Sexual Reform and spoke at its international congresses. In short, no woman had a greater influence on the development and direction of early sexology.

Hirschfeld himself was the most active reformer of all early sexologists. Indeed, his detractors often accused him of putting reform ahead of science or even dismissed him as a mere propagandist. This charge was unjustified, but from the beginning of his career to its end, sexual reform remained his goal, and he himself summarized the meaning of his entire work in the motto *Per scientiam ad justitiam!* (Through science to justice!).

For Hirschfeld, the most important concern was rational sex legislation. France and other Catholic European as well as South American countries had, as a result of Napoleonic reforms, long decriminalized sexual behavior between consenting adults. However, Germany still retained its sodomy law, victimizing untold numbers of homosexuals who became victims of blackmail and worse. Indeed, early in our century, Germany's most important industrialist, Friedrich Krupp, was forced to commit suicide when his homosexuality was exposed. Soon thereafter members of the highest government and court circles found themselves embroiled in sensational trials for proven or alleged homosexual conduct. Thus, the continued lack of legal reform proved to have very serious consequences. Hirschfeld appeared as an expert witness in these trials, which renewed his crusading spirit. He redoubled his efforts to educate the general public, and he persuaded the German intellectual elite from Albert Einstein to Thomas Mann to sign his repeated appeals to the national legislature. In vain—the dominant political parties never mustered the necessary courage to go against public prejudice, and the demand for reform became ever more strident.

Inevitably, therefore, Hirschfeld became a controversial figure. As a Jew with socialist and pacifist sympathies who promoted a questionable, or even disreputable new science, he had no hope of winning honors from the establishment. Nevertheless, before the Nazis finally forced him to flee into exile, he had successfully walked the narrow, perilous path of the reformer, keeping an equal distance from reactionaries and revolutionaries, and always appealing to reason as the best hope for the oppressed and the oppressors alike. Thus, he not only made enemies, but also many friends. He was personally acquainted with many great historical personalities, from Henrik Ibsen to Jawaharlal Nehru, and as a lecturer, he traveled extensively all over Europe, eventually even around the world. Moreover, as a popular educator, he involved himself in the production of documentary and dramatic films and even appeared on the screen himself together with famous actors. In short, Hirschfeld's life as a sexological pioneer was not only exemplary in its integrity, but at the same time as rich in color and drama as any work of fiction. A whole series of Hollywood movies would be needed to do this drama justice.

As we can see in our historical exhibition, even Hirschfeld's purely professional achievements were impressive. His list of publications alone is enormous. But there was more: as early as 1897, he had founded the Scientific-Humanitarian Committee, the world's first "gay rights" organization. In 1908, he edited the first *Journal for Sexology* (Zeitschrift für Sexualwissenschaft), and in 1913 he started, together with Bloch, Albert Eulenburg, and others, the first Society for Sexology (Ärztliche Gesellschaft für Sexualwissenschaft und Eugenik). In 1919, he opened the first Institute for Sexology in Berlin, and in 1921 he convened the first International Congress for Sexual Reform on a Sexological Basis in the same city. Finally, in 1928, he organized, with the help of J. H. Leunbach and others, a World League for Sexual Reform in Copenhagen, and together with Havelock Ellis and Auguste Forel, he became one of the first three presidents. This league held further congresses in London, Vienna, and Brno, Czechoslovakia; it came to an end only after the triumph of Fascism in Europe. Ironically, as much as the Nazis hated Hirschfeld and all he stood for, some prominent party members secretly were his patients. In fact, this may have been one of the reasons why his institute, possibly together with incriminating papers, was destroyed only three months after Hitler became chancellor.

In any case, this destruction signaled the end of all reform and a return to openly reactionary policies. The scientific study of sex or of any other social issue was no longer acceptable. The Nazis had no interest in reaching the goals so ardently pursued by Bloch, Max Marcuse, Helene Stöcker, and Magnus Hirschfeld—the emancipation of women, equal rights for both sexes, people's rights over their own bodies, sex education, or the rational treatment of sexual minorities. Since sexology had provided the arguments for these and other demands, it had to be elim- inated in all countries that came under Nazi domination.

We must understand, however, that the European tragedy also illustrated a larger struggle that continued to rage world-wide. The earlier-mentioned increased "impor- tance of sexuality in life" as a problem for Europeans had also been felt for some time in distant continents as the result of various colonial policies. Thus, beginning in the 19th century, the world experienced not only a "moderni- zation," but also a "Westernization" of sex. For many formerly tolerant societies this was not at all beneficial. Once sex research and sex reform had become necessary in Europe, they also became all but inevitable elsewhere, and thus the whole drama was reenacted on an international scale. Ironically, often only Western sexologists were able to provide the antidote of Western science against the poison of Western prejudice.

Perhaps the best example of a man devoted to this beneficial counter-action was the great French lawyer René Guyon. In 1908, the very year of the first sexological journal, he was called to Bangkok to help with the codifica- tion of laws for the Kingdom of Siam. After the work was completed, he decided to stay, adopted Thai citizenship and a Thai name—Pichan Bulayong. He advanced to the posi- tion of legal advisor to the Ministry of Justice and finally even became a justice of the Thai Supreme Court of Appeals. Combining the best traditions of the French Enlightenment with great respect for the Buddhist heritage of his adopted country, he devoted his life to the fight against repressive Western sexual attitudes.

In his major, and only partially published work, *Studies in Sexual Ethics* (9 vols), he developed a rational basis for radical sexual reform [10]. Finding little to criticize in the traditional Asian and African cultures, his demands were directed mainly to Europe and the Americas. Indeed, Guyon went further and, in a separate essay, ridiculed the League of Nations for introducing pernicious puritanical ideas into many non-Christian countries [11]. In contrast, he praised Hirschfeld's World League for Sexual Reform, whose sensible proposals had been completely ignored by the international politicians in Geneva. For Guyon, the

Reform League reflected the best European legacy, while the League of Nations represented the worst. Neither was he content with its successor organization, the United Nations, whose much-celebrated "Universal Declaration of Human Rights" contained nothing about sexual rights. He wrote a critical essay, had it privately printed in Bangkok, and sent it to all sexologists of whom he had heard, including Alfred C. Kinsey [12]. (Soon thereafter Kinsey published his report on the human female and experienced considerable puritanical pressure of his own [13]. Although he had raised no practical demands, his scientific findings alone proved highly unwelcome and he lost his previous financial support. The much older Guyon died a few years later).

I mention Guyon and his correspondence with Kinsey mainly to show that the struggle for sanity and objectivity in sexual matters had become world-wide and that most of the sexological pioneers knew each other or, through their work, developed at least some indirect connection. This is also true of Guyon's debt to the earlier German sexologists. As already indicated, he was familiar with Hirschfeld's World League for Sexual Reform and repeatedly quoted him and his colleagues. On the other hand, unbeknownst to Guyon, the League had already, at its Vienna congress in 1930, called for a "Magna Charta of Human Sexual Rights." Among these were the equality of the sexes, the right to sexual self-determination, and the "right to one's own body." They further embraced the rights of sexual minorities, including disabled persons and prisoners, the rights of unmarried mothers and their children, indeed even "prenatal human rights." The complete list appeared in the League's journal in early 1933, but shortly thereafter the journal had to cease publication [14]. Once Hitler had invaded France, Guyon's writings could also no longer be published. Those already printed were banned by the Pétain government.

How closely the national and international issues of sexual reform are interwoven, and how this reform, in turn, depends on the objectivity of an international scientific effort, is finally perhaps best illustrated by Hirschfeld's fate in exile. After all, he was the greatest sexologist of his time, and both his triumphs and his defeats remain highly instructive. Unfortunately, not only was his institute destroyed, also his papers were lost, and his collaborators and disciples left only scanty reminiscences to provide some general clues. No biography has yet been written, and thus our present knowledge about him is sketchy at best.

Fortunately, today for the first time I can round out an important part of the sketch—thanks to another great sexologist: Dr. Harry Benjamin, who, at the age of 98, is still living in New York. On the occasion of this congress, he has made his own hitherto unpublished correspondence with Hirschfeld and other material available for quotation.

Harry Benjamin was born in Berlin, came to the United States in 1913, and knew all early sexologists personally, from Havelock Ellis to Magnus Hirschfeld and Sigmund Freud. He himself was a pioneer in the scientific study of transsexualism. He was also—and this is especially relevant in the present context—the acting American representative of the World League for Sexual Reform, and he was instrumental in bringing Hirschfeld to the United States.

Throughout the 1920s, Hirschfeld had been under attack from the Nazis, and as their numbers grew, his work became increasingly difficult. His lectures were regularly disrupted by Nazi goon squads, and by 1930 any public appearance had become impossible. Harry Benjamin arranged for a lecture invitation by the New York Medical Society, and Hirschfeld immediately accepted. His visit was greatly helped by his friend, the poet and writer George Sylvester Viereck, who published a series of interviews with him in newspapers from coast to coast. In these papers Hirschfeld was introduced to the American public as the "Einstein of Sex," a characterization that finally prompted him to demand in jest that Einstein rather be called the "Hirschfeld of physics." In any case, he was warmly received everywhere, visited Detroit, Chicago, Hollywood, and San Francisco, addressed various professional audiences, and even spoke on the radio. In March 1931, he sailed from California to Japan. The trip eventually took him around the world, lecturing and introducing sexology as a new science wherever he went. He never returned to Germany.

Hirschfeld later described his trip in a book, which was published in Switzerland and even translated into English [15]. Although written for a popular audience, the report is also useful for the professional, because it reveals the interdependence of European and non-European studies of sex, the process of mutual education that took place at every new stop between visitor and host. The Asian countries, eager as they were to meet a Western scientific pioneer, had much to teach him. Thus, he became an eager student again. There was simply no room for sexological imperialism.

In Japan, for example, he found a congenial, thoroughly modern scientific climate, but also a society which had wisely retained much of its older, sensible sexual attitude. Several Japanese colleagues had visited Hirschfeld in Berlin, and his first host in Tokyo was the dermatologist Professor Keijo Dohi, a disciple and friend of Albert Neisser. Dohi had also published the first Japanese journal of sexology, entitled *Sex*, and was just organizing a National Congress of Dermatology to which he invited Hirschfeld as a speaker. Hirschfeld also met Dr. Yamamoto in Kobe and leaders of the Japanese Women's Movement, such as the Baroness Shidzue Ishimoto and the writer Fusaye Ishikawa. He also met the personal physician of the emperor and finally even the emperor himself. The newspapers *Asahi Shimbun* and *Osaki-Ahasi* sponsored series of public lectures, and thus, from a personal point of view, the visit could not have been more gratifying.

By the same token, however, it also had its sobering moments. Indeed, one of them inadvertently cast a sudden, revealing light on the whole glory and misery of European sex research. Let us remember that Hirschfeld had devoted a lifetime and a long list of publications to the study of homosexuality and to the reform of antihomosexual laws. All this tireless work had made him the world's greatest expert on the subject, but in Japan he had to recognize this expertise was a peculiarly Western skill developed in response to unreasonable social pressure, a knowledge that would be superfluous under ideal circumstances. One day, Professor Myaki, a psychiatrist at the University of Tokyo, asked him: "Tell me, my dear Hirschfeld, how is it that one hears so much about homosexuality in Germany, England, and Italy and nothing of it among us?" Hirschfeld's profound insight into the issue forced him to answer—one imagines, with a deep sigh—"That, my dear colleague, is because it is permitted by you and forbidden by us" [16].

What was said here about homosexuality was, of course, also true of sexuality in general. One heard so much about it in Europe, because it had become a problem. Many of its expressions had been forbidden, restricted, or frustrated, and, as a result, one had found oneself with a host of social evils. There was no hope of escaping from them but through objective understanding and subsequent rational reform. As mentioned before, it was "the enormous importance of sexuality in European life," its ubiquitous presence as a social and intellectual challenge, that led to the birth of sexology. The accelerating Westernization of the globe soon internationalized many Western sexual problems and thus made more and more countries also receptive to Western ideas of how to deal with them. In addition, once it had been developed, sexology also offered many insights that were useful in themselves and applicable everywhere. Moreover, to the extent that sexologists contributed to medical knowledge, they directly helped people with problems of disease, somatic sexual dysfunction, infertility, and birth control. Finally, sexological warnings against the hasty adoption of Western sex laws and customs were appreciated by thoughtful local lawmakers and administrators.

For all these reasons, Hirschfeld's appearances were eagerly anticipated throughout Asia. Especially in China, where he spoke in most major cities and at all Chinese national universities, the audiences were very large. At Sun Yat Sen University in Canton over 1,000 students appeared for a lecture.

Hirschfeld also lectured widely in India, where he found a tremendous response from both Hindu and Moslem audiences. He also met many of the leaders in the fight for Indian independence, whom he supported wholeheartedly. In Allahabad, he was the guest of Jawaharlal Nehru, in whose house he occupied the room usually reserved for Gandhi, and he also met Nehru's daughter Indira, who was a 15-year-old girl at the time. Nehru wrote in Hirschfeld's diary:

It has been a pleasure to renew the acquaintance with Dr. Hirschfeld, whom I met in Berlin four years ago. Germany and India have developed many cultural bonds, and to Germany India is beholden in many ways. A German savant like Dr. Hirschfeld is therefore welcome in our country, and even though we may be engrossed in our struggle for emancipation, we cannot forget that our independence must lead us to a fuller life and to greater contacts with the thinkers of other countries [17].

Now that Indian independence has long become a reality, Nehru's wish for increased international scientific contact has also been fulfilled. Indeed, our own science in particular will soon bring its best authorities from all over the world to Bombay to lecture at our next World Congress. It will then be a source of great satisfaction for all of us to remember that this city has hosted such lectures before. Indeed, in 1931 Bombay was introduced to sexology by its greatest pioneer. Hirschfeld lectured there very extensively. How popular these lectures were can be gleaned from the letter to a local newspaper, requesting a more convenient scheduling:

To the Editor of "The Chronicle":
Sir—Dr. Magnus Hirschfeld, Director of the Institute of Sexology, Berlin, has been giving to Bombay audiences very interesting and highly instructive lectures on sex problems. But the time chosen for these lectures is so awkward and inconvenient to a large number of people interested in the subject that . . . they are not able to avail themselves of the humanitarian services that the learned Doctor is rendering. . . . In view of the fact that problems like those of sexual reforms and Birth-Control are little or hardly discussed in this city or rather country of ours, it will be no small gain to us, if we are enabled to drink deep into the cup of this branch of human knowledge. . . .

Nanalal N. Talaty [18]

Interestingly enough, not only looking forward to Bombay, but also looking back to our previous congress in Jerusalem, we find that Hirschfeld had prepared the way. Indeed, we find that the international recognition of our science was already once a living reality, and that only European fascism and the Second World War interrupted a logical and otherwise inevitable development. We also find that Hirschfeld's trip around the world occurred at the very historical turning point, when hope turned to despair, and when the well-deserved and growing success of sexology was brutally cut short.

This unique moment of precarious balance between satisfaction and anxiety, when the pride in past accomplishments began to be overshadowed by fears for the future, is captured in a hitherto unpublished letter, which Hirschfeld wrote to Harry Benjamin shortly before returning to Europe. I will quote several key passages here:

March 16, 1932

My dear colleague:
In Palestine, where I spent the last few weeks, the vivacious Jews indeed left me not a single quiet hour. . . . Quite apart from my overdue lectures at Hebrew University in Jerusalem, in Tel Aviv and Haifa, etc., etc., I could hardly survive all the invitations, so that I am now glad to have at least two days for myself aboard this ship. . . .

Apparently, in the meantime, Hirschfeld had also made an attempt to return to the United States for still another visit, because he continues:

Now about my American lecture tour. . . . I think it will be possible to produce a good income, even in America. Just in case, I once again list the main topics: . . .
   a) Sexology - A New and Important Science
   b) Love, Sex and Marriage
   c) Sex Pathology (Sufferings of Love)
   d) Natural Laws of Love
      (Sexual Reform on a Scientific Basis)
   All lectures with slides. . . .
   I am reluctant to return to Germany, where every third voter has given his vote to Hitler. . . . Still, I think my home is my home, and to renounce it is not easy for me. All the more I am looking forward to America which, in spite of its misguided system of Prohibition, has impressed and pleased me most of the many countries I have seen on my trip around the world. This is because of its colossal strength, its marvellous productivity, its creature comforts and its intensity of living. Certainly, the old, high civilization of Asia (especially of China and India) also has its charms, as do the beauty and erudition of Europe, but most of all I love the youthful, future-oriented tempo of America. In any case, at the moment America offers the best chances and perspectives for scientific work [19].

However, Hirschfeld did not want to sail on directly to New York. Still waiting for the Nazi menace to pass, he first traveled in various European countries and even helped organize another congress of the World League for Sexual Reform in Brno, Czechoslovakia. It turned out to be the last, and the following spring his worst fears were realized: on May 6, 1933, the Nazis plundered his institute in Berlin, destroyed the collections, and burned the books. Hirschfeld saw newsreel footage of the events in a Paris movie theater. A month later, still badly shaken, he wrote to his friend George Sylvester Viereck. This letter, also made public today for the first time, reveals that already more than one man and his work was affected:

Paris, June 9, 1933

My dear George Sylvester:
   Many thanks for your sympathetic letter. I have suffered terribly, our beautiful Institute has been closed by the authorities, the largest part of my books and collections destroyed. Since we last saw each other in New York, I have not returned to

Germany, because I saw it all coming. . . . After the
burning of my books and portrait bust . . . I preferred to go to France, because the German emigrants
here—in Paris alone there are over 20,000—are protected against extradition . . . etc. and are being
helped by men like Gide, Herriot, Coilent and many
other individuals and organizations. . . . My health
is not good; the terrible tensions have taken their
toll. In spite of this (perhaps even because of it), I
feel again and again drawn to America, because my
English is better than my French. Thus, I hope to
become effective more easily, especially through
publications. Intellectual work is now a necessity for
me, if I want to find some measure of peace. . . .
P.S. Your books were burned as well, the *Wandering
Jew* even with a special "fire incantation" [20]:

Unfortunately, even the news from the United States was
not very encouraging. A planned lecture tour fell through,
because the American manager proved unreliable. The
economic situation showed no sign of improvement, and thus
even Hirschfeld's American friends had to struggle harder
than ever to survive. As a temporary measure, therefore,
he used what little material he still possessed to open
another sexological institute in Paris. When Harry Benjamin
sent him congratulations, Hirschfeld replied:

IV, 29, 1934

My dear friend Harry,
    I accept your congratulations to the start of our
Institute . . . in Paris, but I am not very hopeful.
It seems that Europe (not only Germany) [is regres-
sing] in all cultural questions —and our science
belongs to these. The power of nationalism, fascism,
racism increases, and I am afraid that a war and
other troubles cannot be avoided in the next years.
    America is our hope, our future; Europe is very
sick, nearly dead. I would like to come to America
and stay there from September 34 to the spring (of)
35, perhaps longer, . . . publish books in English,
give courses and lectures etc. etc. . . . My health is
now better [21]. . . .

Only two months later, in June 1934, Hitler moved
against some of his own supporters and had the entire SA
leadership murdered in the so-called "Röhm affair." As
mentioned earlier, some prominent Nazis had secretly been
Hirschfeld's patients. Perhaps even files from Hirschfeld's

ransacked institute had been used against them. In any case, Hitler now appeared even more dangerous, and only America promised to be entirely safe. Harry Benjamin had, in the meantime, started a second practice in California and once more encouraged Hirschfeld to join him, together with his long-time assistant Karl Giese:

July 11, 1934

Dear esteemed friend:

. . . If I were you . . . I would definitely come here to Los Angeles or San Diego or Santa Barbara. Of course, you cannot count on a medical practice . . . but with your already available income and occasional earnings . . . you could live better and with less worry than in Paris.

Even if the Hitler people break each other's skulls, Germany is lost for us as the civilized country of our youth and our work. So much for that. . . .

I believe the only right thing is to bring Karl Giese along with you and as much as possible of your collection and library. Perhaps it can then develop into an Institute here, but I would not make definite plans in this regard [22]. . . .

It is tempting to speculate about the course of American sex research, if this plan had succeeded. Even a modest institute would have given California a headstart. After all, Kinsey's institute in Indiana was not established until more than ten years later. Furthermore, Hirschfeld's personal papers, which are now entirely lost, would have been preserved and would now give us some sorely needed further insight into the history of our field. It is tragic, therefore, that Hirschfeld's wish to settle in the United States was not fulfilled. His health failing again, he moved instead to Nice, where he died, within a year, on his birthday, May 14, 1935. He had just reached the age of 67.

It was only after the Second World War that Kinsey and other American researchers revitalized sexology. Thus, Hirschfeld's and Benjamin's judgment proved correct: the United States did indeed pick up and reignite the torch. Elsewhere, some of the older sexologists also became active again—for example in England, where Norman Haire published his *Journal of Sex Education*, and even in India, where A. P. Pillay edited an *International Journal of Sexology*. Both of these journals carried articles by pre-war sexologists like René Guyon, Helena Wright, Ernst Gräfenberg, and Coenrad van Emde Boas. European sex research now also found recognition in official departments of sexology at universities like Prague, Hamburg, Frankfurt, Kiel, and Leuven (Belgium). Finally, nine years ago, an International Congress of Sexology was reconvened in Paris. Among its organizers was Hans Lehfeldt, a German-American immigrant, who had witnessed the early growth of our science in Berlin.

Today, at the opening of this congress, we have a special reason for pride, because we have succeeded, where our pioneers failed 50 years ago. Indeed, as revealed by a previously unknown correspondence between Harry Benjamin and Havelock Ellis, the World League for Sexual Reform planned an international congress for 1933 in Chicago [23]. The plan had to be abandoned mainly because of the worldwide economic depression. As Harry Benjamin wrote in one of his letters: "Times are not at all too favorable."

Our present situation is not entirely dissimilar. In many ways, times are again unfavorable, but then they always are. The scientific study of sex will never find progress easy. Without any special advocacy, simply through their sober and painstaking work, sexologists pose a challenge to any status quo. It is the nature of this work to create a basis for sexual reform wherever it is needed, and it is still needed in most countries of the world. In view of this, all possible divisions among ourselves become secondary. We labor in an interdisciplinary field, and we will never agree on a single methodological approach. Neither should we, since sex must be studied in both its biological and social aspects. Thus, both the sciences and the humanities are inevitably involved.

It is also shortsighted to create a dichotomy between a "medical model" of human sexuality and other modes of understanding. Our pioneers, Bloch, Moll, Hirschfeld, Max Marcuse, and their colleagues tried to free the study of sex from the narrow medical preconceptions of their time; they themselves were physicians, and even Havelock Ellis, their English comrade-in-arms, had medical training. In reality, they did not attack medicine, but the prevailing, distorted version of it. They wanted a medicine that was both more modest and much broader in scope. As physicians in Berlin at the turn of the century, they still tried to live up to the ideals of their venerable fellow Berliner Rudolf Virchow—perhaps the greatest physician of the 19th century. For Virchow, medicine was "in its core a social science," and over a hundred years ago, he wrote of medicine, what can and should also be said of sexology:

If medicine is really to fulfill its great task, it must interject itself into the great political and social life; it must name and remove the obstacles to the normal course of life processes. Should we ever reach this goal, medicine will, as it must, become the common property of all men; it will cease to be medicine, and it will become part of the general, then unified body of knowledge which is identical with the ability to act [24].

These prophetic words also describe our goal. Once our science becomes common property, it will cease to be sexology. It will become part of a larger body of enabling knowledge which will finally unite theory and practice. Then even the distinction between sexology and erotology will disappear. Studying sex passionately and making love wisely will be the accomplishment of all men and women.

NOTES

1. Haeberle, Erwin J. "The Jewish Contribution to the Development of Sexology." In Zwi Hoch and Harold I. Lief (eds.), *Sexology—Sexual Biology, Behavior and Therapy: Selected Papers of the 5th World Congress of Sexology,* 397–414. Amsterdam: Excerpta Medica, 1982. Also in *The Journal of Sex Research,* 18, no. 4:305–23.

2. Dalma, Juan. "Leonardo de Vinci, precursor de psicologia, neuro-fisiologia, biodinamica de las poblaciones, sexologia" in *Boletín de la Academia Nacional de Ciencias,* Córdoba, T., 1972, 49:79–112.

3. Malthus, Thomas R. *Essay on the Principle of Population,* 1798, 1830, (ed.) Antony Flew. London: Penguin, 1970.

4. Morel, B. A. *Traité des dégénérescences physiques, intellectuelles et morales de l'espèce humaine.* Paris, 1857.

5. Galton, Francis. *Hereditary Genius.* London: Macmillan, 1869.

6. Kaan, Heinrich. *Psychopathia sexualis.* Leipzig 1843. In Krafft-Ebing, Richard von, *Psychopathia sexualis.* Stuttgart, 1882.

7. Kunz, Hans. "Zur Methodologie der Sexualwissenschaft" in *Zeitschrift für Sexualwissenschaft,* 1923, 13, no. 1:21.

8. Bloch, Iwan. *Handbuch der gesamten Sexualwissenschaft in Einzeldarstellungen, vol. 1: Die Prostitution.* Berlin: Louis Marcus, 1912.

9. Bloch, Iwan. *Der Ursprung der Syphilis.* 2 vols.

Jena: G. Fischer, 1901 and 1910.

10. Guyon, René. *Etudes d'Ethiques Sexuelles,* vols. 1–6. St. Denis: Dardaillon, 1929–38? Vols. 7–9 unpublished at Kinsey Institute. Vols. 1–2 also in English translation. *The Ethics of Sexual Acts,* New York: Alfred A. Knopf, 1934, and *Sexual Freedom,* New York: Alfred A. Knopf, 1940.

11. Guyon, René. *La Societé des Nations aux mains des puritains.* Unpublished manuscript at Kinsey Institute.

12. Guyon, René. *Human Rights and the Denial of Sexual Freedom.* Bangkok: self published, 1951.

13. Kinsey, Alfred C. *Sexual Behavior in the Human Female.* Philadelphia: W. B. Saunders, 1953.

14. The Charta was the work of Rudolf Goldscheid and is quoted in full by Magnus Hirschfeld, "Was will die Zeitschrift 'Sexus'?" in *Sexus,* 1933, 1, no. 1.

15. Hirschfeld, Magnus. *Men and Women—The World Journey of a Sexologist.* New York: Putnam's Sons, 1935.

16. Ibid., 30.

17. Ibid., 192–93.

18. Undated newspaper clip in possession of author.

19. Unpublished letter in possession of author. Translated from German original.

20. Ibid.

21. Unpublished letter in possession of author. Originally written in English, slightly corrected by author.

22. Unpublished letter in possession of author. Translated from German original.

23. Unpublished correspondence in possession of author.

24. *Virchow's Archiv.,* 1862, 22:56.

2

International Sexological Congresses before and after World War II

H. Lehfeldt

It has been my good fortune to participate in a number of international sexology meetings, both before and after World War II. I want to share with you some of my personal experiences at these meetings. Their significance can only be understood in the light of the political and social climate prevailing at the time.

The first congress took place in the late 1920s when the Russian revolutionary regime was firmly established. Birth control and abortion had been legalized, as Lenin had advocated as early as 1913. By 1921, five contraceptive clinics had been opened in Moscow. The International Socialistic Congress, convened in Brussels in August 1928, proposed a more timid approach, resolving that contraception be dispensed to married women only!

In Austria in the 1920s, eight birth control clinics were active. At the gynecologic clinic of Vienna University, women received contraceptive counselling but abortion was illegal.

In Germany, under the Weimar Republic (1919–1933), dispensation of contraceptive devices to unmarried women was considered an obscene act and was liable to prosecution. It was in 1927 that a more liberal attitude began to prevail. Abortion remained illegal and was punishable by jail or penitentiary for both the physician and his patient. However, "medical indications" were often used as a legitimate reason for the termination of a pregnancy. The "Bund für Mutterschutz" (Federation for the Protection of

Mothers) established by Helene Stöker, opened sex counselling clinics in Germany which, from 1924 on, dispensed contraceptives. In Berlin, K. Bendix organized birth control clinics for the "Krankenkassen" (Health Insurance for Workers) in 1928. In the same year, the "Gesex" (Society for Sex Reform) opened a clinic for sex counselling and contraception in Berlin under the direction of F.A. Theilhaber, F. Hirsch, and myself.

In England, the termination of pregnancy was considered a crime; physicians performing an abortion faced prosecution and loss of their medical licenses. In the early 1920s, birth control clinics were established by Mary Stopes, who used cervical caps for contraception, and by Norman Haire, who used diaphragms and Gräfenberg intrauterine devices (IUDs).

In the United States, the Comstock Law, then in force, prohibited abortion and contraception; contraceptive devices were banned as obscene matter. When Margaret Sanger, disregarding the law, opened her first contraceptive clinic in the Brownsville section of Brooklyn, New York, she was sentenced to 30 days in jail.

In France, pioneers in the field of sexology, such as the eminent gynecologist Jean Dalsace and others, lost their hospital affiliations for opening sex counselling clinics. Magnus Hirschfeld had founded his Institute for Sexual Sciences in 1919 in Berlin and similar institutes were started in Königsberg, Prague, and Vienna.

The first international sexology congress was organized by Magnus Hirschfeld, in 1921 in Berlin.

In 1928, in Berlin also, Margaret Sanger gave a postgraduate course for physicians. There, I discussed Gräfenberg's first paper on intrauterine contraception [1,2].

Organized by Magnus Hirschfeld and Norman Haire [3], the third international sex reform congress took place in London in 1929. This meeting produced a wealth of interesting papers. Bertrand Russell lectured on "Taboos of Sex Knowledge," Mary Stopes on "Birth Control," Ernst Gräfenberg on the "Intrauterine Method of Contraception," A. Gens on "The Demand on Abortion in Soviet Russia," Hannah Stone on "Birth Control as a Factor in the Sex Life of Women," and George Bernard Shaw on "The Need for Expert Opinion in Sexual Reform" [4]. Let me quote a short passage from Shaw's presentation:

Everybody is a sexual reformer: that is, everybody who has any ideas on the subject at all. The Pope, for instance, is a prominent sexual reformer; and the Austrian nudists are sexual reformers. If you had a general congress of all the sexual reformers, not merely the members of one particular Society, but all the people who are demanding sexual reform: Nudists and Catholics, birth controllers and self-controllers, homosexualists and heterosexualists, monogamists, polygamists, and celibates, there would be some curious cross-party divisions. The Pope would find himself on nine points out of ten warmly in sympathy with Dr. Marie Stopes. And it is quite possible that the most fanatical Nudists and the most fanatical homosexualists might have in common the strongest objection to polygamy and divorce. . . .

One year after the London conference, Margaret Sanger [5] organized a very important congress on birth control in Zurich. At this time, gynecologists knew little about the different contraceptive techniques available then, such as the diaphragm, the cervical cap, or the IUD. A small number of birth control clinics were active in some countries.

Hannah Stone reported that 19,000 patients had received contraceptive counseling in her clinic in New York City, staffed by 15 physicians, five nurses, and two social workers. In the 26 birth control clinics active since 1923 all over the United States, contraceptive advice had been given to 37,000 married women. We should remember that birth control counselling was unlawful at that time, unless there was a medical, social, or eugenic indication.

In England, 16 clinics were active and had advised 45,000 women.

In Germany, a questionnaire sent out by Margaret Sanger and Hannah M. Stone did not receive sufficient replies to provide valid statistics. However, data collected by the seven clinics of the Berlin Krankenkassen showed that 2,700 women had been counselled on contraception in the course of two years. The technique most widely used in all clinics was the vaginal diaphragm combined with contraceptive jelly. At the Zurich conference, Hannah Stone reported on 15,000 diaphragm users, and Norman Haire on 8,000. The pregnancy rate was 5 percent.

A lively and sometimes heated discussion followed Gräfenberg's presentation—the third report on his IUD— covering a total of 10 years' experience. By then, he had inserted 1,300 devices. His original device had been a silkworm star; later he changed to the ring made of silver. The pregnancy rate for silkworm stars was 3.1, for silver rings 1.0 per woman-year. Norman Haire came out strongly for the Gräfenberg ring while Leunbach (Denmark), who had originally endorsed the method, now opposed it. W. Pust (Germany) reported that 140,000 of his own IUDs had been sold. He always fitted his patients first with the celluloid cervical cap devised by him and inserted the Pust IUD only if the cap had been tolerated well. At the time of the Zurich conference, 500,000-600,000 of his caps had been sold.

Another speaker in the discussion was the Dutch gynecologist Th. van de Velde, famous as one of the few university teachers to speak out publicly on the controversial subject of sexology, and the author of a popular-science book on sexology which was a bestseller. Courteously, but nonetheless categorically, he opposed the IUD. Discussing the Gräfenberg ring he said:

> I am totally unable to get it into my head that no complications arise in such cases. On the other hand, it must not be forgotten, that Dr. Gräfenberg is one who has proved himself to be a most highly capable scientific worker in other fields, and that he continues to be one. . . . If the method is to be tried . . . it should be undertaken only by some few very experienced and skillful gynecologists with a deep sense of responsibility.

Violent opposition against all IUDs and all gynecologists using the method was voiced by the Swiss gynecologist W. Frey.

Felix A. Theilhaber (Berlin) reported on 1500 Pust IUDs worn without major side effects. Yet, he had serious reservations about IUDs in general: as advocated by Gräfenberg, any pregnancy occurring with an IUD *in situ* must be terminated; leaving the IUD in place might cause serious harm to the mother. In the absence of supporting scientific data, Theilhaber was convinced that German medical experts simply would not accept Gräfenberg's belief as an indication for performing an abortion. He concluded that the IUD method might be neither as dangerous as stated by Frey nor as harmless as implied by Pust and Gräfenberg.

In Germany, a few universities had started birth control clinics. By coincidence I found out that the hospital clinic of Berlin University was testing the Gräfenberg ring. A patient of the Gesex clinic brought us her admission card from Berlin University which showed that she had been inserted with a ring and the date of insertion. With this evidence in hand I approached Walter Stoeckel, head of the university hospital and the editor of the *Zentralblatt für*

Gynakologie, the leading German periodical in this field. My offer to write a report on the Zurich conference for his journal was answered with a letter from Stoeckel saying that the subject was of no interest to his readers. Nevertheless, I submitted my report and had the satisfaction of having it accepted and published. I should mention that it was no minor achievement to have a ten-page report on a controversial subject printed in such a prestigious journal, especially one written by a young and unknown sexologist-gynecologist [6]. Another report on the Zurich conference written by A. M. Durand-Wever [7] appeared in a medical journal.

In retrospect, this conference assumes great historical value because it was instrumental in promoting birth control in America and England.

Also in 1930, after the Zurich conference, the Fourth Congress of the World League for Sexual Reform took place in Vienna [8]. There, the German writer Ernst Toller, the psychoanalysts F. Wittels and W. Reich, and others discussed "Sexual Misery." The themes of "Contributions to the History of Sexual Morality" and "Sexuality and Legislation" were discussed by Magnus Hirschfeld, Judge Ben B. Lindsey (author of "Companionate Marriage"), F. Halle, and others. Another topic discussed by the distinguished panel was "Birth Control and the Rights of Children."

The Fifth Congress of the World League for Sexual Reform took place in Brno, Czechoslovakia. Three of the organizers were: Norman Haire, Magnus Hirschfeld, and J. H. Leunbach.

Turning to the post-World War II period, the first important meeting devoted to birth control and sexology was the Sixth Conference of the International Planned Parenthood Federation (IPPF) in February 1959 in New Delhi, with Margaret Sanger presiding [9].

Starting in 1960, K. H. Mehlan, director of the Institute for Hygiene at the University of Rostock (East Germany), organized international postgraduate conferences on contraception and abortion. His first congress [10] was attended by scientists from 17 countries on three continents, including Lady Rama Rau (Bombay), Helena Wright (England), Conrad van Emde Boas (Holland), among many others.

These Rostock meetings provided the first opportunity for Western scientists to obtain first-hand information on the safety of legal abortion as practiced in Hungary, Yugoslavia, and Czechoslovakia. Christopher Tietze and I, the U.S. delegates to the 1960 conference, published the findings of our Eastern colleagues [11]. They showed that skillfully performed legal abortion is not more dangerous than a tonsillectomy and has a lower mortality rate than pregnancy and childbirth.

In June, 1962, the IPPF held its Third Conference in Warsaw, Poland [12]. After I had presented data from the contraceptive clinic of Bellevue Hospital, New York, on the first 5,000 women on oral contraceptives, I was severely criticized by the Soviet delegate (a woman) for using such "dangerous" drugs. No Soviet woman would ever be exposed to such a health risk, she declared. Needless to say ever since, oral contraception has been widely used in the Soviet Union.

At the Sixth World Congress on Fertility and Sterility, June 1966 in Stockholm [13] I listened to an interesting theory regarding sex determination in cases of artificial insemination, presented by my late friend Sophia Kleegman (United States). According to her, selective timing of insemination might allow parents the choice of having a male or a female baby.

The first important international sexologic meeting after World War II was the Symposium Sexologicum Pragense, in June 1968 [14]. It was organized by Josef Hynie (Prague), an eminent endocrinologist and sexologist, who had also worked in Magnus Hirschfeld's Institute for Sexology in Berlin. Hynie became the first scientist in Europe to be awarded a professorship in sexology. Among the delegates to the symposium were sexologists from East and West Germany and various other European countries, including a large delegation from the Soviet Union. I had the honor of representing the United States. The conference opened with a solemn procession of the chief delegates down the hall of the main auditorium of Charles University.

Hynie read the opening address in Latin, followed by representatives of other nations addressing the audience in their respective languages. It was a gathering in beautiful surroundings, in a festive and relaxed atmosphere. It was particularly valuable for providing the Western participants with an opportunity for free exchange of scientific information, especially with Soviet delegates who rarely attended meetings outside their own country. It was the time of the "Prague Spring." A few months later, Czechoslovakia was invaded by the Soviet Union.

In January, 1974, the First International Scientific Congress of the Family Planning Association of Sri Lanka took place in Colombo [15].

The Fifth International Congress on Psychosomatic Obstetrics/Gynecology was held in Rome, in 1977 [16], the Sixth in West Berlin, in 1980 [17].

The series of international conferences devoted exclusively to sexology were initiated by the Society for the Scientific Study of Sex (SSSS), during the presidency of Jack Lippes. My proposal in 1973 to the Board of Directors of the SSSS to organize a conference in Paris had been unanimously accepted, and I was charged with the organization. It was not an easy task. My close friend Jean Dalsace, French member of the SSSS and a pioneer sexologist, had died. His friend Albert Netter, an academic scientist, was the first to inform me that sexology was not a science! He gradually relented, though, and collaborated with us. There were innumerable problems, controversies, and misunderstandings before the first international conference of the SSSS opened in Paris, in July 1974. It became a great scientific success, had a huge attendance, and ended with Lippes' and my names entered in the Golden Book at a reception for us at the City Hall of Paris. Similar conferences followed at intervals of one to two years in different countries.

In 1976, John Money, then president of the SSSS, organized the Second International Conference in Montreal, Canada, together with Robert Gemme (Montreal).

The Third Congress, devoted to Medical Sexology and organized by Romano Forleo, took place in Rome, in October 1978; I acted as honorary president. At the close of the congress it was decided to create a World Association for Sexology (WAS), a special body for the organization of future international meetings.

This new association was responsible for the Fourth and Fifth Sexology Conferences, in Mexico City in 1980, and in Jerusalem in 1981.

The Sixth World Congress for Sexology, which unites us here in Washington, was organized by a cooperative effort of WAS and other sexologic associations.

I would also like to mention the meetings organized by the International Academy of Sex Research which holds conferences every year in a different country. Between 1980 and 1982, meetings were held in Tucson, Arizona, Haifa, Prague, and Copenhagen. Their 1983 meeting is scheduled for November at Arden House in Harriman, New York.

The greatly increased frequency of sexology meetings over the last decades, compared with their infrequency before World War II, is proof of the world-wide progress of scientific sexology. In fact, nowadays so many sexology congresses are held in so many different parts of the world that it has become practically impossible to attend all of them. I know this from my own experience. In the distant past, I was not able to attend *all* the meetings mentioned in today's recapitulation. Some of the ones I had to miss are included for their historical value, or because I helped in organizing them or participated *in absentia* with a paper read for me by another participant.

Only a few of the pre-World War II congresses published proceedings, and these are hard to find. I hope that my reminiscences and the summary of meetings devoted to sexology and related subjects may have some historical interest and be useful for reference.

NOTES

1. Geburtenregelung (Population control). Lectures and discussions at postgraduate course for physicians, Berlin, 1928. Berlin: K. Bendix, 1929.
2. Lehfeldt, H. Geburtenregelung (Population control). Report on postgraduate course for physicians, Berlin, 1928. Hippokrates, 1929, Stuttgart/Leipzig. 2:190–95.
3. *Proceedings of the Third World Congress of the World League for Sexual Reform,* N. Haire (ed.). London, 1929. London: Keagan Paul, Trench, Trubner & Co., Ltd., 1930.
4. Ibid. 432.
5. Sanger, M., and H. M. Stone. The practice of contraception. In *Proceedings of the Seventh International Birth Control Conference,* Zurich, 1930. Baltimore: Williams Wilkins Co., 1931.
6. Lehfeldt, H. VII Internationaler Kongress für Geburtenregelung (Seventh International Congress on Population Control), Zurich, 1930. *Zentralblatt f. Gynäk.* 1931, 55:110–19.
7. Durand-Wever, A. VII Internationaler Kongress f. Geburtenregelung, Zurich, 1930. *Die Mediz. Welt,* 1930, 40:1–7.
8. Sexualnot und Sexualreform (Sexual misery and sexual reform). In *Proceedings, Fourth Congress of the World League for Sexual Reform,* Vienna, 1930. Vienna/Leipzig: Elbemühl, 1931.
9. *Proceedings of the Sixth International Conference of the IPPF,* New Delhi, 1959. London: International Planned Parenthood Federation, 1960 (?).
10. "Internationale Abortsituation." In K. H. Mehlan (ed.), *Proceedings of the International Workshop on Abortion and Related Problems, Including Contraception, Rostock, 1960.* Leipzig: Georg Thieme, 1961.
11. Tietze, C., and H. Lehfeldt. Legal abortion in

Eastern Europe. *JAMA,* 1961, 175:1149–54.

12. *Proceedings of the Third Conference of the IPPF.* K. V. Earle and J. Rettie (eds.), Warsaw, 1962. International Congress Series No. 71, 1973. Amsterdam: Excerpta Medica Foundation, 1963.

13. *Proceedings of the Fifth World Congress on Fertility and Sterility.* B. Westin and N. Wiqvist (eds.). Stockholm, 1966. International Congress Series No. 133. Amsterdam: Excerpta Medica Foundation, 1967.

14. Symposium Sexuologicum Pragense. Lectures delivered at the international congress, Prague, 1968. J. Hynie, and K. Nedoma (eds.), Universita Karlova, Praha, 1969.

15. *Proceedings of the First International Scientific Congress of the Family Planning Association of Sri Lanka,* Colombo, 1974. S. Chinnatamby and N. D. W. Lionel (eds.), Family Planning Association of Sri Lanka, Colombo, 1975.

16. *Abstracts of the Fifth International Congress of Psychosomatic Obstetrics and Gynecology,* Rome, 1977. H. J. Prill (ed.), Rome, 1977.

17. *Abstracts of the Sixth International Congress of Psychosomatic Obstetrics and Gynecology,* Berlin (West), 1980. H. J. Prill and M. Stauber (eds.).

3

Food, Fitness, and Vital Fluids: Sexual Pleasures from Graham Crackers to Kellogg's Cornflakes

J. Money

SEXUAL DEGENERACY THEORY

The antihedonic cult of medical antisexualism that today is labeled Victorianism originated early in the eighteenth century. It filled the void left, in the aftermath of the Inquisition, by the loss of demon-possession theory. Degeneracy caused by masturbation possession replaced demon-possession as the explanation for virtually all of the afflictions, social and personal, of humankind.

The campaign against masturbation commenced with the publication by an anonymous British clergyman of a tract with a long descriptive title: *Onania; Or the Heinous Sin of Self-Pollution, and all its Frightful Consequences, in both Sexes, Considered with Spiritual and Physical Advice to those who have Already Injured themselves by the Abominable Practice*. The first American edition was published in Boston in 1724.

The medicalization of Onania was effected in the 1750s by the Swiss physician, Simon André Tissot, in *A Treatise on*

Supported by USPHS Grant HD 00325 and the William T. Grant, Jr., Foundation.

Adapted from a forthcoming book to be published by the Johns Hopkins University Press.

the Diseases Produced by Onanism. This extremely influential book, originally in Latin, went through many editions in French before its American translation was published in New York in 1832.

This timing synchronized perfectly with the rise to fame of the Reverend Sylvester Graham as a health-reform lecturer in Philadelphia. To food and fitness, Graham added sexual abstinence as the third great principle of his do-it-yourself system of health maintenance and disease resistance. Crowds flocked to hear his promise of how they could resist getting cholera, despite the deadly epidemic that was spreading from Europe to America.

Graham's name is enshrined for posterity in Graham crackers, so named because he was the apostle of whole-grain flour, or Graham flour, as the ultimate health food. The sugar in today's Graham crackers would make him turn in his grave.

In 1834, Graham published *A Lecture to Young Men*, in which he expounded Tissot's theory of degeneracy caused by onanism. It was not only the loss of vital fluid that Graham inveighed against in onanism, but also what he considered the far greater danger of concupiscence and lust, both of which together caused moral as well as physical degeneracy. Proper food and fresh-air exercise to help combat this degeneracy, were part of his system of treatment. The ultimate aim was total abstinence or, if married, extreme continence. There was no place for erotic pleasure in Graham's conception of good health.

Graham's public career spanned less than ten years. By his late forties, he was burned-out. In 1851, at the age of 57, having failed to regain his health, despite repudiating his own dietic system by taking meat and alcohol, he died. His health precepts did not die with him, but were carried forward by many followers, one of whom was James Caleb Jackson (Nissenbaum 1980).

In 1859, Jackson opened a health resort, called "Our Home on the Hillside," in Dansville, New York. There he developed the first dried breakfast cereal, and called it "Granula." In 1881 he sued John Harvey Kellogg, M.D. for marketing a similar product under the same name. Kellogg changed the name of his product to Granola.

Kellogg had been chosen by Ellen Harmon White, prophetess of the newly established Seventh-day Adventist sect in Battle Creek, Michigan, to receive medical training in the East. In 1876, at the age of 24, he became superintendent of the Adventists' new Health Reform Institute, later known as the Battle Creek Sanitarium. The young Kellogg was an ardent advocate of Graham's health tenets, namely, diet, exercise, and sexual abstinence. Practicing what he preached, he did not consummate his marriage and had no progeny. He spent his honeymoon writing *Plain Facts for Old and Young, Embracing the Natural History and Hygiene of Organic Life*, probably the most extreme statement of Victorian antisexualism ever published. Its multiple editions and revisions spread across the Pacific, and were published well into the present century.

Kellogg became famous as an abdominal surgeon, and was active in following the new science of biochemistry as applied to medicine. By contrast, he disregarded the revolutionary findings of Pasteur and Koch that established germ theory, and thus preserved, intact, his own doctrines on diet, exercise, and antisex.

He found an inventor's great personal satisfaction in developing new health-food cereals. His greatest discovery was the flaking of cereals, which culminated in 1898 in cornflakes. They joined the list of Kellogg's health foods that prevented sexual degeneracy. In a quite literal sense, therefore, cornflakes were invented as an antimasturbation food and extinguisher of sexual desire—but only provided they were not contaminated with sugar. John Harvey's younger brother, Will Keith Kellogg, added the sugar, and won the legal right to use the family name on the product. The rift between the two brothers split their wealth and made W. K. Kellogg a multimillionaire. John Harvey Kellogg remained a hedonic pauper, devoid of sexual pleasure, advocating erotic renunciation, until he died at the age of 91 in 1943.

VITAL SPIRITS: SEMEN VERSUS HORMONE

The sexosophy of antisexualism that became synonymous with Victorianism, and is still today extensively adhered to, had very ancient origins in what may be called proverbial sexosophy. Equating the conservation of semen with the conservation of strength is an ancient bit of proverbial sexosophy. The term for semen in Sanskrit is *sukra dhatu*, which translates as "white matter." In addition to matter, *dhatu* may also translate as "relic" or "metal", which allows the possibility that the white matter is also sacred and precious.

Logically, it would have been odd if farmers in the dawn of civilization, once they had discovered and adopted the practice of castrating the male animals of their herds, did not comprehend that early loss of the testicles prevented sexual maturation of the body and made the behavior more tame. To be tame might be equated with being less strong, rather than less violent.

It would be an easy next step to recognize that castrated animals produce no semen, and then to reach the wrong conclusion that human beings who lose too much semen would weaken themselves and become more like eunuchs who had been castrated as boys. This belief has an ancient history and is geographically widespread. Today, in Asia and parts of Africa, for example, it is a common belief among men who complain of a problem in the sexual functioning of the penis. In Europe and America, it is part of the folklore of sports medicine that competitors should abstain from having sex before a big event.

The error in the folklore that loss of semen is equivalent to becoming weak and unmanly, like a castrate, is easy to explain historically. It stems from the centuries when absolutely nothing was known about hormones. Until about a hundred years ago, it was not known that, when the testicles are cut out, the body loses the testosterone, also known as the male sex hormone, that they secrete invisibly into the bloodstream. The ancients knew that without testicles an animal is sterile, and also unable to ejaculate semen. But they did not know that almost all of the fluid of the semen is produced in the prostate gland, and that only the sperms are made in the testicles. Thus, it was easy to arrive at the wrong conclusion that, because castration causes loss of semen, semen itself must be the vital fluid that must be conserved in order to be virile, strong, and healthy.

This wrong conclusion could have been exploded on the basis of common sense observation alone, by toting up a few simple statistics to compare the working power and strength of men who saved their semen, and those who did not. Statistics, however, is a twentieth century way of solving problems. Our forefathers did not think that way. They looked to the prestige and authority of their predecessors for answers to problems.

Their wrong conclusion could also have been proved wrong, had anyone had the wisdom and insight to understand the significance of some of the first experiments involving what in the 1700s were called vital spirits, fluids or humors, and are now called hormones. No such luck! John Hunter (1728–1793) himself did not spell out, in full, the implications of his experiments. Using chickens, he transplanted the testicle of a rooster chick into the abdominal cavity of a hen, and discovered that, if the transplant took root, then the hen chicken would take on some of the bodily and behavioral characteristics of a rooster (Jorgensen 1971).

The existence of sex hormones was not proved until the end of the eighteen hundreds. It was as recently as the 1920s that they were extracted in pure chemical form, and the 1930s when they were synthesized and marketed for use in treatment.

Without absolute proof about the existence of sex hormones, wrong ideas about the power of semen persisted and became virtual science fiction. One wrong idea was that the body purifies semen from only the most precious vital spirits in the blood. Another error was that semen is made from neurine robbed from nerve tissue. Another error even went so far as to warn boys against masturbation because it drained away brain fluids down the spinal cord.

It was always necessary to gloss over girls and women in formulating theories based on the dire effects of the loss of semen. Since women could not lose semen, their ills and afflictions had to be based on menstruation and the wandering of the womb (hysteria).

SEXUALLY TRANSMITTED DISEASE

When Tissot medicalized the masturbation-possession theory of the anonymous author of *Onania*, he was quite explicit in acknowledging his debt, even as far back as Hippocrates, to his forebears with respect to the doctrine of semen loss.

It is quite possible, also, that Tissot recognized, as explicitly as the medical concepts of the day permitted, that medicine needed an explanation for what nowadays we would call the epidemiology of sexually transmitted diseases. The only terminology for these diseases available to Tissot was the social vice, which for him was part of the same plague as the solitary vice of masturbation. Both were caused by sexual excess. Sexual excess meant excessive loss of semen, and excessive concupiscence. Each influenced the other and together they debilitated and degenerated their victim.

Tissot, and later his followers, did not clearly distinguish between semen and any other fluids, except urine, that passed through the penis. The opaque, yellowish pus of gonorrhea and the clear glairy exudates of other infections or "strains" were regarded as evidence that sexual excess led to the various symptoms of the disease known as "spermatorrhea." In women, the corresponding disease was leukorrhea. Syphilis was not recognized as a separate disease, but there was apparently some recognition of the degeneracies it could induce, long-term; and of those that could be transmitted to the offspring of a sexually degenerate mother, that is, a syphilitic prostitute.

The logic, or rather the illogic of all this diagnostic chaos was the idea that loss of too much semen, especially in the solitary vice, could produce all the symptoms and diseases of the social vice. Thus did masturbation become blameworthy as the cause of all infectious genital and urinary discharges in both sexes. Since syphilis was not distinguished from these infections that produced discharges, masturbation was also held accountable for its advanced-stage degenerative symptoms, and for the sins of the fathers (and mothers) being visited on the offspring in the form of birth defects.

EROTIC IMAGERY: CONCUPISCENCE

Tissot borrowed from the anonymous author of *Onania* in formulating his sexosophy of degeneracy caused by loss of semen in solitary and social vice. Neither author made reference to the sexosophy of demon possession nor to the idea that onanistic theory filled the gap left by the demise of demon-possession theory. Both theories were all-purpose, general-utility sexosophical explanations of a wide range of social and individual afflictions.

Demon-possession sexosophy, unlike onanistic sexosophy, had been equally applicable to both sexes. Historically, accusations of witchcraft were leveled more often at women than men. Women's nocturnal copulations with demonic incubi and succubi were considered more dangerous to men than were their counterpart in men to women. Yet, it was, of course, adolescent boys and men, not girls and women who had actual wet dreams culminating in orgasm and discharge of semen. Both sexes however, could be accused of lascivious dreams in which, by witchcraft, they copulated with a servant of Satan. It was the erotic content of the dream that constituted the crime for which a witch, male or female, was burned at the stake.

The idea that erotic imagery in thoughts, fantasies, and dreams is the crime, or at least the sin, was taken up by the crusaders against onanism. For them it solved the problem of why loss of semen in solitary vice should be more dangerous and degenerative than in social vice. In either case, abstinence and the conservation of semen was also a sign of the conservation of moral purity. Indeed, moral purity became equated with abstinence or, at least continence. Above all, moral purity meant renunciation of concupiscence, the sin of sexual desire in imagination, thoughts, fantasies, and dreams. Masturbatory loss of semen was particularly condemned because it was associated with masturbation fantasies of explicit concupiscence and lust. Wet dreams also were condemned as evidence, spilling over into sleep, of concupiscence and lust undisciplined while awake.

Wet dreams and semen loss left women unaccounted for in degeneracy theory. Concupiscence and lust saved the day and allowed degeneracy theory to apply to females as well as males. To achieve moral purity, women also were required to relinquish concupiscence and the wickedness of erotic imagination and desire.

According to the doctrine of the Inquisition, women were so sinfully incapable of resisting concupiscence, including the imagination of copulating with Satan or his demons, that the redemption of their immortal souls required the sacrifice of their mortal bodies by burning them alive.

The price that women had to pay to be rescued from the fires of the Inquisition was the renunciation of all claim to concupiscent sexuality and eroticism, and the assimilation of an antithetical new doctrine of women's preternatural moral purity, erotic apathy, and sexual inertia. This new doctrine reached its zenith by the mid-nineteenth century. It declared that women copulated not out of lust, but in order to be relieved of their husband's attentions, and to fulfill the obligations of maternity.

Concupiscence was the sinful imagination or mental portrayal of lust and copulation, regardless of whether men or women were the sinners. From being the sin of demon possession, it became historically recycled as the sin of masturbation possession. It would be recycled yet a second time, after masturbation had become morally decriminalized in the present century. Its new name is the crime of pornography possession. Its condemnation and persecution are militant, politically tyrannous, and still very much in vogue.

From demons to masturbation to pornography, the representation of eroticism and lust in mental imagery and fantasy has continued to be condemned and accused as the cause of degeneracy and depravity, both personal and social. Depravity and degeneracy, in turn, are accused of being the cause of the afflictions of both the individual person and the society. The reasoning is circular. Circular reasoning disobeys the rules of sexology as science. It is perpetuated as the rhetoric of negative sexosophy.

NOTES

Graham, S. *A Lecture to Young Men.* Providence: Weeden and Cory, 1834. Facsimile reprint edition, New York: Arno Press, 1974.

Jorgensen, C. B. *John Hunter, A. A. Berthold, and the Origins of Endocrinology.* Odense: Odense University Press, 1971.

Kellogg, J. H. *Plain Facts for Old and Young, Embracing the Natural History and Hygiene of Organic Life.* Burlington, Iowa: I. F. Segner, 1888. Facsimile reprint edition, New York: Arno Press, 1974.

Nissenbaum, S. *Sex, Diet, and Debility in Jacksonian America: Sylvester Graham and Health Reform.* Westport: Greenwood Press, 1980.

Tissot, S. A. *A Treatise on the Diseases Produced by Onanism.* Translated from a New Edition of the French, with Notes and Appendix by an American Physician. New York, 1832. Facsimile reprint edition in *The Secret Vice Exposed! Some Arguments Against Masturbation,* C. Rosenberg and C. Smith-Rosenberg (advisory eds.). New York: Arno Press, 1974.

4

Integrate Sexology:
The Functions of Sex Role in Cultural History

E. W. Klimowsky

Iwan Bloch and Albert Moll were among the first medical professionals who approached the subject of sexology in its relation to culture and cultural history. Magnus Hirschfeld in 1926 generalized the subject in his fundamental two-volume treatise "Geschlechtskunde" (Sexology).

In a number of books and articles [1,2], I have shown that throughout the Graeco-Roman history (ca. 900 BC–AD 300) and that of the Western World (ca. AD 1000 to the present time) sex roles changed from marked masculinity to increasingly feminine traits in men, and from very feminine to increasingly masculine traits in women. This concept should be the aim and object of my proposed "integrate sexology."

In the Greek geometric age (ca. 900–700 BC) as well as in the corresponding Western Romanesque era (ca. AD 1000–1200), in the visual arts, the bodies of men and women were initially represented almost alike, in a triangular shape. Socially, a woman had no status at all; she did not belong to one of the three "ordines"—prayers, fighters, and workers (*oratores, bellatores, laboratores*).

In the Greek archaic age (ca. 700–480 BC) as well as in the corresponding Western European Gothic era (ca. AD 1200–1400), in all varieties of arts—visual, verbal, and musical—rising feminine traits in men and vice versa in women became slowly but irresistibly apparent. Therefore, a body-consciousness produced life-size sculpture instead of the earlier statuettes.

The beginning of the Gothic age marks the time of women troubadours (*trobairitz*). They were addressed by the troubadour as "midon" (my lord) and they demanded loyalty and faithfulness from their troubadours; if he turned to another midon, she blamed and even scolded him.

The structure of the body-tenure and the corresponding clothing-shape followed a clear zigzag, especially stressed for women by a protruding belly, symbolizing permanent pregnancy.

A noteworthy blend of masculine and feminine traits became alive together with the fierce struggle between those traits, finding visual expression in the widespread scenes where the woman subdues the man. Especially popular were the following: a man is thrashed by a woman; the woman, personified as Phyllis, rides on the back of a man, personified as the philosopher Aristotle; Yaël or Salome or Judith decapitating the national enemy; Dalila shearing the hair off Samson's head; the head of John the Baptist being presented on a silver platter to Salome according to her demand.

In the relatively short period of classical art in Greece and the Renaissance art in the West, the types of culturally productive men and and women disclose a nearly balanced manifestation of intermixed masculine and feminine traits.

The body-build, especially its breast region, was presented almost alike for women and young men. Standing or seated male figures, especially youths and youthful deities, become indistinguishable in pose from females. In the subsequent period, this remarkable feature becomes even more pronounced.

In this classical time, the feminized body-build coincides with the rejuvenation of the whole body. In the representation of grown-up men, especially of the gods, drastic changes take place: the beard disappears in favor of a youthfully shaven face; the limbs and stature make the bodies flourish in the prime of their youth. Finally, many deities become boys, even babies. So Heracles is venerated as a child strangling the snakes which his mother, Hera, has sent to kill him; Dionysos becomes a small boy trying to snatch a few grapes; even Zeus is venerated as a baby in his cradle in a cave, where the Curetes dance around him.

An effective means of expressing a woman's state of mind and its changes was the presentation of the nude female in the fifth century BC. "The subtlest rhythms of the female body are noted with an eager delicacy unsurpassed by Correggio or Clodion" [3].

The corresponding expression in the literary arts were the theatrical achievements by Euripides (480–406 BC) in whose gender identity the feminine traits had reached an unprecedented height, so that he was called "the discoverer of the female soul."

Another field in which change became manifest was medical theory that became recognizable in fifth and fourth century BC writings. It was a long time before the treatment of illnesses was freed from purely masculine theoretical and methodological fetters and could be devoted to the feminine knowledge which had been won in the course of decades and even centuries of observation of sick persons, and of the natural remedies destined to cure.

According to the Pythagorean doctrine (ca. 580–497 BC), the world is composed of basic symbols, among them the square and the oval. Their ideal relation was the harmony (symmetria) on which thought, behavior, and even dietary prescriptions were to be based.

The body-build of men and women, as reflected in the visual arts, clearly stressed any sexual differences. For the masculine costume, the penis was proudly shown and emphasized by a cap ("cod-piece") which, for festive occasions, was decorated with multicolored ribbons and jewels.

In medicine, this situation is exemplified especially by the two following phenomena: (1) Theophrastus Paracelsus (1493–1541) initiated a new concept of theory and practice: man and woman are quite different and have, therefore, to be correspondingly treated on the lines of chemically oriented biology including pharmacotherapy. (2) The moment of mating, that is, when the matrix attracts the male semen, was believed to be the beginning of a natural struggle. If the semen was masculine, a boy would be born; should the semen be feminine, a girl would be produced.

Since the feminine traits of men (including, of course, medical men) increased, their practical attitude toward obstetrics slowly began to prevail; they now became ready to render their services to women in labor. Until then, this had been the exclusive domain of more or less experienced midwives. The self-educated surgeon Ambroise Paré (1517–90) invented a sling to support the abdomen of the birth-giving woman and enabled her to give birth to as many as 20 children.

At that period, many models of birth-chairs were invented.

Other examples of that change in sex self-consciousness are the androgynous portraitures drawn by Leonardo da Vinci (Johannes, Philippus, Matthaeus in the "Last Supper," the angel in the rock grotto and the masculine head of "the Night" at the sepulchre of Lorenzo de Medici in Florence). King Francois 1 of France, who was acquainted with Leonardo, had himself portrayed androgynously, one half as Mars and the other half as Diana.

The rise of feminine trends in male sex roles also aroused intensive interest in the anatomy and physiology of the human body, including the measurements made by Michelangelo, Leonardo da Vinci, and Albreht Dürer. In the field of psychology, in the attempt by Leonardo da Vinci to study and understand embryonic connections with the womb of the mother.

The struggle between masculine and feminine elements in the male erupted in full force in the persecution of the witches, who were the incarnation of all the opposition to and hatred of those feminine elements in the masculine gender. In the Western world it became a hotbed of very real persecution of hundreds and thousands of "witches."

In Greek and Western Baroque alike (300 to 150 BC and AD 1600 to 1740), and even more so in the subsequent Rococo, the traits of the opposite gender gained the upper hand in the sex roles of men and women.

The body-build as reflected in the proportionate length and breadth of exemplary original Greek statues changed in the direction of femininity. Measurements on masculine statues of suprasternal height, symphysis height, trunk length, bi-acromial diameter, chest circumference at inspiration, hip circumference, arm length to tip of medial finger, were made at my suggestion in the National and Acropolis Museums of Athens by a team composed of an archaeologist (Barbara Philipaki) and the anthropologist Prof. Dr. M. Papamiltiades. The results were that from the second fifth of the sixth century BC until the last decade of the fourth century BC, an undulating increase of the pelvis as compared with the bi-acromial diameter, had been on the minds of the antique sculptors. Within 270 years, the ideal anatomical structure went from an exaggerated male ideal to a nearly feminine one and sometimes—as with the Kouros from Marathon—even exceeded the proportion between the pelvis-breadth to that of the bi-acromial diameter, like that of the Knidian Aphrodite.

FEMINIZATION IN THE MASCULINE GENDER ROLE

During this same time period, one observed a corresponding feminization of masculine figures in art.

1. "A soft graciousness now becomes the chief character-
    istic. The expressions of the faces show a dreamy

gentleness, often with an emotional note" (Richter, Greek Art) [4].

2. The Tanagra figurines with their juvenile sweetness of girls and young women, and above all the standing, lying, sleeping or aggression-repudiating hermaphrodites, expressed the new ideal. Their body-build is slim, with girlish breasts and masculine genitals.

3. Corresponding with the change in the ideal body-build, is the deep alteration relating to the understanding of children and their behavior and social position; children, who for Aristotle had been merely ugly dwarfs.

Among the indicators of a change in sex roles and even of gender identity is the sensitivity to pheromones directly or artificially emanating from the human body. The study of the far-reaching effects of this phenomenon in Graeco-Roman and modern times will become an important clue for integrate sexology.

In 1709 the softest art material, porcelain, was put into use by newly founded china factories in Meissen, Vienna, Sèvres, and other places. Objects and styles are of extremely feminine sweetness.

The steady rise of feminine traits in male sex roles made itself felt just recently. According to the BBC of 18/3/1983, the ban on men's training as midwives was lifted. Women could, however, have a female midwife, if they wished.

The neo-classical age in Greek and modern Western civilization (second to first century BC and AD 1790–1820) excelled in the short-lived but—until today—highly valued equipoise of the traits of both genders in one and the same individual.

In Roman and modern Romanticism (AD 50–200 and AD 1790–1850) the traits of the opposite gender in both men and women rose to an until-then unsurpassed height.

The second half of the nineteenth century, until the First World War, was characterized by the continuous attempts of the beginning feminist movement to occupy its place in society. There were also unabated and sometimes vehement counter-attacks from the masculine side: Schopenhauer and Nietzsche as philosophers, Ibsen and Strindberg as dramatists.

Similarly, in the visual arts, especially painting, there was a host of presentations of one or more women as slaves or otherwise sexually humiliated captives (Ingres, Giacometti, Slevogt, Moore, Picasso), or even with a cut throat, or as prostitutes.

That man is afraid of woman has been shown by the painters Edward Munch and Alfred Kubin ("The deadly leap") in their pictorial presentations.

There was quite an important group of first-rank painters, mostly adherents of expressionism, who saw themselves both as a man and as a woman. In his painting "Pygmalion," the surrealist Paul Delvaux in 1939 converted the sculptor of a female beauty into a sculptress trying to animate the torso of a young man.

The masculine opposition to feminine naturalism took the form of "cubism" and had two aims: to convert the subservience of impressionist concepts into abstract lines, and to concentrate those abstract lines and their contents into premodeled structures. This is evident in the works of Picasso, Braque, and Brancusi.

Many women adopted masculine behavior: sitting or standing with widely spread legs or taking small daughters into the polling booth to teach them the exercise of women's voting rights.

Since about 1920, hairstyles have become one of the indicators of changes in sex roles: after the First World War, the cropped hair of women; much later, the long hair of men. At approximately the same time, clothes were all cut on the same pattern.

Within the framework of the urgent desire of men and women to make themselves independent of age-old fetters, two trends succeeded:

1. To separate the bodily union from its biological consequences (that is, contraception);
2. To destroy the social fetters which bodily union of man and woman had cast upon them, by the social acceptance of sexual contact outside of marriage.

In view of even the limited selection of features just mentioned, the new socio- and integrated sexology here proposed is long overdue. Only in that way can two important achievements be reached:

1. The "arbitrary" sex attributes will lose their "arbitrariness"; and
2. Sexosophy (the philosophy of sex) will become a full-fledged science.

NOTES

1. Klimowsky, Ernst W. *Das mann-weibliche Leitbild in der Antike,* 135–50. Munich: Verlag Uni-Druck, 1972.

2. Klimowsky, Ernst W. *Geschlecht und Geschichte,* 111. Verlag Niggli und Verkauf, 1956.

3. Clark, Kenneth. *The Nude,* 149. London: Penguin Books, 1965.

4. Richter, Gisela M. A. *Greek Art,* 127. London: Phaidon Press, 1959.

PART II

Childhood Sexuality

It is astounding in 1983 to realize how little is known about childhood sexuality. This lack of information has both potential clinical and theoretical significance. With recent trends toward earlier sexual activity, knowledge of childhood attitudes toward sexuality, of course, assumes practical significance. Numerous psychoanalytically oriented clinicians assume that early childhood experiences and attitudes influence adult behavior.

Until comparatively recently, the only information concerning childhood sexuality was based upon observations of psychoanalytic therapists. This information was based on selected clinical samples and also frequently was based on the memories of adult patients in psychotherapy. Adult memories are subject to considerable distortion regarding childhood experiences. It is also risky to extrapolate data about the general population from highly selected clinical samples. Other psychoanalytic hypotheses accepted as factual have not stood the test of empirical investigation. In this regard, it is of note that both Goldman and Borneman found minimal evidence to support the analytic hypotheses of a latency period of sexual development. It is also of interest to note the difficulty that both groups of investigators had obtaining adult permission to study children's attitudes. Again, social mores are shown to influence scientific inquiry.

5

An Overview of Children's Sexual Thinking: A Comparative Study of Australian, English, North American, and Swedish 5-15-Year Olds

R. Goldman and J. Goldman

INTRODUCTION

We define sexual thinking as "thinking about" the varied observations and experiences of sex and sexuality children encounter in the course of their development. In this sense they are sexual thinkers from birth, from the first encounter with mother's breasts, to the dawning recognition of their own and their parents' sexuality, through to their direct experience of sexuality during adolescence. Children's awareness and perceptions of sex and sexuality would appear to be a vital aspect of their development.

The theories of Freud, Piaget, and Kohlberg have contributed to this area, and having previously investigated children's religious thinking in terms of Piagetion theory [1], we felt that an investigation of children's sexual thinking would provide the opportunity to test out some of these theories. It might also provide some guidelines for sex educators in terms of what children at various ages perceive about sex, the cognitive strategies they might use in explaining sex and sexuality and, more importantly, what they appear to be capable of understanding, given early sex education.

Despite Piaget's early contact with Freudian theory and practice and Piaget's own training as a biologist [2], he concentrated his investigations of children's developing cognition upon the physical and mathematical sciences and only rarely studied children's biological (including sexual) thinking [3]. In fact, we could report it to be one of Piaget's blind spots repeated by the Geneva school generally despite its varied investigations in many different cultures [4]. Nevertheless, like Freud, Piaget posited some brilliant hypotheses about children's sexual cognition, particularly during the artificialist stage of cognitive growth [5].

Our study should be seen not only in terms of theory but also against certain world-wide trends in the sexual development of the young: earlier physical maturing (the secular trend in physical growth), the earlier sexual experience of the young, the delayed age of marriage, and greater risk of teenage pregnancies and veneral disease [6]. These phenomena raise questions about how prepared and knowledgeable are the young in facing these risks and what practical programs should be provided by society to help them.

Research Aims

In addition to examining the hypotheses of various theorists and seeking guidelines for practical policies, our aims were fourfold. First, to measure the extent of children's knowledge and ignorance about sexuality in the basic years of schooling. Second, to see if there were any discernible stages of sexual cognition with increasing age. Third, to identify what cognitive strategies and processes children use to explain biological and sexual functions, particularly in their own growing and changing bodies. Fourth, to observe the capacity of children for sexual understanding where sex education is systematically available from an early age.

The Research Method

A face-to-face clinical interview was designed and conducted on a same sex basis. After pretesting the interview blank with Australian children, we finalized six major sections containing some 63 questions, with many contingent questions to secure fuller responses. Each interview took between 40 minutes and one hour.

The six sections covered how children perceive old age, the aging process, and growing up; mothers' and fathers' roles in the family and the basis of marriage; differences between the sexes at birth and during adolescence, including sex preferences for friends; conception and birth, including length of gestation, the birth exit, sex determination, and not having babies; children's views on sex education, when, what, and by whom, and included was a ten-word sexual vocabulary list. The last section covered how children perceived nakedness and the wearing of clothes [7].

The Sample

The sample of children aged 5–15 was made up of alternate year cohorts, aged 5, 7, 9, 11, 13, and 15 years from Australia, England, North America, and Sweden.

Each cohort was controlled for age, sex, intellectual ability (based upon teachers' assessments), and socio-economic status (based on Treiman's Standard International Occupational and Prestige Scales [8].

To ensure what we define as "best conditions for sexual development" all children interviewed had to be living in a two-parent situation and had at least one younger sibling. In our view they would then have observed mother and father roles, and experienced the arrival of a new baby into the family. Family size ranged from two to nine children, and 65 percent of the total sample had at least one other sex sibling.

Selection of children was made in each country from public school systems, using elementary and high school registers (except in Sweden where schooling does not begin until seven years; consequently five-year-olds were drawn from state kindergartens), once the permission of district inspectors or superintendents had been gained. Depending on the size of the school, in the age groups selected, every second, third, or fourth child was chosen. Known as systematic sampling, it is equally acceptable to statisticians as random sampling. After ensuring only Caucasian children remained, to exclude diverse migrant and cultural groups and to make each country comparable with the others, the children who met "the best conditions" were then chosen.

School principals sent out letters to the parents of those children finally selected, asking permission for the interview, and enclosing a sheet describing the project, which was named "Children's Conceptualisation of Development."

Political and Other Aspects of the Sample

Australian school practices and child rearing have been dependent upon the British model, although in the last

20 years North American assumptions about schooling and child development have become increasingly influential.

Accordingly, to establish some tentative Australian norms in terms of sexual thinking, we decided to take comparative samples of American and English children, to see what similarities and differences might be evident between these three areas, each having some distinct similarities of language and culture.

Sweden was selected for other reasons. In health and sex education, Swedish school curricula are markedly advanced compared with the cautious and controversial approach in Australia, the United States, and Britain. For over 20 years, sex education has been compulsory in all schools in Sweden for all children from the age of eight. It therefore serves as a contrast group to the English-speaking areas, especially in terms of the fourth aim to assess the capacity of children to understand sexuality if taught from an early age.

It must be reported that no problems were experienced in gaining the approval of administrators and school principals in Australia, England, and Sweden. In the United States, however, we encountered considerable questioning, resistance, and refusals in our attempts to gain access to schools. By a misfortune of timing, we arrived in the United States only a few weeks before local Board of Education elections were to take place. Superintendents were plainly fearful that knowledge of our project might provide ammunition to vocal minority groups. The Anaheim experience was frequently cited.

Nevertheless, we gained access to some U.S. schools, but had also to sample schools across the Niagara River in Ontario, Canada, to ensure sufficient numbers. Hence, we had to combine U.S. and Canadian children across all age groups to provide a North American sample.

Symptomatic of these political and cultural problems were the different refusal rates of parents in giving approval for their children to be interviewed. These were Sweden 5.3 percent, Australia 16.3 percent, England 20.1 percent, and North America 23.6 percent.

The regions selected were urban-suburban within reasonable travelling distance of the universities used as bases; Melbourne, Australia, Berkshire in England, Stockholm in Sweden, and both upper New York State in the United States and southern Ontario in Canada.

Because of regional and political factors, we cannot claim to have used "national" samples, but rather descriptive samples of child populations not untypical of the countries involved. We therefore describe the study as a comparative descriptive study based upon regional clusters of schools, stratified for socio-economic status and other factors, and within schools systematic sampling from class lists of children who met the required criteria.

Criteria for Evaluating the Results

Some results were coded into categories rather than quantified by scores. But most were scored on previously constructed criteria based on a numerical hierarchy. Some of these such as length of gestation, led to a natural three point scale (between eight and ten months or "realistic," scoring three, between six and eight months and ten and twelve months, "semirealistic," scoring two, and any other estimate, for example, three weeks or five years as "unrealistic," scoring one.

A biological realism scale for many items was devised with the assistance of several biologists and psychologists. Piagetian scores on a 0–5 point scale were also devised for many items, some overlapping with biological realism scores. And a modified Kohlberg six point scale was used, particularly in the section on clothes and nakedness [9].

All responses were scored by the two investigators independently on appropriate criteria. A satisfactory level of scorer reliability was achieved ($r = 0.75$ to 0.98).

The Results

How Children Perceive Sex Differences in Babies

Before we present the more global findings, we have selected one item from the 63 major questions to illustrate the study, "How children perceive sex differences in babies." Other items are reported elsewhere [10].

The question asked was "How can anyone know that a newborn baby is a boy or a girl?" Apart from nonsense answers such as "I have a baby sister," or "I like boy babies better," a biological realism six-point scale used indicated a progression from unrealistic to realistic recognition of sex differences in the newborn, as children increased in age. Younger children in Sweden were more realistic much earlier, and younger children in the North American sample were the least realistic.

Initially children seized upon irrelevant physical factors such as hair ("If it's longer, it's a girl"), color of eyes, the size of the baby, and the clothes ("Mum puts it in a dress, so it must be a girl").

Next came authoritarian and artificialist explanations. The doctor, nurse, the priest or mother tells you, or official color tags, clothes or bedclothes (the inevitable blue or pink) are the indications, or a boy or girl name is sufficient reason for identity.

Children then develop semirecognized physical differences but expressed them in rather vague descriptions: "They're different down there, some kind of different bottom." "Boys stand up to the wee-wee and girls don't." Physical differences are later more clearly recognized, but even then it is a long time before children progress from the use of pseudonyms to describing the sex organs by their correct names. Here is a North American boy aged 13: "Down between your legs, where they go to the locker room." (Q: How do you mean?) "It's embarrassing, but the boy doesn't have a slit down the middle but has a round tube." (Q: What is that?) "A penis." An Australian boy, aged seven: "You can tell by its penis it's a boy." (Q: What if it's a girl?) "She's got something, don't know what it's called. I call it a hamburger."

The English-speaking children at five to seven years are strongly unrealistic, providing mainly irrelevant physical factors, authoritarian, or artificialist answers. By the age of nine a growing number, the majority in the Australian sample, have achieved a realistic recognition and by eleven years the English and North American children have caught up. Seventy-one percent of Swedish seven-year olds can correctly identify sex differences; by comparison, the English figure is 40 percent and the North American 30 percent.

What is most noticeable about the responses about newborn babies and, later, pubertal differences, is the widespread use of pseudonyms for the sex organs. More than 60 pseudonyms were used to describe the penis and more than 40 to describe the vagina (occasionally called "the virginia"). These could be categorized as associations with urination or excretia, analogies such as a "hot dog" or "a muffin," names of people such as "Joey" or "Fanny," anatomical descriptions or those with animal or bird associations, "a pecker" or "a beaver." The widespread use of these pseudonyms is accompanied by the frequent reference among older children to the correct terms as "rude," "dirty," or "naughty." Others clearly did not know the names nor what they signified.

The Swedish results merit two observations. The first is that there appear to be no cognitive or developmental factors which would prevent children perceiving sex differences realistically from an early age. The second observation, linked with findings from many other items in this study, is the absurdity of the Freudian theory of a latency period. Children are overtly curious about sexuality and the sex organs between five and twelve years of age and obviously try to penetrate the taboos around them. The Swedish results would indicate "the latency period" as perhaps a temporary aberration of central Europe in the late nineteenth century. For too long Freud's latency ideas have been responsible for the view of children as non-sexual beings during latency and the mistaken idea that sex education should be delayed until puberty.

Some Major Findings of the Study

For statistical reasons, the results of more than 40 items should be examined separately. However, some cumulative evidence does indicate trends about which we will make some tentative generalizations.

Twenty-three major items were combined into total scales. These were the Piagetian scales, the Biological Realism scales, and the Sexual Vocabulary scales. An examination and analysis of these do provide an overview of children's sexual thinking not possible by the analysis of individual items.

The Piagetian scales, based upon the levels of preoperational, concrete, and formal operational thinking about sexuality support Piaget's theory that with increasing age, children in all the countries sampled proceed from pre-logical to logical thinking. There were no significant differences between countries in the scores on these six items. North American children scored slightly better, with Swedish children close behind. These items, however, have a somewhat "social" bias and may well be explained by evidence of the generally more advanced social development of the North American children.

The Biological Realism scales (six items) however, reveal considerable differences between the samples. The Swedish scores over the whole sample are the highest, the Australian and English scores are close together, and the North American scores are the lowest. When Analysis of Variance (ANOVA) is applied, the differences between countries are highly significant.

Similar results can be found from an analysis of the Sexual Vocabulary scales (ten items), the Swedish scores high, and the North American scores significantly low. Due to some justifiable criticism since first publishing these results, an alternative method of scoring the Sexual Vocabulary has been used. The results, however, support the previous findings—the significantly high scores of the Swedish children, and the highly significant low scores of the North American children.

Further generalizations from many separate items support these observed differences. We can report considerable time-lags between Sweden and the three English-speaking countries in what makes up the universe of children's sexual thinking. Low-level thinking and poor problem-solving in the area of sexuality are evident. If the Swedish scores represent the norm of what is possible for children to cognize sexually, the other samples reveal a retardation factor or time-lag in understanding. In some items there is a two-year retardation of the Australian and English children, and up to a three-year retardation in the North American children's sexual thinking. Although there is no demonstrable causation, it is interesting to observe that Sweden has the earliest and most systematic sex education in its school system, and the North American regions sampled appear to have the later and least provision for sex education in their schools.

The evidence from the Swedish sample indicates that the retardation observed in the English-speaking children of this study may be due to cultural and educational differences and that children are capable of understanding quite complex biological concepts much earlier than was first thought. Only two of the concepts examined—the cause of childbirth at a particular time, and the sex determination of babies—were judged to be appropriate at the high school level only.

Retardation in sexual thinking is postulated as due partly to inadequate communication and adult inhibitions about using correct terminology and descriptions with children, the consequential usage of sexual pseudonyms by children, and the need to find suitable explanations for sexuality without adequate information. False analogies in sexual thinking appear to cause confusion and assist retarded thinking.

In the absence of adequate and systematic sex education, children invent their own explanations for biological and sexual processes often in the form of mythologies; medical mythologies being the dominant explanations in early to middle childhood.

Sex education is seen as essential by the vast majority of children and should in their view be provided in elementary schools, whereas the provision actually given to the majority appears to be in high schools only—apart from Sweden—and often late in secondary schooling. In the English-speaking countries a sizeable proportion of teenagers report having received no sex education at school, while some of these also report no help from their parents. A considerable shortfall exists between what the children want to know and what they claim to have received, which in their view is provided too late.

The home remains the most cited major source of sex information in the person of the mothers, with teachers and the media as secondary major sources. Children have considerable confidence in asking sex questions of mother, little confidence is asking them of fathers, friends, or teachers, unless the latter are specialist teachers in sex education or related subjects. The indications are that parents, particularly mothers, need assistance in helping them to be more effective sex educators of their own children. Attention should also be directed to encouraging fathers to become more involved in their children's sex education.

The best conditions for well-developed sexual thinking would, as reflected in evidence from our study, appear to be upbringing in a family with at least one other-sex sibling in a family of three children or more, a well-informed active mother who works or studies, and a systematic school sex education program in the elementary school to follow the early years at home. Since the decreasing size of families makes several of these conditions inaccessible to the majorty iof children, supplementary sex education through other social agencies, schools in particular, becomes a pressing social need.

Kohlberg's theory of three levels of development in moral thinking (preconventional, conventional, and postconventional) was supported by some of the results, but with few teenagers revealing postconventional moral thinking about sexuality. On the whole the young subscribe to "conventional" sexual judgments.

Several of Freud's theories about children's sexual thinking receive some support from our study. One such is his cloacal theory, similar to "the digestive fallacy," that young children perceive conception to occur by the mother swallowing certain foods, which leads to plumpness and the inflated stomach. The food becomes the baby and it is born through the anus. Freud's latency period, however, is completely contradicted by our evidence in item after item.

A BRIEF DISCUSSION

In the light of earlier maturing (the mean age of menstruation in Australia is 12.5 years, similar to the other countries studied), earlier sexual activity and the social and health risks attendant upon these factors, our study would indicate a widespread state of ignorance about sexuality in the young.

It is plain that the English-speaking countries have failed, and continue to fail, the young in providing them with basic information, knowledge, and guidance necessary to cope with their earlier maturing. Adolescent girls are particularly ignorant in these countries about menstruation, about the sexual parts of their own bodies, about contraception and venereal diseases. Boys and girls both share considerable ignorance in knowledge about conception, which is the great taboo area. If correct information about how babies are made and how they are prevented is withheld, we have a sure recipe for early sexual unhappiness.

The North American results are the most disturbing of all. In terms of dating and early sexual activity, the North American children sampled appear comparatively to be both socially precocious and sexually ignorant, a combination guaranteed to provide social and sexual difficulties.

If all schools were allowed to provide sex education, our study would indicate the greatest need to be a conceptual structure for children's sexual thinking to provide clear sequential guidelines for programs, parents, and teachers. We are currently working on this to be presented next year in our book *Readiness for Sex Education* [11].

NOTES

1. Goldman, R. J. *Religious Thinking from Childhood to Adolescence.* London: Routledge and Kegan Paul, 1964. New York: Seabury Press, 1967.

2. Cowan, P. A. *Piaget with Feeling.* New York: Holt, Rinehart and Winston, 1978.

3. Piaget, J. *Biology and Knowledge.* Edinburgh: Edinburgh University Press, 1971 (First published in French, 1967).

4. Modgil, S. *Piagetian Research: A Handbook of Recent Studies.* Windsor: NFER, 1974.

5. Piaget, J. *The Child's Conception of the World,* 367. London: Routledge and Kegan Paul, 1951 (First published 1927).

6. Hunt, W. B. "Adolescent Fertility, risks and consequences." *Population Reports, Series J.* U.S. Department of Health, Education, and Welfare, 1976, 10:157–76.

7. Goldman, R. J., and J. D. G. Goldman. *Children's Sexual Thinking* (Chapter 3). London, Boston and Mel-

bourne: Routledge and Kegan Paul, 1982.

8. Treiman, D. J. *Occupational Prestige in Comparative Perspective.* New York: Academic Press, 1977.

9. Goldman, R. J., and J. D. G. Goldman. "Children's perceptions of clothes and nakedness." *Genetic Psychol. Monographs,* 1981, 104, no. 2:163–85.

10. Goldman, R. J., and J. D. G. Goldman. "What children want to know about sex." *Australian Science Teachers Journal,* 1981, 27, no. 2:61–69.

Goldman, R. J., and J. D. G. Goldman. "Sources of sex information for Australian, English, North American and Swedish children." *Journal of Psychology,* 1981, 109: 97–108.

Goldman, R. J., and J. D. G. Goldman. "Children's concepts of why people get married." *Australian Journal of Sex, Marriage and Family,* August 1981, 2, no. 3:105–18.

Goldman, R. J., and J. D. G. Goldman. "How children perceive the origin of babies and the roles of mothers and fathers in procreation." *Child Development,* 1982, 53:491–504.

11. Goldman, R. J., and J. D. G. Goldman. *Readiness for Sex Education.* London, Boston and Melbourne: Routledge and Kegan Paul (to be published 1984).

6

The Value and Significance of Comparative Studies in Childhood Sexuality

R. Goldman and J. Goldman

INTRODUCTION

Our recent research comparing children's sexual cognition from five to 15 years in Australia, England, North America, and Sweden illustrates the value of comparative studies in childhood sexuality [1].

As Australians we lack an established series of norms for children and we have tended to accept British and American norms in our assumptions about child-rearing, developmental stages, and educational practices. Because Australia is a derivative culture, its two major sources being Great Britain and the United States, a comparison of Australian children with their assumed normative peers in those countries helps us in Australia establish some basic norms.

This research therefore, with its comparative perspective, provides some valuable information about the state of children's sexual knowledge, and the converse, their sexual ignorance. We discovered a great deal about children's strategies of thinking about sexuality, how they solve the mysterious problems presented by sexuality, inventing myths and hypotheses about procreation, gestation, and birth.

The work of Dr. Bernstein on "the origins of babies" provided us with one particularly important area of children's sexual thinking which we partially replicated [2]. The comparison of our North American sample results with Bernstein's results may be of special interest. Her sample taken from around the Berkeley campus was entirely made up of children from upper socioeconomic status (s.e.s.) families. Ours was taken more randomly through public school registers, controlled for the whole range of ability and s.e.s. Our results revealed the same sequences of thinking about the origins of babies as she discovered, but with considerable age discrepancies. The more typical North American sample scored lower and slower than the more able children who were mainly of university professors or with fathers of higher educational achievements. Nevertheless, the sequences were confirmed not only in our North American sample, but also in our other sampling, suggesting a generalized sequence at least among developed industrial democratic type countries.

Sweden was included in our study as a contrast group. While there are certain cultural commonalities which Sweden shares with us, in the realm of sexuality there are three distinct differences. One is the more enlightened attitude to sexual matters, including homosexuality, illegitimacy, availability of contraceptives to the young, and de facto marriage, all supported through legislation.

The second difference is the universal compulsory provision of sex education for all children in all schools from eight years onwards, and also extending down into the state-provided kindergartens. The third, which is not always recognized, is that since these sex education programs have existed for more than 25 years, most parents of present-day Swedish children are themselves the products of both enlightened legislation and early sex education.

The Swedish sample, therefore, helped us to evaluate the cognitive potential in children's sexual thinking; that is, the ages at which children are capable of understanding sexuality, if sexual taboos and prevarications are diminished and if early systematic sex education is introduced universally into the school system.

For example, we found only two of the 63 items of sexual knowledge explored in our study that were not understood in the elementary school years in Sweden. These were the process by which sex is determined at conception, and the causes of birth at the end of the gestation period.

Thus, if we consider the Swedish sample to be the norm for sexual thinking, then on total results the Australian and English samples revealed a two-year retardation. The North American sample showed up to a three-year retardation in their sexual thinking.

Although no simple cause and effect connection can be argued, of the two countries the United States and Sweden at the lower and upper ends of our scoring scales, the

United States has the least and longest delayed sex education due to intense minority opposition provision, and
Sweden has the fullest and the earliest due to almost universal consensus support.

Classifying Comparative Studies

Comparative studies have a long tradition, but in sexuality
such studies are still rather rare. We can extrapolate from
independent studies some comparative data and recognize
certain apparent universalities in sexual development. One
example is earlier sexual maturing from Tanner's work in
Britain [3], Ljung in Sweden [4], and Harper and Collins
in Australia [5]. Another is the onset of earlier sexual
activity in the young from Venner in the United States [6],
Schofield in Britain [7], and Collins in Australia [8].

The problem with these studies, all of considerable
value, is that the data are not entirely comparable, the
samples are not usually matched and the investigations have
occurred at different times. Thus, normative trends can
only be estimated and their significant contributions are
somewhat weakened.

We have so far used the term "comparative" studies,
rather than "cross-cultural," simply because the research
literature provides ambiguous definitions. Comparative
studies are generally classified as "cross-national" or
"cross-cultural."

Cross-National Studies

Most studies into children's sexuality to date are best
described according to Jahoda [9] as cross-national studies.
These generally use samples from western industrialized
countries, possessing high standards of living and in
particular having a well-developed compulsory school system
from elementary to secondary. An example of this is
Williams' study of sex-trait stereotypes in France, Germany,
and Norway [10]. Two others can be seen in presentations
at this Congress such as Borneman's study of Australian,
German, and Swiss children [11] and our own, briefly
presented today.

Lloyd [12], however, has modified Jahoda's definition
claiming that national groups may contain many cultures and
subcultures, and within Europe there may be considerable
differences that may affect sexuality and its development in
the young. Even within one country where cultural, religious, and language differences may be minimal, it can be

said there are various cultures or sub-cultures expressed in diverse socio-economic status or regional groupings.

Our own study, to make comparisons more rigorous, used only White Anglo-Saxon Protestants (WASP) samples in the English-speaking countries. In all countries, including Sweden, the samples were Caucasian and largely Protestant also. We would hope replication studies with different ethnic, racial, and religious groups would yield valuable insights into the relationship between sexual development and distinct cultures, within reasonably homogeneous societies. But many more studies would be significant if diverse groups within such a heterogeneous society as the United States or the European Common Market could be sampled.

Cross-Cultural Studies

Countries or cultures may within their own grouping be fairly homogeneous, but many varying cultures may co-exist within a continent, for example, Asia or Africa. Cross-national studies are where a number of countries may have considerable cultural commonality, but cross-cultural studies are where countries or groups have certain racial commonalities but are divided by very different and diverse cultures.

Such cultures tend to be classified as "developing," that is, not as developed or as industrialized as western democratic societies. Ford and Beach's *Patterns of Sexual Behaviour* [13] is a classic cross-cultural as well as cross-species study, and by analysis the authors have been able to categorize societies sexually on a continuum as restrictive, semi-restrictive, and permissive. Some cultures, they point out, in their child-rearing practices forbid children watching the birth of animals, while in others boys of four to five years old are removed from their homes to bachelor accommodations to prevent them from witnessing the sexual intercourse of parents.

By far the most numerous cross-cultural studies have been cognitive [14], and the great majority of these have been Piagetian studies [15]. But very few cross-cultural studies have been devoted to the sexuality of children. Some of the earlier descriptive studies were by anthropologists, who in describing a culture sometimes included observations of sexual customs and behavior in the young. The most famous is Margaret Mead's study of Samoa [16], although recently an Australian academic has published criticisms of her methods and conclusions [17].

A few cross-cultural studies have been used to test

Freudian theories, such as Stephens [18] on castration fears and studies of Kibbutzim children in Israel to test the Oedipal hypothesis.

The Objectives of Comparative Studies

The objectives of comparative studies can be classified into five categories:

1. The comparison of norms within one society with norms of other societies of a similar culture (cross-national).
2. The sampling of societies with similar cultures, where one variable is seen to be distinctive of one of them (cross-national).
3. The search for possible universalisms throughout all societies (usually cross-cultural).
4. The testing of hypotheses to test the validity of various theories about human behavior (cross-cultural).
5. The generating of new hypotheses in the sampling of very diverse cultures (cross-cultural) [19].

Relevance of Comparative Studies to
Childhood Sexuality Studies

These objectives are relevant to our understanding of childhood sexuality in various ways, which in our view illustrate the value and significance of comparative studies, both cross-national and cross-cultural:

1. Norms of sexual development and behavior are notably absent even in developed and resource-rich countries. Says David Finkelhor: "We know more about sexual deviance than we do about sexual normality or ordinariness" [20].
2. Where one variable is notably different, useful interpretations and practical consequences can be deduced. Scandinavian countries are particularly useful as "control" samples for the developed countries of Europe, North America and Australasia.
3. While Ford and Beach have highlighted differences between cultures relating to courtship behavior, rites of passage, pre-marital sex and the restrictions on children observing sexuality, certain sexual universalisms may possible exist which would further our understanding of child rearing, child development and child education in all countries and cultures.

4. Many theories of sexual development need rigorous examination which only cross-cultural studies can validate or invalidate. Among these are Freud's stages and related theories about Oedipal relationships in the family, communal theories of child-rearing, and field dependency theory as applied to sexual development [21].
5. Societies greatly dissimilar to that experienced by investigators do provoke new theories to explain what is observed and thus generate new hypotheses. This has certainly occurred and led to the questioning of certain societal assumptions about sexual deviancy such as masturbation, homosexuality, and pubertal behavior.

In conclusion, as Cole and Scribner have written "cross-cultural research is like virtue—everybody is in favor of it, but there are widely differing views of what it is and ought to be" [22]. Applied to investigations of childhood sexuality this comment is thought-provoking.

NOTES

1. Goldman, R. J. and J. D. G. Goldman. *Children's Sexual Thinking*. London, Boston and Melbourne: Routledge and Kegan Paul, 1982.
2. Bernstein, A. C. "The Child's Concepts of Human Reproduction." Ph.D dissertation, University of California, Berkeley, 1973.
3. Tanner, J. M. *Education and Physical Growth*. London: University of London Press, 1961.
4. Ljung, B. O., A. Bergsten-Brucefors, and G. Lindgren. "The secular trend in physical growth in Sweden." *Annals of Human Biology,* 1974, 1:245–56.
5. Harper, J. H. and J. K. Collins. "The secular trend in the age of menarche in Australian schoolgirls." *Australian Paediatric Journal,* 1972, 8:44–48.
6. Venner, A. M., C. S. Stewart, and D. L. Hager. "The sexual behaviour of adolescents in middle America." *Journal of Marriage and the Family.* November 1972, 34: 696–705.
7. Schofield, M. *The Sexual Behaviour of Young People*. Penguin, Harmondsworth, 1968.
   Schofield, M. *Promiscuity*. London: Gollanez, 1976.
8. Collins, J. K. "Adolescent dating intimacy: norms and peer expectations." *Journal of Youth and Adolescence,* 1974, 3:317–27.
9. Jahoda, G. "A cross-cultural perspective in psychology." *The Advancement of Science,* 1970, 27, no.

1:57–70.

10. Williams, J. E. et al. "Sex-trait stereotyping in France, Germany and Norway." *Journal of Cross-cultural Psychology,* 1979, 10:133–56.

11. Borneman, E. "Progress in Empirical Research on Childhood Sexuality." Postgraduate course. Washington, D.C.: Sixth World Congress of Sexology, 1983.

12. Lloyd, B. B. *Perception and Cognition from a Cross-cultural Perspective.* Penguin, Harmondsworth, 1972.

13. Ford, C. S., and F. A. Beach. *Patterns of Sexual Behaviour.* New York: Harper and Row, 1951.

14. Berry, J. W. and P. R. Dasen. *Culture and Cognition: Readings in Cross Cultural Psychology.* London: Methuen, 1965.

15. Modgil, S. *Piagetian Research: A Handbook of Recent Studies.* National Foundation of Educational Research, 1974.

16. Mead, M. *Coming of Age in Samoa.* New York: W. Morrow, 1928.

17. Freeman, D. *Margaret Mead on Samoa: the Making and Unmaking of an Anthropologic Myth.* Canberra: ANU Press, 1983.

18. Stephens, W. N. *The Oedipus Complex Hypothesis: Cross-cultural Evidence.* Glencoe, New York: Free Press, 1962.

19. Strodtbeck, F. "Consideration of meta methods in cross-cultural studies." *American Anthropology,* 1969, 66:223–29.

20. Finkelhor, D. *Sexually Victimized Children.* New York: The Free Press, 1979.

21. Witkin, H., R. B. Dyk, H. F. Faterson, D. R. Goodenough, and S. A. Karp. *Psychological Differentiation.* London: Wiley, 1974.

22. Cole, M., and S. Scribner. *Culture and Thought: A Psychological Introduction.* New York: John Wiley, 1974.

7

Progress in Empirical Research
on Children's Sexuality

E. Borneman

Anyone old enough to remember public reactions to the first
Kinsey Report and professional reactions to Masters' and
Johnson's first attempts at measuring and filming human
sexual activities will know how difficult it is to introduce
new techniques of sexological research. No field of sexology is beset with more objections of this sort than research into children's sex lives. They reach the height of
absurdity with the denial that there is such a thing as
children's sexuality.

Of course, paedologists mean something different by
children's sex lives than do laymen. We do not limit the
term to having intercourse. In our vocabulary, a child's
sex life is the child's entire life as a sexual being. In this
sense, it may even be permissible to speak of prenatal sex
life.

We believe, anyway, that the study of children's sexual
activities provides salient clues to questions of adult sexuality that cannot be answered by the study of adult sex
life itself. But our work is extremely difficult because
adults, as a rule, feel obliged to protect their children
against any sexual inquiries. They begin to acknowledge
nowadays that adult volunteers can be questioned on all
aspects of their sex lives, but they refuse to let their
children be questioned. To film and measure children's
sexual activities, as Masters and Johnson have done with
adults, is impossible in most countries of the Western

world. The result is not only ignorance but a plethora of false information.

When my first research team began its work some 40 years ago, we believed, for instance, that a boy's first ejaculation indicated that his semen had become fertile. We believed, too, that a girl could not be impregnated before she had had her first menstruation. We accepted these assumptions because they seemed obvious. It never occurred to us to question or test them.

Then we heard of a girl of nine who had been raped and borne a child prior to her menarche. Naturally, we assumed that the girl had simply failed to comprehend her first menstrual symptoms. Then we heard of a second and a third case of premenstrual impregnation. Gradually we came to wonder whether the psychosomatic shock of rape might not cause premature ovulation. Having looked into a dozen cases of raped minors, we now believe this to be true. Apparently girls can be impregnated prior to their first natural menstruation.

The point is not very important, but it made us wonder how many of the unquestioned tenets of children's sexual physiology were really valid. We found that the first ejaculation was by no means a dependable sign of fertility. Many boys are still infertile after months of nightly ejaculations, and others have fertile seed long before their first ejaculation.

The next point we were curious about was the first orgasm. We had read of almost one hundred reports of orgasms or paraorgasms among infants and pre-school children. We found six children under two years and seven under four years who seemed to be able to produce bodily states which we would have termed orgasmic had they occurred in a grown-up. Our difficulties began when we told the parents that we wanted to film their children's masturbation activities and were eager to measure their bodily reactions. It then turned out that even the most "progressive" parents were not willing to let us proceed. This meant that we had reached the limits of what was permissible in physiological research on children's sexuality at that time. So we began to look for other ways of getting at the truth.

We had heard that certain neo-Reichian groups in Germany and Austria were allowing their children to be present during parental intercourse. We had also heard that these children were by no means satisfied with a spectator's role and wanted to participate in their parents' sexual activities. We found this to be true. We also found that the children were healthy and stable. But again, we were not allowed to employ cameras and microphones because the parents were afraid of legal complications.

Our fourth attempt to learn something about children's sexual reactions was a series of interviews with male and female prisoners sentenced for (a) incest, (b) intercourse with children. We found, to our own surprise, that these people were not only willing but eager to talk to us. We visited 12 prisons and spoke to 18 persons sentenced for incest and to 16 sentenced for intercourse with children and juveniles under 14. We also spoke to 12 male homosexuals sentenced for intercourse with boys under 18. Since we were not able to check the correctness of their statements we summarize them here without identifying ourselves with them:

1. Boys are capable of full erection from birth on.
2. Boys and girls are capable of orgasmic satisfaction long before their first ejaculation or menstruation.
3. In contrast to the many testimonies cited by Florence Rush and other adherents of the "children are always victims" school of thought, children are generally the initiators and not the victims of intercourse with grown-ups.
4. The use of force in sexual activities between adults and children is as harmful as any other use of force against children (for instance, hitting them).
5. Where sexual intercourse takes place as a result of the child's initiative, and where no one gives the child a bad conscience, intercourse between adults and children causes no mental harm.
6. Where negative effects have been observed, they are not the results of intercourse itself but of adults' suggestions that intercourse is evil and harmful.

Since we were unable to prove or disprove these assertions, we turned to secondary material. We asked all child analysts known to us to let us have their notes on children's dreams, and we copied from the literature of psychoanalysis all published children's dreams, hoping to extract information on children's sex life from them. Some of our findings are quoted in the summary at the end of this paper.

The last stage of our research began in 1960 and consisted of taped conversations with 4,367 children and juveniles. The task we had set ourselves was to devise a system of questioning which would not be recognized as sexological and should therefore give no offense to parents. For this purpose we employed "forbidden" children's riddles, songs, verses, and games of the sort represented in England and the United States by items of the following kind:

Miss Big Tits, Superstar,
Wears a dirty look-thru-bra.

Shirley Temple, curly hair,
Pulled her drawers up to there.

I am a mechanical rocket,
My tail goes bang,
My balls go clang,
And now I explode in your pocket.

Penicillin says the doctor,
Penicillin says the nurse,
Penicillin says the lady with the alligator purse.

Jack and Jill went up the hill
To fetch a pail of water.
Jill forgot to take the pill
And now she's got a daughter.

Little Miss Muffet
Sat on a tuffet,
Drawers all tattered and torn.
It wasn't the spider
That sat down beside her—
It was her old man with his horn.

These rhymes are characterized by the fact that children use them only in the presence of other children. Another characteristic is that their circulation is limited to a specific age group. Each type of verse apparently gets to be interesting to a given child when it has reached a certain stage in sexual development. The moment this stage is over, the child's interest turns to another type of rhyme. We found that each verse or riddle has a particular line on which the message depends, and each of these lines contains a particular word on which the whole structure rests. If you find this word, you have the clue to the power that it exerts over the child's imagination.

We were able to isolate three major points on which the meaning hinges: The first point deals with food, sweets, eating, drinking, sucking, swallowing, and internalizing in any other manner. It corresponds roughly to Freud's oral phase, but it occurs one to two years later than the period deemed by modern analysts to be "oral."

The second point deals with dirt: dirty words, dirty activities, dirty animals (pigs, bugs, fleas), excrement, enemas, farting, and so on. It obviously corresponds to Freud's anal phase, but again it occurs one to two years later.

The third point deals with genital activities. We have recorded an inordinate amount of verses about brother-sister incest and a fair amount about parental intercourse—all of them between age six and seven, again a year or two after Freud's phallic-oedipal phase.

We were unable to find evidence for Freud's thesis of a latency period, and we found that verses with outright genital themes occurred both before and after puberty.

My friend, the late psychoanalyst Igor A. Caruso, suggested that the two years' delay in oral, anal, and oedipal rhymes might be explained by the fact that children learn to speak between the first and second year so that the child voices its sexual obsessions with a retardation effect of 12 to 24 months.

Now to our methods of recording, transcribing, and interpreting our samples. At the beginning we made many mistakes. We tried, for instance, to ask grown-ups whether they could recall any "indecent" or "obsene" rhymes which they had known during their childhood. For reasons which I will explain when I come to our findings, this endeavor turned out to be wholly abortive because adults unconsciously censor such verses and reproduce them in mutilated form. The method also yields false information about the first and last occurrence of the verse in the course of the informant's childhood.

Our second method was to ask parents: "What rhymes does your child know, and which of them does it try to hide from you?" This did not work because parents misinterpreted their children and tried to protect them. It also failed because children succeed very well in bluffing their parents and keeping their knowledge of such verses strictly to themselves.

Our third method was to gain access to children through nursery schools and school teachers. This did not work because the children took us to be spies from the enemy camp and treated us with the suspicion and distrust normally reserved for nursery and school teachers.

At last we dared to turn directly to the children—in playgrounds, at swimming baths, in parks, and on the streets. But here, too, we made mistakes by asking foolish questions like "Do you know any rhymes or riddles that you would not use in your parents' presence?" This made the children clam up, of course, and got us nowhere.

For a while we gave up asking any questions and limited ourselves to recording snatches of children's games from a distance. But this led to poor sound quality and raised more questions than it answered.

One day, when we were sitting in a park, playing back our last tapes, we found the answer, for the kids simply gathered around us and wanted to hear what we were playing. They laughed themselves sick. I asked: "Do you know this one?" And one of the boys said: "No, but I know another one, and it goes like this!" We switched to recording and were in business. From that day on, we always opened the conversation by playing back old tapes.

Another trick we acquired round about this time was to take domestic animals with us to the parks and playgrounds—a dog, a cat, a tortoise, a rabbit, a little lamb. The kids would gather at once and ask questions: "Is she yours?" "What's his name?" "How old is it?" Then we would play one of the countless rhymes about cats, dogs, lambs or rabbits, and the children would tell us all the variants they knew.

Sooner or later, of course, the adults intervened, called the cops or the park attendants and asked what in the world we were up to. Most of us were arrested at least once and got used to carrying thick wallets full of documents identifying us as members of a research team. But the experiences were painful, and so we began to train children in handling tape recorders. This worked extremely well. Most adults underrate the technical intelligence of children and tend to patronize them. From then on we left the entire field work to the children and youths.

Regardless of whether we conducted the questioning ourselves or whether we left it to the children, we concluded each recording session with the question: "Is there anything else you want to tell us?" It turned out that these open-end sections provided the real dynamite. Although the word "sex" never occurred in our questions, the kids understood the tenor of our research and volunteered more sexual information than we had dared hoped for.

I now come to a summary of our findings during 30 years of research. It includes my own observations as a child psychologist in various children's wards, my team's enquiry into the orgasmic potency of infants, our investigations into the fertility of raped minors, our research on the fertility of boys prior to their puberty, and our interviews with parents who allowed their children to participate in their marital intercourse. It also includes the findings of our talks with men and women sentenced for incest and for intercourse with minors. It finally sums up our analysis of close to a thousand children's dreams and our interpretation of oral, anal, and genital children's rhymes. It also draws on the open-end-sections of our taped conversations with 4,367 children and juveniles.

The age groups and numbers of these latter informants were as follows:

Age	Informants	Age	Informants
2 - 3	175	11	302
4	199	12	323
5	222	13	337
6	246	14	345
7	268	15	358
8	275	16	361
9	284	17	373
10	299		

Since we started this stage of our work in 1960 and maintained contact with about 8 percent of our test group (399 informants), it was possible to carry out longitudinal studies on the following number of informants of the following age groups:

No. of Informants	Current Age (years old)	No. of Informants	Current Age (years old)
28	25	22	15
23	24	20	14
29	23	14	13
19	22	21	12
26	21	11	11
25	20	13	10
18	19	16	9
24	18	17	8
27	17	12	7
15	16	10	6
		9	5

Since it would be impossible to sum up 30 years' research in a few pages, we have selected 14 points to represent our findings in concentrated form:

1. Human sexuality differs from that of other primates in that it consists less of bodily activities than of mental ones—desires, fantasies, disappointments, anxieties. In this specific sense, the child's sex life resembles

that of the adult human much more than adult human sex life resembles that of the adult ape.

2. Freud's theory of the oral phase as the first and original one in sexual development is almost certainly erroneous. We agree that sexual development in the human is a process based on libidinal concentration in specific erogenous zones—first the oral, then the anal, then the genital area. But we insist that prior to the oral phase, the entire skin surface of the newly born is a single erogenous zone. We believe that this pre-oral phase is of far greater importance than the oral one because it provides explanations for a number of neuroses and deviations never so far classified. It allows radically new methods in the therapy of psychosomatic skin disorders. We have called this initial phase of infant sexuality "the cutaneous phase" from the Greek word for "skin" (*kytos*) and its Latin derivative (*cutis*). One of the implications of this discovery is that Freud's thesis of the genital phase as the terminal one may also be false. We have come to doubt whether genital primacy, Freud's synonym for sexual maturity, has ever existed as a provable reality. We tend to think that it was a fiction right from the start, and we believe to have observed that the sexually-mature person of our day is a cutaneously oriented person whose entire body surface is libidinally sensitive. Such people are neither genitally fixated nor are they obsessed by the need for orgasmic performance. The embraces they seek are not exclusively of the genital kind and are not limited to partners of the opposite sex. We call such persons "trans-genital" because they have left the genital phase behind them and have now moved into a state of mature cutaneous receptivity. We believe, in short, that Freud's model of an oral-anal-genital sequence is only a segment of libidinal development. It is false because it overrates the principles of primacy and of dominance. It shuts its eyes to the possibility that an equal distribution of rights and duties may exist between the erogenous zones just as it exists between human beings or between human societies. The cutaneous phase, the only one free from the dominance of one erogenous zone over all others, may therefore be assumed to stand both at the beginning and (on a higher plane) at the end of human sexual ontogenesis.

3. We have become convinced that today's ruling view on the grave consequences of parental absence during the first year of life is defective. We have investigated

the parental relations of almost one hundred children in nursery schools and child homes who remained stable, confident and cheerful in spite of temporary separation from their parents. We found that in each case the child was loved and accepted by its parents who, however, were quite frank in expressing priority for their marital life. If, as it happened in a number of cases, the father was transferred to a post in another country or another city and the wife followed him to establish a home, the child seemed to accept the parents' temporary absence without depression, despair, or shock. Bowlby's well known observations of separation anxiety apply only to children of parents that are insufficiently in love with each other or have given the child from birth on the illusion of having to come first in the affections of both parents. We therefore believe that separation anxiety is not produced by the separation itself but only by the separation from parents with insufficient affection for each other and excessive devotion to the child. The better the parents' mutual relationship, the greater the child's ability to do without them for a while.

4. We have become convinced that Freud's oedipal theories are founded on a reversal of the cause-and-effect relationship. The oedipus complex is a product of the nuclear family and goes back to parental rivalry for the child's affection. We found next to no evidence of oedipal leanings among children raised in *kibbutzim* or extended families. Where the male role in propagation is unknown or is being ritually denied, oedipal leanings between daughter and father (or between father and daughter) cannot develop because the father does not know which one of the community's children is his, while the daughter does not know which one of the many men in the communal men's house is her father.

5. We have become convinced that Freud's theory of the "primal scene" and its traumatic effect is wrong. Freud's many descriptions of this scene follow the same pattern: The child hears sighs and groans from the parental bedroom, opens the door, finds dad lying on top of mom or kneeling behind her while she's on all fours. Dad obviously is doing her some kind of violence. Mom moans. The child is shocked. A few days later it discovers mom's blood-stained sanitary towels in the bathroom and knows for sure now: What mom and pop are doing when they lock the bedroom door is something horrible. Result: The child either becomes impotent or frigid or neurotic or sadistic or

masochistic. Generations of analysts have swallowed this without ever asking themselves how many people all around the globe can *afford* to have separate bedrooms for parents and children. The majority of human beings, from the stone age to the present, would have become neurotic if the primal scene theory were valid. The fallacy, as so often, is that Freud presents a segment of the event and pretends that it stands for the whole. Children can very easily be traumatized by their parents' intercourse—but only when the child discovers the truth *belatedly* and by *accident*. Most children have seen their parents cuddling, embracing and kissing—but they have never been allowed to see what the cuddling, embracing, and kissing is meant to lead up to. Thus, what traumatizes the child is not the sight of the sexual act but the fact that it has never seen it in its proper emotional context. What causes the shock is not that the child has seen too *much*, but that it has seen too *little*.

6. The ancient question why mammals' rate of reproduction in captivity is only a fraction of that in the wild has long been answered: Mammals can only reproduce effectively if, during the imprinting stage of childhood, they can observe their elders mating. Undoubtedly the human species is biologically programmed in the same manner. If our moral laws prevent us, during the genetically prescribed period of imprinting, from observing the mating activities of our elders, we suffer a number of irreparable displacements in the choice of our sexual objects. One of them is addiction to pornography. If children, during the imprinting stage, are not allowed to use their five senses in observing the mating procedures of their species, and if they are encouraged to acquire their sexual knowledge belatedly via words and pictorial images (*graffiti* in school toilets, sex education at home and at school, sex photos and sex films in their leisure hours), they inevitably develop a fixation on words and pictures. They no longer strive for an active partner with desires of his or her own but learn instead to prefer a substitute for the real thing. This is the etiology of addiction to pornography in restrictive societies.

7. The child has no natural sense of "obscenity" and no natural sense of "shame." It derives its knowledge of these matters from other children who have learned it from other adults. It infers what it is supposed to feel and think not only from the spoken words of its

elders but primarily from their unconscious expressions—face, body, gestures, stance.

8. Human infants are born with the gift of communicating without words. That is why they understand their parents' body language long before the parents begin to learn the body language of their baby. Children begin to forget this innate knowledge only when they learn to talk. Most children, however, retain a rudimentary knowledge of body language up to adolescent age and can therefore read adults' secret thoughts and feelings very much better than adults can read those of their children.

9. Our restrictive attitude to sexuality produces two periods of traumatic repression—the first during the third year of life (Freud called it "infantile amnesia"), the second during puberty (we have called it "pubertal amnesia"). The first blocks most memories of sexual activities prior to the third year of life. The second one reduces the recall of pre-pubertal sex acts. In both cases, the repression of sexual memories is so powerful that it sweeps away a good many non-sexual memories as well. One of the results of the first amnestic period is that few people can recall anything that happened prior to the third year of their life. The most significant result of the second amnestic period is that parents can turn to their children to tell them in all honesty: "When I was your age, I *never* used dirty language." Or: "When I was young, I'd never *heard* of such horrible rhymes." Or: "When I was young, I *never* did such wicked things!" Even the children themselves, the moment they have entered puberty, begin to deny that they have ever taken part in pre-pubertal sex acts. Among our test persons were four who had been photographed by their parents during infantile sex games. When the children, in their teens now, were confronted with these snapshots they furiously denied that they were the kids depicted. Only under hypnosis did they recall the acts, and then, of course, in great detail and with remarkable precision. Neither infantile nor pubertal amnesia occurs in societies that erect no taboos on children's sexual activities. In cultures where parents make no secret of their sex life, no infantile amnesia can be traced. In societies where children are allowed to experiment sexually with one another, no pubertal amnesia develops.

10. Children who develop manual skills at an early age also masturbate earlier and more efficiently than their more

backward contemporaries. We suspect that nature has invented infant masturbation as a bonus to reward manual efforts—just as sexual intercourse among adults probably serves as nature's incentive to encourage communication between individuals. Some later forms of masturbation are veiled accusations against parental indifference and emotional starvation. They seem to argue: "If you don't care for me, I'll have to care for myself!"

11. Children's sexual activities, especially their attempts to show their genitals to each other, cannot be explained as quests for genital satisfaction—as infantile substitutes for adult coitus—but must be understood as a search for identity: "I am *not* like you. I am *not* a boy. I am a *girl*. I am I." These attempts to discover one's sexual ego are of great importance in stabilizing the growing child.

12. During the last decade we have observed a marked tendency to sex role reversal in children's play behavior. Games traditionally played only by girls are now being played increasingly often by boys, while traditional boy's games are being taken over by girls. Traditional boy's rhymes are being adapted by girls, girls' rhymes by boys. In intersexual games, where boys used to take the initiative, girls are now the initiators. Where we had massive evidence of penis envy only a decade ago, we now find frequent evidence of bosom envy. More and more boys of school age show themselves to be jealous of girls' ability to bear and nurse children.

13. Although the process of accelerated growth, earlier menstruation, earlier puberty, and earlier ejaculation has slowed down during the last decade, it still creates sexual problems because it is accompanied by a process of delayed mental maturity. In Europe we call this process "neotenia", a term coined by the anthropologist Julius Kollmann in 1885. This does not mean that the mental powers of the human species are dwindling, but it means that the total quantity of human knowledge grows so rapidly that each generation needs more time to master it. This also applies to the growing difficulties of sexual orientation in an increasingly complex world. While our body matures earlier from generation to generation, our mind matures later. Almost all sexual problems of our day arise from this growing gap between physiological and psychological maturity.

14. My team and I have therefore learned to distinguish

between *generative* maturity (the ability to beget and bear children) and *sexual* maturity (the ability to satisfy another human being and to be sexually satisfied by the other one). Responsible sexual behavior is not governed by generative, but by sexual maturity —and sexual maturity is a wholly psychological process without any counterpart in a physiological matrix. Morphological, endocrinological, and other somatic phases of generative development cannot be proved to exert a direct influence on the psychosexual processes of maturation. With the exception of pathological phenomena, physiosexual processes exert no measurable influence on psychosexual ones.

BIBLIOGRAPHY

Books

Borneman, E. *Unsere Kinder im Spiegel ihrer Lieder, Reime, Verse und Rätsel (Studien zur Befreiung des Kindes,* vol. 1). Olten (Switzerland) and Freiburg (Western Germany): Walter Verlag, 1973. 2d ed., Berlin: Ullstein Verlag, 1980.
—————. *Die Umwelt des Kindes in Spiegel seiner "berbotenen" Lieder, Reime, Verse und Rätsel (Studien zur Befreiung des Kindes,* vol. 2). Olten (Switzerland) and Freiburg (Western Germany) Walter Verlag, 1974. 2d ed., Berlin: Ullstein Verlag, 1980.
—————. *Die Welt der Erwachsenen in den "berbotenen" Reimen deutschsprachiger Stadtkinder (Studien zur Befreiung des Kindes,* vol. 3). Olten (Switzerland) and Freiburg (Western Germany): Walter Verlag, 1976. 2d ed., Berlin: Ullstein Verlag, 1981.
—————. *Reifungsphasen der Kindheit (Sexuelle Entwicklungspsychologie,* vol. 1). Frankfurt (Western Germany): Verlag Diesterweg, 1981. Aarau (Switzerland): Verlag Sauerländer, 1981. Vienna (Austria): Verlag Jugend und Volk, 1981.

Articles

Borneman, E. "Verbotene Kinderreime und das Geschlechtsleben des Kindes." *Betrifft Erziehung,* 1976, 3:38—40.
—————. "Busenneid bei Knaben." *Päd.* Extra, 1976, No. 23/24:19—25.
—————. "Ausbruch aus dem Käfig der Kindheit." *Psychologie und Gesellschaft,* 1977, 1, no. 2:7—30.

—————. "Die Urszene. Das prägende Kindheitserlebnis und seine Folgen." *Warum,* 1977, 3:34–37; 1977, 4: 34–37; 1977, 10:8–13.

—————. "Erziechung und Sexualerziehung." *Betrifft Erziehung,* 1977, 10, no. 4:32–37.

—————. "Von der Einsamkeit des Kindes in der Welt der Erwachsenen." *Sexualpodagogik,* 1977, 3:11–15. Discussion: No. 1 and 3, 1978.

—————. "Oben und Unten im Kinder—und Jugendreim." *Musik + Medizin,* 1978, 11:35–44.

—————. "Zur Frage eines Lehrbuchs der sexuellen Entwicklungspsychologie." *Sexualpodagogik,* 1979, 3:38–30.

—————. "Analytische Entwicklungspsychologie." *Disput,* 1979, 2, no. 7:27–32.

—————. "Puberale Amnesie." *Psychoanalyse* (Salzburg), 1980, 1, no. 1:62–76.

—————. "Die Zärtlichkeit des Kindes. Zu einer klassenlosen Sexualität." *Neue Sammlung,* 1981, 1:36–44.

—————. "Leibfeindliches Lernen." *Westermanns Podagogische Beitroge,* 1981, 33, no. 6:238–40.

—————. "Lehrer und Schule im Spiegel von Bank—und Wandkritzeleien." *Erziehung Heute,* 1981, 11/12:30–32.

—————. "Psychohygiene in der Schule." *Korntner Schulversuchsinformationen,* 1981, 2:17–24. Also in: *Kindheit,* 1982, 4:131–46.

PART III

Diagnostic Evaluation
of Erectile Complaints

A serendipitous finding that healthy males have erections during rapid eye movement sleep opened the door for investigations concerning the etiology of sexual complaints. Karacan originally suggested that the presence or absence of nocturnal penile tumescence could be used to differentiate organic from psychogenic erectile problems. Considerable research followed from Karacan's original hypotheses. Current data suggests that nocturnal penile tumescence recording is useful in the differential diagnostic evaluation but far short of an absolutely reliable measure. Other investigators concerned with the high cost of nocturnal penile tumescence recording in a fully equipped neurophysiology laboratory have experimented with alternative technologies. These alternative approaches include measuring erectile responses to vibration and erotic imagery. A consensus as to the most effective diagnostic procedures has yet to be reached. Clinical investigators in many disparate centers have begun to develop protocols for the evaluation of erectile problems. Many of the papers in this section concern these recommended diagnostic approaches. The male with his simpler physiology still eludes complete understanding. Many males with suspected organic erectile problems have been subjected to extensive organic evaluations without finding a definitive answer concerning etiology. It is well known that females have a lubrication response during rapid eye movement sleep. However, technological problems have prevented such studies from gaining wide clinical acceptance.   Therefore, the papers in this section are concerned mainly with the diagnostic evaluation of male complaints.

8

Psychophysiological Assessment of Erectile Dysfunction

J. Bancroft

In recent years the importance of physical factors in causing erectile failure has become increasingly recognised [1,2]. Considerable attention is now being paid to diagnostic procedures which distinguish between organic and psychogenic causation, including measurement of penile blood pressure [3,4], nocturnal penile tumescence or NPT [5], artificial erection [6], angiography [7], and xenon washout techniques [8]. Of these, the only non-invasive technique which assesses normal erectile function is the measurement of NPT, and the relevance of this nocturnal response to erotic responsiveness is still not clear. The only report so far which uses measurement of erections to erotic stimuli as a possible diagnostic procedure is that of Kockott et al. [9]. In this chapter we report further evidence for such a procedure, incorporating in addition a noninvasive photometric method of measuring penile blood flow.

METHOD

Penile erection was measured as increase in penile diameter using a mecury-in-rubber strain gauge. Pulsatile flow in

---

The research reported in this paper is based on collaboration with a number of colleagues including Christopher Bell, Robert Csillag, David Ewing, David McCulloch, Ronan O'Carroll, and Pamela Warner.

the dorsal artery of the penis was measured using a reflectance photometer and light source fixed to the dorsum of the penis by adhesive felt. Other measures of pulsatile flow in the ear, heart rate and systolic and diastolic blood pressure were also recorded, but will not be reported further in this chapter.

These measures were recorded in response to erotic fantasy and erotic film shown on a television screen. This testing, which lasted for approximately one hour, was carried out on two occasions.

An example of an erectile response and the measures taken from it are shown in Figure 8-1. Full details of the method, and results from normal subjects are reported by Bancroft and Bell [10].

SUBJECTS

Three groups of men have been studied using this method; impotent men with diabetes (n = 26, mean age 41.7 ± 8.4), without diabetes (n = 25, mean age 40.5 ± 11.6), and normal volunteers (n = 22, mean age 39.1 ± 10.1).

Figure 8–1. Erectile response showing changes in penile diameter and penile pulse amplitude, and variables measured. Those reported in the paper are the maximum diameter change and pulse amplitude "difference"; that is, c–b, each being the mean amplitude for maximum and minimum for 10 and 5 seconds, respectively.

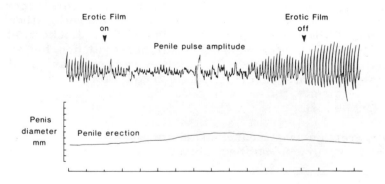

RESULTS

Between-group Comparison

A comparison of these three groups has been based on three equal-sized groups (n = 19), matched for age, and excluding in the case of the non-diabetic impotent men, those whose impotence was clearly due to organic disease.

Erection

The mean increases in penile diameter to erotic film and fantasy are shown in Table 8–1. In response to film, the groups of normal and non-diabetic impotent men were not significantly different from one another but both produced significantly greater erectile responses than the diabetic impotent group. In response to fantasy, the normals were significantly different compared to the diabetics.
Eighty-two percent of the normal subjects produced at least one erection greater than 10 mm increase in diameter; the proportion of the non-diabetic impotent men was 50 percent and of the diabetic men, 23 percent.

Penile Blood Flow

Pulse amplitude "difference" (i.e., difference between the maximum and minimum amplitude during erotic stimulation) is shown as means in Table 8–1. A significant difference is confined to that between the normal and diabetic men, though in response to fantasy the non-diabetic impotent men also showed significantly greater change than in the diabetics.

*Temporal Relationship between Penile
Flow and Penile Diameter Change*

One striking finding in the study was that, whereas typically the penile pulse amplitude increased in parallel with the penile diameter, other temporal relationships were observed. In particular, a dissociated pattern was common, in which pulse amplitude either decreased as erection developed or increased only after the erotic stimulus had ended or the erection had started to subside. An example of such a response is shown in Figure 8–2. This type of erection was significantly more frequent in the non-diabetic impotent group. We are particularly interested in this pattern as it may reflect the effects of psychological inhibition. Erections of this type tend not only to be smaller

TABLE 8-1. Psychophysiological Responses to Erotic Film and Fantasy--Comparison of Three Groups of Men

		Normal (N) n = 19	Non-Diabetic Impotence (I) n = 19	Diabetic Impotence (DI) n = 19	Analysis of Variance (d.f. 2,54) and Sheffe Tests)
Mean Max. Erection to film (mm/increase/diam.)	Mean	9.3	8.3	4.2	F = 7.65 N v DI p = < 0.005
	S.D.	±2.9	±5.3	±4.1	p = < 0.005 I v DI p = < 0.05
Mean Max. Erection to fantasy (mm/increase/diam.)	Mean	4.4	2.7	0.8	F = 7.72 N v DI p = < 0.05
	S.D.	±4.2	±2.2	±0.9	p = < 0.001
Penile pulse Amplitude					
'Difference' in response to film μv	Mean	1729	1061	474	F = 7.87 N v I p = < 0.005
	S.D.	±1431	±1212	±449	p = < 0.1 N v DI p = < 0.005
'Difference' in response to fantasy μv	Mean	1188	876	346	F = 9.22 N v DI p = < 0.001
	S.D.	±1250	±715	±354	p = < 0.001 I v DI p = < 0.01

Figure 8–2. This response in a 30-year-old man with probable psychogenic impotence shows a decrease in penile pulse amplitude as a small erection develops and an eventual increase in pulse amplitude as the erection is subsiding. This is an example of a "dissociated response."

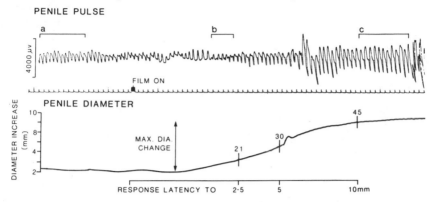

but also slower to develop. A further type of response, in which pulse amplitude increased without any erection, was found more commonly in the diabetic impotent group.

Within-group Comparison

The non-diabetic impotent men were then divided into two groups, based on history and physical examination, those with probable psychogenic causation (n = 17) and those in whom organic factors were likely to be of primary or equal importance (n = 8). The psychogenic group showed significantly greater erectile response to film (mean increase in diameter 8.8 ± 5.1 and 2.5 ± 1.5 $p = < 0.005$) but did not differ significantly in their pulse amplitude change.

The diabetic men were first divided into those with probable psychogenic factors (n = 9) and those with only the diabetes to account for their impotence (n = 17). These two groups did not differ significantly in their erectile responses (mean increase in diameter 5.5 ± 4.0 and 3.6 ± 2.9, N.S.) but did differ in pulse amplitude change, the psychogenic group showing significantly higher "difference" scores ($p = < 0.01$).

The diabetic men were then categorized according to the presence of two diabetic complications, autonomic neuropathy and retinopathy, both likely to be relevant to erectile function. The presence of autonomic neuropathy was based on well established tests of cardiovascular reflexes [12,13]. Six diabetics had no evidence of autonomic neuropathy, 13 showed parasympathetic damage only and in seven both parasympathetic and sympathetic damage. The "no damage" group produced significantly greater erections than the combined parasympathetic and sympathetic damage group (p = < 0.05), the "parasympathetic damage only" group not being significantly different from either. These groups did not differ, however, in their penile pulse amplitude change.

The diabetic men were also categorized as having no retinopathy (n = 8), background retinopathy (n = 9), and severe (that is, exudative or proliferative) retinopathy (n = 8) on the basis of fundal examination. These three groups did not differ significantly in the degree of erection, but the "no retinopathy" group did show significantly greater penile pulse amplitude change than the severe retinopathy group (p = < 0.025).

These results therefore suggest that the effects of autonomic neuropathy are shown more in the degree of erection produced than the degree on increased penile arterial flow, perhaps because damage to the control of venous outflow or arteriovenous shunts is the main effect. Retinopathy, on the other hand, as an indicator of small vessel damage, is reflected more in terms of penile arterial blood flow.

Comparison of Results from Psychophysiological Testing and Measurement of NPT

In a further study, 31 men were subjected to recording of NPT (on two consecutive nights) in addition to the psychophysiological testing described above. These men included 12 with diabetic impotence, 11 with non-diabetic impotence, and eight normal subjects (full details of this study will be reported in Shapiro et al. [14]).

Preliminary analysis shows that by taking a mean erectile response to erotic film of five mm or greater, all subjects in this category, with one exception, showed nocturnal erections of greater than five mm increase in diameter (that is, 15.7 mm increase in circumference). The exception was one normal subject, aged 26, who showed a mean response to film of 7.6 mm, and produced NPT response greater than three mm but less than five mm increase in diameter. Of those subjects with mean erectile responses to film of less than five mm (which included none of the normal men) seven out of 14 produced at least one NPT response greater than five mm increase in diameter. This included four diabetic men with probably psychogenic factors contributing to their impotence.

DISCUSSION

Psychophysiological testing, as described in this paper, has diagnostic significance and is much easier and cheaper to use than the laboratory measurement of NPT. One third to one half of impotence subjects may be screened out by this method, making NPT testing unnecessary.

For the remainder, additional information is likely to result by combining psychophysiological testing of this kind with other diagnostic tests. Measurement of penile blood flow may well have specific relevance for certain types of organic impotence (for example, peripheral vascular disease) as well as offering some interesting possibilities for studying the neurophysiological mechanisms of erection, the pharmacological effects of various drugs and the mediating mechanisms involved in psychological inhibition of erection.

NOTES

1. Wagner, G., and R. Green. *Impotence. Physiological, Psychological, Surgical Depression and Treatment.* New York: Plenum Press, 1981.

2. Bancroft, J. *Human Sexuality and its Problems.* Edinburgh: Churchill Livingstone, 1983.

3. Abelson, D. Diagnostic value of the penile pulse and blood pressure. A Doppler study of impotence in diabetics. *J. Urology,* 1975, 113:636–39.

4. Velcek, D., K. W. Sniderman, E. D. Vaughan, T. A. Sos, and E. C. Muecke. Penile flow index utilizing a Doppler pulse wave analysis to identify penile vascular insufficiency. *J. Urology,* 1980, 123:669–73.

5. Schiavi, R. C., and C. Fisher. Assessment of diabetic impotence: measurement of nocturnal erections. *Clinics in Endocrinology and Metabolism,* 1982, 11:3, 769–84.

6. Virag, R. L'Exploration multidisciplinaire de l'impuissance. Résultats preliminaires d'une étude portant sur 339 cas. *Contraception-fertilité-sexualité,* 1982, 10:873–78.

7. Michal, V. Arterial disease as a cause of impotence. *Clinics in Endocrinology and Metabolism,* 1982, 11:3, 725–48.

8. Wagner, G., and A. Uhrenholdt. Blood flow measurement by the clearance method in the human corpus cavernosum in the flaccid and erect states. Vasculogenic Impotence. In A. W. Zorgniotti and G. Rossi (eds.), *Proceedings of the First International Conference on Corpus Cavernosum Revascularization,* 41–46. Springfield: Thomas, 1980.

9. Kockott, G., W. Feil, R. Ferstl, J. Aldenhoff, and U. Besinger. Psychophysiological aspects of male sexual inadequacy: results of an experimental study. *Archives Sexual Behavior,* 1980, 9:477–94.

10. Bancroft, J., and C. Bell. Psychophysiological assessment of penile erection, a new approach. I. Methodology and results in normal subjects. Unpublished data.

11. Bancroft, J., C. Bell, D. Ewing, D. McCulloch, and P. Warner. Psychophysiological assessment of penile erection, a new approach II. Erectile Function in Diabetic and Non-diabetic Impotence. Unpublished data.

12. Ewing, D. J., and B. F. Clarke. Diagnosis and management of diabetic autonomic neuropathy. *Brit. Med. J.,* 1982, 285:916–18.

13. Ewing, D. J., and J. Bancroft. The evaluation of the autonomic nervous system in impotent males. *International Angiology.* In press.

14. Shapiro, C., R. O'Carroll, and J. Bancroft. Comparison of erectile responses to erotic stimuli and during sleep. In preparation.

9

Organicity in Cases of Male Erectile Dysfunction Referred to Sexual Therapy

P. Alarie and E. Beltrami

DEFINITION OF THE PROBLEM AND EPIDEMIOLOGY

Characteristics of the Sample

Our sample consisted in seventy-three men. Forty-eight were married, 18 percent single, 15 percent divorced, 5 percent widowers and 14 percent of unknowned marital status. Eleven percent were in their twenties, 18 in their thirties, 31 percent in their forties, 33 percent in their fifties, 7 percent in their sixties and 1 percent in their seventies. This distribution by decade is very similar to the distribution in the sample of four-hundred and fifty four men studies by Schmidt, 1983 [1]. But if we consider only the patients finally diagnosed as suffering from organic etiology, they have a tendency to be concentrated towards the higher end of the scale: 46 percent in their fifties and 13 percent in their sixties.

Characteristics of Referring Professionals

Sixty-seven percent of the sample were referred by full-time sex therapists with the following backgrounds: masters degree in sexology (22 percent of all referrals), psychiatrists (31 percent of referrals), social workers (7 percent of referrals), and one psychologist (3 percent of referrals). Sixty percent had been referred to the sex therapist by family doctors with the diagnosis of "psychological impotence." Twenty percent were referred directly to the clinic by general practitioners, a few cases were sent for organic investigation. Twelve percent of the patients were referred by specialists in the field of urology, endocrinology or vascular surgery. They were either suspected of an organic pathology without a definitive diagnosis, or they knew the pathology but not if it was the cause of the erectile dysfunction.

Epidemiologic Considerations

Epidemiology of organic erectile dysfunction is difficult to assess. Old text books referred to 10 percent organic "impotence" versus 90 percent "psychogenic;" but no research substantiates this data. The recent scientific literature has a tendency to increase the percentage of organic impotence. Schumaker 1981 [2] stated that men suffering from erectile dysfunctions were harboring much more medical pathologies than normal subjects: seventy-two percent! However the specific etiologies of these pathologies were not defined. Specialized clinics, either in urology or endocrinology, claim to find a high percentage of organic cases. But this can be anticipated since patients referred to a specialist usually have a serious reason to consult in this specific field. Often they are referred with a precise diagnosis by their family doctors. Schmidt 1983 [1] found 33 percent with organic pathology. But this was only a diagnostic impression after the first interview and no definitive data was given on the true ratio once the complete investigation was terminated. In the presence of such incomplete data, we considered it important to proceed until a final diagnosis was clearly proven.

In fact, the main point of this clinical study is to know if the traditional medical examination on dysfunctional men is sufficient to establish a precise diagnosis, and if not, how many patients reach the nonmedical sex therapists with a misdiagnosed "psychological impotence"?

METHODS OF INVESTIGATION

Definition of Male Erectile Dysfunction
(previously called impotence)

We chose the classification of Diagnostic Statistical Manual (D.S.M.) III [3] which defines this symptom as a "persistent and recurrent inhibition of excitement phase in sexual activity, being manifested by an incapacity, partial or complete, to obtain or to maintain an erection sufficiently rigid to complete the sexual act. This inhibition is *primary* if a satisfactory erection has never been obtained. It is *secondary* if there had been a previous normal functioning."

Structured Interviews

All patients investigated had been previously seen by a sexologist and a general practitioner. But as no standard format was used by referring professionals, this information was not considered in our clinical study. Our team consisted of a medical doctor specially trained in the sexual field, a psychiatrist-sexologist and several medical specialists in the areas of urology, neurology, endocrinology and vascular medicine. A private laboratory performed the nocturnal penile plethysmography. Thirty-one percent of our sample underwent a psychiatric assessment. During the medical examination done in the course of our study, all patients passed a structured interview specific to erectile dysfunction (Alarie and Gagnon 1982) [4]. The following factors were considered: the time of onset, related circumstances, marital harmony, the percentage of stiffness of erection, as well as the maximum time of erection, the frequency of sexual desire, and some characteristics of ejaculations. This subjective interview had a specific goal which was to evaluate the vascular, neurological, hormonal and urologic status of the patient.

Sexually Oriented Medical Examination

The seventy-three patients were submitted to a medical examination specific to erectile dysfunction. The *vascular system* was checked for murmurs, blood pressure of the four limbs, time of capillary filling, status of vascularization of inferior limbs, and special attention was given to the aorto-iliac zone. The systolic pressure of the inferior limbs (measured by Doppler effect) which was compared to the radial systolic pressure, was routinely measured. We found this procedure (when positive) highly indicative of an aorto-iliac vascular pathology. *Hormonal* status was also evaluated with special attention to body hair distribution, skin pigmentation, galactorrhea or gynecomastia and testicular measurement. From an *urologic* point of view, the flaccid penis was measured in the office, special attention was given to possible curvatures of the penis, and the patient was asked to measure at home the penile circumference during and before the maximum erection he could achieve in the best possible situation. The *neurological* status was assessed with emphasis on the lumbar and sacral portion of the spinal cord. The "five genital reflexes" and the "volontary contraction of the pelvic floor muscles" as described by Per Orlov Lundberg [5] were checked.

Nonspecialized Laboratory Investigations

All our seventy-three patients underwent a *basic laboratory* biochemical and hormonal evaluation which, following the recommendation of Lundberg 1977. Wagner 1981 [6], Smith 1981 [7], Stuntz 1983 [8], Montague 1981 [9], Marshall 1975 [10], Sparks 1980 [11], Thorner 1977 [12], Weideman 1981 [13], Buvat 1982 [14], included: complete blood count, *blood* glucose, urea, creatinin, uric acid, calcium, phosphorous, electrolytes, cholesterol, triglycerides, total proteins, albumin, direct bilirubin, alkaline phosphatase, Lactic Acid Dehydrogenase (LDH), Serum Glutamic Oxaloacetic Transaminase (SGOT), Serum Glutamic Pyruvate Transaminase (SGPT), Gamma GT, Creatnine Phosphokinase (CPK), *urine* analysis and culture, Venereal Disease Research Laboratories Test (VDRL), and plasmatic concentration of the following hormones: total testosterone, prolactine, follicle stimulating hormone (FSH), Luteinizing hormone (LH), Thyroid Stimulating Hormone (TSH), total T_4, free T_4, and the percentage of Thyroxine Binding Globulin (TBG).

For diagnosis of *diabetes mellitus,* we performed either an oral glucose tolerance test or two (two hour post-glucola) glycemias. For the sake of precision, some cases had determinations of their glycolysated hemoglobin (HBAIC) to evaluate the presence of any subtle trace of an active diabetes. These tests were chosen on the basis of the work of National Diabetes Data Group 1979 [15], Gabbay 1976 [16], Koenig 1976 [17], and Bates 1978 [18].

Specialized Investigation Procedures Sexually-Specific

Noninvasive vascular studies: a Doppler measurement of bilateral systolic blood pressure in the arteries of the *penis* (dorsal, cavernous, glans) was taken by our cardiovascular consultant and compared to the *brachial* systolic pressure, in accordance with the studies of Abelson 1975 [19], Gaskell 1971 [20], Kedia 1981 [21], Kempczinski 1979 [22,23], Montague 1981, Engel 1978 [24], Karacan 1978 [25], Gaylis

1978 [26]. For the diagnostic criteria we chose to follow Kempczinski and use the Penile Brachial Systolic Gradient (PBSG). A gradient equal or inferior to 20 mmHg was considered normal if the patient was under 40 years of age; a gradient inferior to 40 mmHg was considered normal over 40 years of age. This evaluation was chosen as the indication for aorto-iliac angiography and selective hypogastric arteriography. It was noted in a few cases that a difference of only 30 mmHg between the two cavernous arteries seemed to be a more indicative clue than the PBSG to the vasculogenic impotence of the pudendal artery and its terminal branches.

Aorto-iliac angiography and selective hypogastric arteriography: these procedures were performed on the basis of a positive finding of the previous vascular noninvasive diagnosis.

Neurophysiologic diagnostic procedures: in the presence of diabetes mellitus, multiple sclerosis or any other form of neurologic disorder, our consultant in neurology measured the latency time of the bulbocavernosus reflex which can detect subtle neurologic disorders in relation to erection. Blaivas 1980 [27], Bors 1959 [28], Buvat 1982 [29], Buck 1976 [30], and Tordjman [31]. An evaluation for peripheral neuropathy was done in all cases.

Urologic diagnostic procedures: in diabetics, multiple sclerotics, alcoholics, and patients with an abnormal bulbocavernosus reflex or abnormal nocturnal penile tumescence, our consultant in urology proceeded to urodynamic studies which included: cystometrography, urethral pressure profile, and urinary flow studies (debimetry). These parameters were chosen to diagnose an autonomic neuropathy related to erectile function or an obstruction to urine out-flow. Buvat 1982, Buck 1979, Tordjman 1982.

Nocturnal penile tumescence: this test was performed over a period of two consecutives nights using two mercury strain gauges. The monitor was a medical monitoring system plethysmograph. This procedure was used to determine the organic or psychogenic etiology or to verify if the organicity discovered was etiologic to the erectile dysfunction. In two patients this evaluation clearly defined that the organic pathology (one case of multiple sclerosis, one of vascular obstruction) was not the cause of the erectile dysfunction. One of them (the vascular case) has already recuperated his full function after a brief sex therapy. In accordance with Fisher 1979 [32], and 1977 [33], Jovanovic 1972 [34], Karacan 1972 [35], 1976 [36], and 1977 [37], Wasserman 1980 [38], Bohlen 1981 [39], Schmidt 1983 [40], Schiavi 1982 [41], Marshall 1981 [42], we would recommend this procedure be used as a screening procedure when possible.

Penile investigation: whenever the patient described a curvature of the penis during erections which was impossible to visualize during usual medical examination, we asked him to take superior and lateral photographs of his erect penis with a Polaroid camera. If there was sufficient curvature seen on the photograph, we sent the patient to have an echography (ultrasound) of his penis to confirm the clinical impression. This was useful in cases of suspected Peyronie's disease or congenital curvature of the penis secondary to hypoplasy of one of the corpora cavernosa.

RESULTS

Cases Diagnosed as being from a Purely Organic Etiology

In this group, a total of seven cases (9.7 percent) were diagnosed. Two had *vasculogenic* causes. The first had a complete obstruction of the common iliac arteries and the second had an ilio-pudendal artery obstruction.

From an *endocrinological* point of view, even though some cases demonstrated levels of testosterone lower than normal, no real hypogonadism was diagnosed by the endocrinologist. Routine tests of thyroid functions disclosed only one which came back with a nonetiologic thyroid dysfunction. But two cases showed prolactinomas as responsible for their sexual dysfunction.

Urologically, all infections and vesical diseases had been properly diagnosed before referral to sex therapy. The referring doctors were right in eliminating these diagnoses. However, two cases of Peyronie's disease had not been diagnosed before referral and also one case of congenital curvature of the penis.

Cases with Organic and Psychological (Mixed) Etiology

One *urological* case had mixed etiology: his Peyronie's disease was responsible for his impotence, but his psychological reaction limited the value of surgery and his function was not restored. He was then referred in sex therapy to complete his treatment.

All the rest of the mixed etiologies were *drug-induced;* two cases because of Inderal+Lasix or Inderal+Hydrodiuril, one secondary to probucol and alcohol abuse, one from Spironolactone and Valium and the last from Aldactazide (Spironolactone+Hydrodiuril). The removal of the medication with subsequent amelioration of sexual function was the criteria for causal relationship.

In summary, 17 percent of all cases (13 cases, 7 purely organic, and 6 of mixed etiology) had been sent to sex therapy with a clear organic pathology that was not previously diagnosed. All the rest (60 cases) were caused by the stressful life events, inadequate life styles, lack of sexual knowledge or psychiatric conditions (eleven cases) and most of them are presently undergoing sex therapy; some of them have already improved.

Organic Pathologies Nonetiologic to Sexual Dysfunction

It is of some interest to note that 55 patients (75 percent) were suffering from pathologies that could have some influence on their sexual functioning.

Pathologies of genital organs: Twenty-six (35 percent) had benign diseases linked to the sexual sphere: the prostate (11), the testicules (4), the penis (3), the bladder (3), infection of the genitourinary tract (3) or infertility (2).

Endocrinologic conditions: Eighteen patients (24 percent) had endocrinologic disorders that could have been causal of their dysfunction: hyperlipemia (8), glucose intolerance (5), diabetes mellitus (3), diabetes insipidus (1), thyroid dysfunction (1).

Cardiovascular conditions: Eight patients (10 percent) had cardiac disease: coronary insufficiency (3), high blood pressure (3), vasculopathy (2). We note that if these conditions *per se* did not directly interfere with their sexuality, the prescribed drugs for their conditions were harmful to their erectile potential.

Neurological conditions: One case of multiple sclerosis with neurogenic bladder and important autonomic neuropathy was nevertheless able to have full erections under certain circumstances; two nocturnal penile plethysmographies confirmed that this neuropathy was not the cause of his occasional impotence. One case of herniated disc, even if located in the sacral spinal cord where the erection centers are situated, was not etiologic. One cerebellar tumor did not affect sexual functioning.

Miscellaneous: Six cases had a syndrome of severe tabagism with three of them suffering from chronic bronchitis. In the digestive system we found one case of hepatitis, one peptic ulcer and one duodenitis. There were also five cases of obesity, five of alcohol abuse, one anemia, and one gout.

Psychiatric Pathologies

If we consider the clear-cut psychiatric problems, we found five *anxiety* states, all playing a part in a psychogenic etiology. Two *couple dysfunctions* were equally associated to a psychogenic etiology. Out of four *depressions,* one was consecutive to an obstruction of the internal carotid artery and was completely relieved after the proper operation. All other three depressions played a psychogenic etiologic role. Two patients were diagnosed as *psychotics* by the referring professionals. One of them had been seen by three urologists and a general practitioner who had not believed his verbal report about the curvature of his penis on the basis that is was part of his delusional ideas. Our instruction to the patient to photograph his erection brought the proof of organic pathology juxtaposed to a psychiatric problem. It later appeared that part of the disorganization of this patient was due to the fact that nobody wanted to believe him on such an important subject. His anxiety decreased when his problem was taken into consideration. The second patient was diagnosed by our team as schizophrenic on the first interview. Later we found that in fact he was suffering from a toxic psychosis because of a chronic drug abuse. When he was convinced to cease drugs, he appeared completely normal and even well-structured and motivated. His erectile dysfunction was treated in sex therapy with success.

DISCUSSION AND CONCLUSIONS

Epidemiologic Considerations

It is of interest to note that all the patients that had an organic cause for their dysfunction were in fact in the 70 percent sent by doctors who ignored the possibility of an organic etiology. In some ways, the full time sexologists were more accurate in suspecting a medical pathology and in referring the subjects to the clinic for investigation. However, if in a sample completely screened by medical doctors we can find 17 percent of organic pathology, we suspect that the ratio is much higher in the general population. In fact, it seems that all the cases suffering from endocrinologic dysfunctions except prolactinomas were probably diagnosed, treated, and not referred. On the contrary, some problems are more difficult to diagnose without specialized procedures: Peyronie's disease, obstruction of the blood flow in the penis, congenital curvatures of the penis, drug-induced erectile dysfunctions, and prolactinomas.

Diagnostic Considerations

It is clear that a sexual specific evaluation is of the utmost importance for the proper diagnosis of erectile dysfunction. Patients were mislabelled as being of "psychogenic" etiology and referred to a treatment doomed to failure and some others were convinced that their organic pathology was causative of their erectile dysfunction when it was not the case. As none of the methods described were invasive and none was the source of pain and discomfort, this is a supplementary argument in favor of a precise investigation. The fact that out of thirteen psychiatric pathologies, two were organic is a good reminder of the importance of a comprehensive investigation.

NOTES

1. Schmidt, C. W. "Common Male Sexual Disorders: Impotence and Premature Ejaculation," Ch. 4, 173–96, 2nd ed. In J. K. Meyer, C. W. Schmidt, and T. N. Wise, eds., *Clinical Management of Sexual Disorders*. Baltimore: Williams and Wilkins, 1983.

2. Schumaker, Sallie, and C. W. Lloyd. "Physiological and Psychological factors of impotence." *The Journal of Sex Research,* 1981, 17, no. 1:40–53.

3. American Psychiatric Association. *Diagnostic and Statistical Manual of Mental Disorders,* 3rd ed. Washington, D.C.: American Psychiatric Association, 1980.

4. Alarie, P., and L. Gagnon. "L'impuissance masculine." *Le Médecin du Québec,* April 1982, 17, no. 4:49–71.

5. Lundberg, P. O. "Sexual dysfunctions in patients with neurological disorders," Ch. 2, 129–140, in R. Gemme and C. Wheeler, eds, *Progress in Sexology, Proceedings of the World Congress of Sexology, Montreal 1976.* Montreal: Plenum Press, 1977.

6. Wagner, G. E. "Methods for differential diagnosis of psychogenic and organic erectile failure," Ch. 8, 89–130, G. Wagner, and R. Green, eds, *Impotence: Physiological, Psychological, Surgical Diagnosis and Treatment.* New

York: Plenum Press, 1981.

7. Smith, A. D. "Causes and Classification of Impotence." *Urologic Clinics of North America,* 1981, 8, no. 1:79–89.

8. Stuntz, R. "Diagnosis and Diagnostic Techniques: Laboratory Studies," in J. K. Meyer, C. W. Schmidt, and T. N. Wise, eds., *Clinical Management of Sexual Disorders.* Baltimore: Williams and Wilkins, 1983.

9. Montague, D. "Clinical Evaluation of Impotence." *Urologic Clinics of North America,* February 1981, 8, no. 1: 103–18.

10. Marshall, J. C. "Investigative Procedures: Male Sexual Dysfunction." *Progress in Endocrinology and Metabolism,* 1975, 48:545–67.

11. Sparks, P., R. A. White, B. Peter, and M. S. Connoly. "Impotence is not always psychogenic." *JAMA,* 1980, 243:750–55.

12. Thorner, M. O. "Prolactin." *Clinics in Endocrinology and Metabolism,* 1977, 6:201–21.

13. Weideman, C. L., and R. C. Northcutt. "Endocrine Aspects of Impotence." *Urologic Clinics of North America,* 1981, 8, no. 1:143–51.

14. Buvat, J., and M. Buvat-Herbaut. "Le point sur . . . dysfonctions sexuelles et endocrinologie, *Cahiers de Sexologie Clinique,* 1982, 8, no. 45:149–58.

15. National Diabetes Data Group. "Assessment Criterias of Diabetes." *Diabetes,* 1979, 28:1039.

16. Gabbay, K. H. "Glycolysated hemoglobin and diabetic control." *New England Journal of Medicine,* 1976, 295, no. 8:443–44.

17. Koenig, J. R., C. M. Peterson, R. Jones, C. Saudek, M. Lehrman, and A. Cerami. "Correlation of glucose regulation and hemoglobin ALC in diabetes mellitus." *New England Journal of Medicine,* 1976, 295, no. 8:417–20.

18. Bates, H. M. "Glycohemoglobin levels and diabetes mellitus." *Laboratory Management,* January 1978, New York.

19. Abelson, D. "Diagnostic value of the penile pulse and blood pressure: A Doppler study of impotence in diabetics." *The Journal of Urology,* 1975, 113:636–39.

20. Gaskell, P. "The importance of penile blood pressure in cases of impotence." *C.M.A. Journal,* 1971, 105: 1047–51.

21. Kedia, K. R. "Vascular Disorders and Male Erectile Dysfunction." *Urologic Clinics of North America,* 1981, 8, no. 1:153–68.

22. Kempczinski, R. F. "Role of the vascular laboratory in the evaluation of male impotence." *Proceedings, Seventh*

Symposium on Vascular Surgery, Palm Springs, 1979, March, California.

23. Kempczinski, R. F. "Role of vascular diagnostic laboratory in the evaluation of male impotence." *The American Journal of Surgery,* 1979, 138:278–82.

24. Engel, G., S. J. Burnham, and M. F. Carter, "Penile blood pressure in the evaluation of erectile impotence." *Fertility and Sterility,* 1978, 30:687–90.

25. Karacan, I., J. C. Ware, B. Dervent, A. L. Altinel, J. I. Thornby, R. L. Williams, N. Kaya, and R. Bradley-Scott. "Impotence and blood pressure in the flaccid penis: Relationship to NPT." *Sleep,* 1978, 1, no. 2:125–32.

26. Gaylis, H. "The assessment of impotence in aorto-iliac disease using penile blood pressure measurement." *Suid-Afrikaanse Tydskrift Vir Chirurgie,* 1978, 16, no. 1:39–46.

27. Blaivas, J. G., T. F. O'Donnell, P. Gottlieb, Jr., and K. B. Labib. "Measurement of bulbocavernosus reflex latency time as part of a comprehensive evaluation of impotence." *Vasculogenic Impotence,* 49–65. Illinois: C. C. Thomas, 1980.

28. Bors, E. H., and K. A. Blinn. "Bulbocavernosus reflex." *Journal of Urology,* 1959, 82–128.

29. Buvat, J., A. Lemaire, J. D. Guieu, and J. P. Bailleul. "Exploration neurologique et urodynamique d'une impuissance." *Cahiers de Sexologie clinique,* 1982, 8, no. 47:283–85.

30. Buck, A. C., P. I. Reed, Y. K. Siddiq, G. D. Chisholm, and R. Fraser. "Bladder dysfunction and neuropathy in diabetes." *Diabetologia,* 1976, 12:251–58.

31. Tordjman, G. "Le point sur...diabète et dysfunctions sexuelles." *Cahiers de Sexologie Clinique,* 1982, 8, no. 47:263–69.

32. Fisher, C., R. C. Schiavi, and A. Edwards. "Nocturnal penile tumescence and erectile disorders." Paper read at *The Eastern Association for Sex Therapy,* March 1977, New York.

33. Fisher, C., R. C. Schiavi, A. Edwards, D. M. Davis, M. Reitman, and J. Fine. "Evaluation of nocturnal penile tumescence in the differential diagnosis of sexual impotence." *Archives of General Psychiatry,* 1979, 36:431–37.

34. Jovanovîc, U. L. "Sexuelle Reaktionen und Schlafperiodic bei Menschen: Ergebnisse Experimenteller Untersuchungen." *Beitrage fur Sexualforschung,* 1972, 51:1–292.

35. Karacan, I., C. J. Hursch, R. L. Williams, and J. I. Thornby. "Some characteristics of nocturnal penile tumescence in young adults." *Archives of General Psy-*

chiatry, 1972, 26:351–56.

36. Karacan, I., P. J. Salis, J. I. Thornby, and R. L. Williams. "The ontogeny of nocturnal penile tumescence." Waking and Sleeping, 1976, 1:27–44.

37. Karacan, I., F. B. Scott, P. J. Salis, S. L. Attia, J. C. Ware, A. Altinel, and R. L. Williams. "Nocturnal erections, differential diagnosis of impotence and diabetes." Biologic Psychiatry, 1977, 12:373–80.

38. Wasserman, M. D., C. P. Pollak, A. J. Spielman, and E. D. Weitzman. "Theoretical and technical problems in the measurement of nocturnal penile tumescence for the differential diagnosis of impotence." Psychosomatic Medicine, 1980, 42:575–85.

39. Bohlen, J. "Sleep erection monitoring in the evaluation of male erectile failure." Urologic Clinics of North America, 1981, 8, no. 1:119–34.

40. Schmidt, C. W. "Nocturnal penile tumescence studies and associated techniques," 2nd ed., in J. K. Meyer, C. W. Schmidt, and T. Wise, eds., Clinical Management of Sexual Disorders. Baltimore: Williams and Wilkins, 1983.

41. Schiavi, R. C., and C. Fischer. "Assessment of Diabetic Impotence: Measurement of Nocturnal Erections." Clinics in Endocrinology and Metabolism, 1982, 2, no. 3:769–84.

42. Marshall, P., D. M. Surridge, and N. Delva. "The role of nocturnal penile tumescence in differentiating between organic and psychogenic impotence: the first stage of validation." Archives of Sexual Behavior, 1981, 10, no. 1:1–10.

43. Marshall, P., D. M. Surridge, and N. Delva. "Differentiating between organic and psychogenic impotence on the basis of MMPI decision rules." Journal of Consulting and Clinical Psychology, 1980, 4:407–8.

10

Erectile Function in Nonimpotent Diabetics

R. C. Schiavi, C. Fisher, M. Quadland, and A. Glover

General surveys have consistently demonstrated a high prevalence of erectile impairment among diabetics [1–5]. Evidence, primarily of an indirect nature, suggests that neuropathic and vascular changes contribute to the pathogenesis of erectile failure [6–9]. In addition, several authors [10–12] have emphasized the important role that psychological factors play in the development and maintenance of diabetic impotence.

The frequent coexistence of organic and psychological determinants creates difficult problems in differential diagnosis. During recent years the monitoring of nocturnal penile tumescence (NPT) during sleep has been used with increasing frequency for the objective assessment of organic impairment in erectile capacity [13]. Karacan et al. [14,15] and Fisher et al. [16], for example, have found that, in contrast to normals and psychogenically impotent patients, impotent diabetics showed decreased tumescent time, decreased duration and frequency of full erections, and a reduction in the maximum increase in penile circumference during REM (rapid eye movement sleep) erections. Although these data support the diagnostic value of NPT assessments, it is severely limited by failure to include nondysfunctional diabetics as controls.

At present there is an almost total lack of physiologic information on the erectile capacity of nondysfunctional diabetic men and no studies that have compared NPT in matched diabetic groups with and without erectile problems. We have reported [17] preliminary results of an NPT investigation on four age-matched groups studied under similar conditions: normal men, diabetics without erectile problems, impotent diabetics, and psychogenically impotent subjects. The focus of this chapter will be on the sleep characteristics and NPT parameters of the sexually normal and dysfunctional diabetics included in this recently completed investigation.

METHOD

Fifty-two men were evaluated in the sleep laboratory during three study nights. Selection criteria were ages 23–26, no evidence or organic disease other than diabetes, lack of significant psychopathology and no current history of drug use other than anti-diabetic medication. The number of subjects in each group were: 13 normals, 12 diabetics free of erectile problems, 11 impotent diabetics, and 16 psychologically impotent men. All subjects had an extensive personal and psychosexual interview and, when not recently available, also underwent a medical evaluation and laboratory tests. Diagnostic categorization was based on clinical evidence alone independent of NPT information.

Methods of procedure and analysis have been previously described in detail. Electroencephalogram (EEG) and eye movements were monitored continuously through the night and sleep was scored according to standardized criteria. Penile tumescence was recorded by means of two strain gauge loops: one placed around the penis about one inch from the base and the other just behind the corona of the glans. During the third study night visual checks were carried out to ascertain degree of rigidity in relation to the recorded increase in penile circumference. This was done by awakening the subject during erections and having both the subject and investigator rate its degree on a 0–10 scale. Penile tumescence was expressed in millimeters of increased circumference as measured by the strain gauge. Quantitative comparisons were made on mean values of degree, frequency and duration of tumescence recorded during the three nights. Deviations from baseline recordings of 81–100 percent of the greatest penile circumference estimated to be full by direct observation were considered to be maximum episodes. Statistical comparisons among groups were made by analysis of variance. If the results on this test were significant, further analysis by the Fisher's Least Significant Difference Test was carried out to identify the source of the statistical difference [18].

RESULTS

Subject Characteristics

The mean ages of the normal, nondysfunctional diabetic, impotent diabetic and psychogenic groups were 27.9, 29, 27.1 and 30 years respectively. The mean age at clinical onset of diabetes was 17.5 years for the nondysfunctionals and 17.6 years for the impotent diabetics. All diabetics were taking insulin at the time of the investigation and were under reasonably good metabolic control. Three nondysfunctional diabetics reported transient erectile problems during past periods of metabolic discontrol but denied erectile difficulties during the six-month period preceding the study. Mean duration of erectile problems among the diabetic group was 4.3 years (range 2–8) and among the psychogenic group 5.6 years (range 1–17). All impotent diabetics described progressive difficulties in gaining and maintaining erections during intercourse and masturbation for at least one year. Diabetic complications were present in four diabetic impotent subjects and in none of the nondysfunctional group.

Sleep Parameters

There were no significant differences among groups in sleep duration, percentage of time awake following sleep onset and number of REM periods (Table 10–1). Significant differences were observed, however, in REM duration (F 5.2 df 3,48 p < .01) and in percentage of sleep time in REM (F 3 df 3,48 p < 0.05). The two diabetic groups were not different from each other but both spent significantly less sleep time in REM than the psychogenic group; impotent diabetics also differed statistically on this variable from normal controls. Latency time to REM onset was prolonged in both diabetic groups; nondysfunctional diabetics spent a significantly longer sleep period before REM than the other three groups (F 2.99 df 3,48 p < 0.05). This information is listed in Table 10–2.

Tumescent Parameters

Selected degree, duration and frequency variables are summarized in Table 10–3. There were significant differences among groups in mean penile circumference increases averaged over all the tumescent episodes (F 6.7 df 3,48 p < 0.005) as well as in the average of maximum penile circum-

TABLE 10-1. Sleep Parameters

| | Diabetics | | | |
	No Erectile Problem (n = 12)	Erectile Problem (n = 11)	Normals (n = 13)	Psychogenics (n = 16)
Sleep Time (Min.)	405±7 (368-447)	371±14 (261-417)	406±10 (337-448)	406±10 (362-472)
Awake (Percentage Time)	5.0±0.7 (2.0-10.5)	6.1±1 (3.7-14.3)	4.6±0.7 (1.2-11.0)	4.4±0.5 (2.8-10.7)
No. REM Periods	3.9±0.2 (2.3-5.0)	3.6±0.2 (3.0-4.6)	4.0±0.2 (3.0-5.0)	4.2±0.1 (3.3-5.3)

Mean of three study nights ±SE. Values within parentheses represent range.

TABLE 10-2. Sleep Parameters

| | Diabetics | | | |
	No Erectile Problem (n = 12)	Erectile Problem (n = 11)	Normals (n = 13)	Psychogenics (n = 16)
REM Time (Min.)	73±6 (36-108)	61±5.5 (32-85.5)	83±5 (53-115)	91±5 (51-134)
REM Time/Sleep Time (%)	17±1 (10-24)	16±1 (7-22)	20±1 (14-27.5)	21±1 (15-29)
REM Latency (Min.)	104±7 (72-165)	90±11.5 (40-170)	81±6 (55-127.5)	77±4 (52-104)

Mean of three study nights ±SE. Values within parentheses represent range.

ference increases recorded during the three nights (F 7.0 df 3,48 p < 0.005). Both the nondysfunctional and the impotent diabetic groups had significantly diminished mean circumferential increases during erectile episodes compared to the normal and psychogenic groups.

TABLE 10-3. Tumescent Parameters

| | Diabetics | | | |
	No Erectile Problem (n = 12)	Erectile Problem (n = 11)	Normals (n = 13)	Psychogenics (n = 16)
Degree				
Penile circumference increase (mm)	18±1 (11-29)	15±2 (4-32)	23±15 (13-31)	25±2 (11-40)
Maximum penile circumference increase (mm)	21±1.5 (16-32)	18±3 (4-39)	27±1.5 (16-35)	29±2 (13-45)
Frequency				
No. total episodes	4.0±0.3 (1.3-5.0)	2.8±0.3 (0.7-4.3)	4.3±0.2 (3.6-5.0)	4.2±0.2 (3.3-5.3)
No. maximum episodes	2.3±0.3 (0.3-3.7)	0.56±0.2 (0-1.6)	2.1±0.4 (0.3-4.3)	2.4±0.4 (0-4.3)
Duration				
Tumescent time (min.)	177±17 (50-277)	101±19 (8-199)	193±8 (150-252)	187±13 (125-303)

Mean of three study nights ±SE. Values within parentheses represent range.

There were also significant differences among the four groups in total number of episodes per night (F 4.2 df 3,48 $p < 0.05$), number of episodes that reached maximum tumescence (F 4.7 df 3,47 $p < 0.01$) and total time spent in tumescence (F 8.1 df 3,48 $p < 0.005$). In these three variables, however, nondysfunctional diabetics did not differ from the normal and psychogenic groups and had values significantly higher than the group of diabetics with erectile problems.

DISCUSSION

The systematic assessment of sleep and nocturnal penile tumescence in diabetic subjects with and without erectile impotence provided information of theoretical and practical significance. For the first time, it was demonstrated that young male diabetics who are free from erectile problems exhibit impairment in REM tumescence similar to diabetic impotent men. The impairment shown by nondysfunctional diabetics, however, is limited to diminished increase in penile circumference during nocturnal erections and does not extend to parameters such as duration and frequency of NPT episodes. The observation that the frequency of maximum erections determined by direct observation of nondysfunctional diabetics, does not differ from the normal and psychogenic groups is in keeping with lack of evidence of behavioral erectile impairment and suggests that the decrease in circumferential changes during REM erections had not yet reached clinically detectable differences in erectile capacity. The diminished penile circumferential changes noted among diabetics suggest that nondysfunctional and impotent diabetics do not constitute discrete clinical categories and that a subclinical erectile impairment may exist in nondysfunctional diabetics. It seems reasonable to conclude that these men may be at risk for the rapid development of erectile failure during metabolic decompensation or when exposed to psychosocial stressful conditions.

The observation that nondysfunctional and impotent diabetic groups do not differ in degree of penile circumference increases has important practical consequences for the use of NPT as an ancillary diagnostic procedure. This is particularly the case in that differences in penile circumference change have been used by several investigators to categorize subjects as organic or psychologically impotent [19]. The findings of the study show that other NPT parameters such as number of total or maximum erectile episodes, although less sensitive, are better discriminators of organic impotence since they differentiate clinically relevant degrees of erectile impairment.

The polygraphic assessment of sleep in conjunction with NPT variables disclosed unexpected information. Diabetic men in both groups spent significantly less sleep time in REM and longer latencies to REM onset. The possibility that metabolic abnormalities associated with diabetes may disturb sleep brain function and REM activity requires further investigation. From a practical standpoint, this observation suggests that sleep-staging needs to be taken into account in the evaluation of NPT data among diabetics. Indeed, in the present study, when tumescent duration was adjusted as percentage of REM time, the decreased time spent in tumescence noted in the impotent diabetics was no longer significant when compared to the other three groups. Lack of consideration of sleep-staging may lead to erroneous diagnostic conclusions by attributing to erectile capacity differences in sleep patterns among various clinical groups.

In conclusion, the results of this study indicated the value of studying sleep-related erectile changes in non-dysfunctional diabetics; it also emphasized the methodological significance of including nondysfunctional diabetics as a comparison group in the parametric evaluation of NPT as a diagnostic method of erectile function.

NOTES

1. Rubin, A. and D. Babbott. Impotence and diabetic mellitus. *JAMA,* 1958, 168:498–500.

2. Schoffling, K., K. Federlin, H. Ditschuneit, and E. F. Pfeiffer. Disorders of sexual function in male diabetics. *Diabetes,* 1963, 12:519–27.

3. Kolodny, R. C., C. B. Kahn, H. H. Goldstein, and D. M. Barnett. Sexual function in diabetic men. *Diabetes,* 1973, 23:306–9.

4. McCulloch, D. K., I. W. Campbell, F. C. Wu, R. J. Prescott, and B. F. Clarke. The prevalence of diabetic impotence. *Diabetologia,* 1980, 18:279–83.

5. Jensen, S. B. Diabetic sexual dysfunction: A comparative study of 160 insulin treated diabetic men and women and an age-matched control group. *Archives of Sexual Behavior,* 1981, 10:493–504.

6. Ellenberg, M. Impotence in diabetes: The neurologic factor. *Annals of Internal Medicine,* 1971, 75:213–19.

7. Campbell, I. W., D. J. Ewing, B. F. Clarke, and L. J. P. Duncan. Testicular pain sensation in diabetic autonomic neuropathy. *British Medical J.,* 1974, 2:638–39.

8. Faerman, I., L. Glacer, D. Fox, M. N. Jadzinsky, and M. Rappaport. Impotence and diabetes: Histological studies of the autonomic nervous fibers of the corpora cavernosa in impotent diabetic males. *Diabetes,* 1974, 23:971–76.

9. Abelson, D. Diagnostic value of the penile pulse and blood pressure: A Doppler study of impotence in diabetics. *J. Urology,* 1975, 113:636–39.

10. Schiavi, R. C. and B. Hogan. Sexual problems in diabetes mellitus: Psychological aspects. *Diabetes Care,* 1979, 2:9–17.

11. Fairburn, C. G., F. C. W. Wu, D. K. McCulloch, D. Q. Borsey, D. J. Ewing, B. Clarke, and J. H. J. Bancroft. The clinical features of diabetic impotence: A

preliminary study. *Brit. J. Psychiatry,* 1982, 140:447–52.

12. Tattersall, R. Sexual problems of diabetic men. *British Medical J.,* 1982, 285:911–12.

13. Schiavi, R. C. and C. Fisher. Assessment of diabetic impotence: Measurement of nocturnal erections. *Clinics in Endocrinology and Metabolism,* 1982, 11:769–84.

14. Karacan, I., F. B. Scott, P. J. Salis, S. L. Attia, J. C. Ware, A. Altinel, and R. L. Williams. Nocturnal erections, differential diagnosis of impotence and diabetes. *Biological Psychiatry,* 1977, 12:373–80.

15. Karacan, I., P. J. Salis, J. C. Ware, B. Dervent, R. L. Williams, F. B. Scott, S. L. Attia, and L. E. Beutler. Nocturnal penile tumescence and diagnosis in diabetic impotence. *Am. J. Psychiatry,* 1978, 135:191–97.

16. Fisher, C., R. C. Schiavi, A. Edwards, D. M. Davis, M. Reitman, and J. Fine. Evaluation of nocturnal penile tumescence in the differential diagnosis of sexual impotence. *Archives of General Psychiatry,* 1979, 36:431–37.

17. Schiavi, R. C., C. Fisher, M. Quadland, and T. Gloger. The diagnosis of erectile disorders. *Proceedings, Fifth World Congress of Sexology.* Z. Hoch and H. I. Lief (eds.), *Excerpta Medica.* Amsterdam: Elsevier Science, 1981.

18. Snedecor, G. W. *Statistical Methods.* The Iowa State University Press, Fifth Edition, 1956, 251.

19. Hosking, D. J., T. Bennet, J. R. Hampton, D. F. Evans, A. J. Clark, and G. Robertson. Diabetic impotence: Studies of nocturnal erection during REM sleep. *British Medical J.,* 1979, ii:1394–96.

11

Diagnostic Methods in Male Impotence

G. Wagner

Doing a sexual history is essential for the differential diagnosis of erectile problems. A given history way well lead to a suggested etiology.

As well as a proper physical examination of the whole body, a careful evaluation of the vascular status, particularly of the lower limits, should be performed. Careful penile palpation is crucial and may demonstrate congenital and acquired malformations as well as Peyronie's plaques. To exclude pathology of the testes, the epidydimis and spermatic cord should be throughly palpated. Serum testosterone, prolactin, glucose, and creatinine determinations should be part of the workup.

The Doppler technique is suitable for studying individual arteries and disclosing arterial insufficiency in any of the arteries leading to erectile tissue. A ten megahertz bi-directional probe is used over the penile arteries. The arterial systolic blood pressure of the penis is measured after a cuff has been placed around the penis. The ratio between penile and brachial blood pressure is calculated. In normals, this ratio exceeds 0.85. In cases of erectile dysfunction based on the so-called "pelvic steal syndrome," a drop in penile blood pressure will occur after exercise. This drop in penile blood pressure is due to shunting of blood flow away from the pelvis to the buttocks and lower limits with exercise. In normals, the ratio between brachial and penile blood pressure will remain constant after exercise.

Genital reflexes can be tested by putting slight pressure on the glans penis, causing a contraction of the bulbo-cavernosus muscle. Alternatively, one can measure the latency of the bulbo-cavernosus reflex employing an electro-myograph (EMG) electrode in the muscle. A surface stimulator stimulates the pudental nerve. Somato-sensory evoked potentials of the dorsal nerve of the penis can be studied to investigate the integrity of cortical, spinal, and peripheral sensory pathways.

Nocturnal penile tumescence recording can also be employed in the differential diagnosis of erectile problems. During normal sleep there are four to six rapid eye movement phases of sleep which are accompanied by penile tumescence. This phenomenon can be studied in a sleep laboratory. The increase in the penis size is measured by two strain gauges. One disadvantage of this method is that volume changes alone are recorded. An external rigidi-tometer should utilized.

An alternative procedure is to measure penile response to penile vibration. This procedure provides a direct evaluation of the afferent and efferent local neural fibers involved in erection. Not all men react to vibration, which means that only a positive response is of diagnostic value.

Direct visual sexual stimulation tests can also be employed. Mercury strain gauges are placed on the penis, and different erotic film strips are shown to the patient. Most men will react to erotic visual stimulation by penile tumescence.

Xenon wash-out from the corpus cavernosum can be utilized to to detect venous abnormalities. A few hundred microcuries of radioactive xenon dissolved in saline is placed in the corpus cavernosus. The disappearance of xenon is monitored by a detector. Xenon washout is first recorded in the flaccid, unstimulated penis. The disappearance of the injected xenon is related to the blood flow through the cavernous tissue. Xenon washout is then recorded after visual sexual stimulation. In normals, the washout should not increase during tumescence. A dramatic increase in washout indicates an abnormal drainage from the cavernous body.

In order to localize an abnormal leakage from the cavernous body, cavernosography is required. A slow infusion of radiocontrast medium into the cavernous tissue occurs while cinema-fluorscopy is conducted. This occurs both in the flaccid and erect state. Contrast shadows are sign of fistula.

Following cavernosography, infusion of normal saline to produce tumescence is performed. Once full volume and rigidity is obtained, the infusion rate is reduced to maintain the erection. This procedure gives a precise measure of the maintenance flow necessary to maintain an erection. A high flow rate means that the patient has an insufficient ability to regulate and diminish the outflow from the cavernous body.

PART IV

Psychotherapy of Sexual Dysfunction

In the 1960s behavior therapists influenced by Hans Eysenck's respondent conditioning model of neurosis began conceptualizing sexual difficulties as being the result of anxiety elicited by sexual stimuli. These therapists began reporting successful results treating such disorders with counterconditioning approaches such as imaginary desensitization and *in vivo* desensitization approaches. These early reports had minimal impact on the clinical practice of non-behaviorists. The situation changed drastically when Masters and Johnson published *Human Sexuality Inadequacy* in 1970. Many clinicians in this and other countries enthusiastically embraced the concept that sexual disorders were the result of performance anxiety, poor marital communication, and sexual misinformation and the idea that most of these disorders would respond to brief intensive symptom-oriented psychotherapy. Concurrent with this increased clinical activity, clinical investigators began controlled outcome studies. The result of this investigation has been questioning of the simplistic conceptual model advanced by the behaviorists and Masters and Johnson, refinements of clinical technique, and the realization that many patients may require alternative treatment approaches.

This section includes an outcome study by Vansteenwegen and associates, a study of ego-analytic sex therapy by Apfelbaum, a discussion of diagnostic criteria by Manara, a discussion of the problems of integrating the disabled into sex therapy by Dunn and associates, a study of biofeedback and erectile dysfunction by Segraves, a discussion of psychotherapy with cases of organic impotence by Perelman, and a study of the wives of men with impotence by Wabrek. This section concludes with an important topic for clinicians, a study of spontaneous remission rates in untreated sexual disorders by Nathan.

12

Ego-analytic Sex Therapy:
The Problem of
Performance-Anxiety Anxiety

B. Apfelbaum

The ego-analytic model is the how-you-handle-it model. The idea is that sex problems are caused, not—as we usually assume—by anxiety, anger, or depression, but by how the person handles these feelings.

Many impotent men have some hatred of women, and it seems to many clinicians that this must be one cause of impotence. But many of our greatest sexual virtuosos have hated women. The difference is that they are good haters. The impotent men are poor haters. The poor hater expresses his anger with a limp penis. The good hater expresses his anger with an erect penis.

The good hater feels *entitled* to his anger. That's an ego-analytic word. If you feel entitled to your anger, then it is not undermining. It can even be strengthening.

Many impotent men are depressed, and it is obvious to all clinicians that depression is one cause of impotence. As sex therapists, we get the impression that when a man gets depressed his erections reflect it. Two years ago I did a quick survey of five analytic therapists I know. I asked them to list the men they had seen in the past year whom they thought of as depressed, and they came up with 23 men. Then I asked them how many of these men mentioned having any erection problems. The total number was zero.

Many depressed men get *relief* from sex. They need it *more* and may even get more out of it. I once had a patient who suffered severe and immobilizing depressions. He was a psychiatrist and he believed that it was sex that kept

him out of the hospital. When he did develop a dysfunction, he was not concerned about the dysfunction as such,
just about having to be hospitalized. The object of sex for
him was reassurance and support, not performance. To the
extent that a man is vulnerable to male-role expectations,
the object of sex is performance; he has to be up for it.
Being depressed threatens him and he cannot perform.

Helen Kaplan (1979,35f) is the only sex therapist who
has noted that many men experience performance anxiety
and have no erection problems. She also has an explanation for this, an explanation very different from mine.
Here is how she puts it:

> The mere thought, "maybe I won't have an erection
> tonight," need not be associated with anxiety of
> sufficient intensity to drain the penis of blood. In
> the secure person who has a good relationship, such
> a thought will not produce impotence, but when there
> is deeper unrecognized anxiety about sex . . .
> unconsciously he needs to avoid a successful per-
> formance.

Kaplan says that these men have an "active role in evoking
the anxiety-provoking thoughts which result in impotence,"
although they are not consciously aware of it. In other
words, her conclusion is that performance anxiety causes
impotence only in those men who unconsciously wish to be
impotent.

I find no evidence to support Kaplan's interpretation,
but she does deserve credit for pointing out that performance anxiety alone is not enough to cause impotence. I
think that the critical missing factor is performance-anxiety
anxiety—the anxiety about having performance anxiety.

This is the anxiety that gets intensified by telling people
that the purpose of sex is enjoyment, not performing.
Many sex therapists and most other kinds of therapists,
and all therapeutically untrained physicians are prone to
scold people for being worried about performing sexually,
to tell them that sex is natural. We are prone to tell
people that being worried about performing is natural.

That at least avoids intensifying the anxiety about
worrying about performing, but it does not relieve it. The
problem, as I see it, is that the impotent man is threatened
by his performance anxiety. He thinks he should not be
anxious. He does not think that anybody else is anxious in
sex. It really scares him. He then tries to hide. He tries
to act as if everything is OK.

The men who are vulnerable to performance anxiety do

not feel entitled to have any feelings that might interfere with sexual performance. They have to act as if every-thing is OK. You could even say that *that* is the cause of their problem. Our solution is to help them to stop acting as if everything is OK.

We developed our solution in our work with that most difficult of all sexual relationships, that between a male patient and a female body-work therapist in individual body-work sex therapy (Apfelbaum, in press), our modifi-cation of approaches to sex therapy using surrogate part-ners. Many people have a romanticized vision of the surro-gate-patient relationship (Apfelbaum 1977). They imagine a serene, seductive, and confident woman who will just soothe away the patient's performance worries. They imagine someone who is immune to the effect of the patient's anxi-eties, anxieties that are intense to begin with, and that are further intensified by the pressures of the therapy itself.

For the patient, the therapy often seems to be his last chance. He has mobilized all his resources for this last effort. At considerable expense, he has travelled to our center and he now has two weeks to show whether he has the real stuff (as he sees it). He is to meet with a woman not of his own choosing, an expert in front of whom he is afraid he will appear as a humiliating failure.

Typically, this is just too much to bypass by the usual distraction techniques: sensate focus, the Hartman and Fithian caresses (popular among surrogates), or the Kaplan technique of having the man conjure up a favorite mastur-batory fantasy. The alternative of gradual desensitization would fare no better in the hothouse climate of a two-week time limited therapy.

The ego-analytic approach is to change the patient's relationship to his anxiety. The first thing we do is to break it down into its components and the next thing is to train the man to *share* these experiences at the moment that they are happening in the body work. For a given patient, performance anxiety may break down into the following components: a feeling of urgency (often expressed nonver-bally through pelvic motions and pubococcygeal (PC) muscle contractions); the feeling that he should not be anxious, that we expect him to be enjoying this "nondemand" rela-tionship, and that any other man would be; feeling like a loser; feeling hopeless; being afraid of disappointing the body-work therapist, of her getting irritated or bored.

Once we have separated out these worries, we then put them into simple statements, like: "Now, I'm feeling ur-gent;" "I'm afraid I'm disappointing you;" "I feel like I should be enjoying this more;" "This doesn't seem to be getting anywhere;" "I'm afraid this isn't going to work," or even a simple statement like: "I'm feeling uncomfortable."

The patient then practices reporting these experiences during the body work and finds, to his surprise, that such reports are often accompanied by surges of erotic feeling. In the process, he learns to pay attention to these small signs of arousal and to differentiate them from anxiety.

It could be said that we are just using another kind of distraction technique. Instead of concentrating on performance, the patient is kept busy noticing and reporting his experiences. But we find that the statements have to be accurate or they do not work. At one point, the patient may say, "I'm feeling urgent," and experience a burst of arousal. At another point, when he is feeling hopeless, he may experiment with saying he feels urgent and nothing happens.

One hidden effect is the impact of this kind of reporting on the body-work therapist. A man who in his initial response to the body work had been largely silent, withdrawn, and preoccupied is transformed into an involved and interacting partner. Instead of desperately trying to act as if everything is OK and trying to reassure the body-work therapist that he is not worried, denying his all-too-obvious tension, he is taking her into his confidence. This relieves the pressure on *her* to act like everything is OK, and to not puncture his denials. She now has something to respond to and this, in turn, makes him feel responded to.

A brief transcript may help to visualize this process. Since we rarely record body-work sessions, we have few such transcripts available. This one is of particular interest because of the unusual severity of the symptom. This 42-year-old Alaskan construction worker was primary impotent, although he was sexually experienced, with multiple partners, and with a previous unconsummated marriage of eight years. He had been through a course of couple sex therapy with his then-wife at another center, but had still not been able to sustain an erection sufficient for penetration. The previous therapists reported that he had demonstrated "massive performance anxiety." His was a longer than average case for us, requiring 17 sessions over a three-week period.

On the transcript the patient is expressive, even chatty. Initially he was quite reserved and taciturn, especially about personal matters, although he was bright and otherwise articulate in a homespun way. He prided himself on enduring conditions of extreme hardship without complaint.

This transcript is from Day Twelve and covers a three and one-half minute time span. There is full nudity, the patient is supine, and the body-work therapist is sitting next to him doing genital stroking, using a lubricant. The patient is holding a list of 18 statements that had been developed in previous sessions. The words in italics are those that he took from the list. As can be seen, he felt free to break up these sentences as he went along, rearranging and interpolating.

At first the patient's tone is flat, and it is clear that he is reading and ruminating.

> P: *I feel like I'm,* I'm still partially *cut-off* or ignoring something, you know, ignoring part of it or something.
> BT: Hmm. I wonder if it could be on the list. I just don't, I don't know what it would be.
> P: Kind of, kind of *out of touch*, a little bit, not like when I'm into a real gripping worry. I already mentioned *that barrier feeling*. I don't know if I feel that now or not. I don't think so. *I feel* kind of *urgent*, kind of *preoccupied* too. *I wish you could help me get out of this mood*. *I don't* really *like this mood*. I don't know if *I feel shy* or *embarrassed*—maybe that is the feeling in there—that I'm in this mood, or *helpless* too, you know. A mixture.
> BT: Mm-hm.

[The patient's tone now begins to become more animated.]

> P: *This mood* that I'm kinda in *seems irrational*, you know. *I'm* kinda, *I'm afraid to ask for anything*, but uh—it's just because *I don't know where I'm at*, in a mood or my feelings or something, you know I'm—*It feels like I'm waiting for some kind of reassurance* or something—or something that makes me feel different or, you know, I'm waiting. I don't know.

[The BT reported that he had a full erection at this point. It began appearing when he read the lines: *I'm afraid to ask for anything, I don't know where I'm at,* and *It feels like I'm waiting for some kind of reassurance*. In the past, this would have been the point at which he was silently straining to produce an erection, or trying to cover his impending failure by telling his partner how much he was enjoying everything she was doing.

Next, in what follows, as he is about to lose his erection as a consequence of internal struggles with his worry about

132 / B. Apfelbaum

losing it, he sustains his aroused state by noticing and sharing this worry.]

> BT: Uh-huh.
> P: I'm starting to feel more though, so it must be something that—but now I get afraid I'll do something wrong [*I'm afraid I might do something wrong*], you know. I'm starting to feel turned on and feel good and now *I'm worried that something will wreck it [this mood].* *I want to get more turned on, but I don't know what to do.* [Long pause.] Yeah, that's the feeling that keeps coming through. *I feel like I should be doing something, but I'm afraid that I might do something wrong* that will turn me off. *I feel like I should do something to stay turned on.*
> BT: Hmm.
> P: Maybe something with you or, you know, or—or the way I'm looking at my feelings or something. But I'm feeling more turned on and this seemed to do it. This seemed to—just going through there seemed to do something there.

By the end of treatment the patient was experiencing full erections lasting 30 minutes or more and had no difficulty with penetration. He also reported no difficulty on one, two, and five year follow-ups. His first posttherapy sex partner was his ex-wife. He said that she expressed so much relief at his being expressive rather than silent in sex that he found this to be highly reinforcing. However, it is not our expectation that any of his posttherapy sexual encounters would much resemble this protocol. We expect that the ways of responding to his anxiety which he learned in the therapy will be internalized. We also expect that he now will be likely to share his worries, but it generally requires very little of that to reduce the tension level for both him and his partner.

REFERENCES

Apfelbaum, B. The myth of the surrogate. *Journal of Sex Research,* 1977, 13:238–49.
Apfelbaum, B. Individual body-work sex therapy: Five case examples. *Journal of Sex Research,* in press.
Kaplan, H. S. *Disorders of Sexual Desire.* New York: Brunner/Maze, 1979.

13

Outcome of Ten Years of Residential and Outpatient Sex Therapy: An Exploratory and Comparative Study

A. Vansteenwegen, M. Luyens, and S. Daelemans

How effective is sex therapy? Everyone refers to the results of Masters and Johnson [1] and everyone adds that these results were never replicated. Arentewics and Schmidt [2] in a very impressive and extremely well-designed study came to different conclusions. Their failure rate was for most dysfunctions much higher. The study presented here is an exploratory postfactum clinical outcome research. It is an overview of ten years of sex therapy in the Clinic for Sexual Dysfunctions [3] of the Communication Center [4,5] University Psychiatric Hospitals, Catholic University of Leuven, Belgium.

For a group of 192 patients, a number of patients, situational and therapy variables were studied. The number of variables in the data enabled us to gain some information about some current questions in sex therapy.

In our Clinic for Sexual Dysfunctions, two formats of therapy were available: an intensive residential three week approach and an outpatient-once-a-week-approach. One group was treated by two therapists, another by one therapist only. So a comparative outcome study concerning type of treatment and type of therapists was carried out. Heiman and LoPiccolo [6] did not find any difference in a daily versus weekly format of therapy. Clement and Schmidt [7] found a trend toward a somewhat better outcome with weekly therapy. They compared also one therapist with cotherapy and did not find differences in outcome.

Yet no replication research is done concerning the *residentiality* variable of sex therapy which was present in 90 percent of Masters and Johnson's treatments. This study was preceded by a review of 82 outcome studies of treatment for sexual problems [9].

We found that behavioral therapy (35 studies, 34.5 percent with controlled design) resulted in 78 percent better or successful outcomes, Masters and Johnson therapy (18 studies, 5.5 percent with controlled design) had favorable outcomes in 77.5 percent. Psychodynamic-oriented therapy (six studies none with controlled design) had a better or successful outcome in 95.5 percent of the cases. In regard to the different dysfunctions, the outcome can be summarized as follows: The percentage of cases with "better" or "successful" outcome were for erection problems (9 studies): 70 percent; for impotence (21 studies) 67.5 percent; for ejaculation incompetence (13 studies) 97 percent; for premature ejaculation (20 studies) 90 percent; for frigidity (8 studies) 79 percent; for anorgasmic dysfunctions (32 studies) 79 percent (secondary [9 studies] 51.5 percent); vaginismus (10 studies) 88.5 percent.

PATIENTS

The treated group consisted of 192 patients; 177 were with their partner in therapy and 15 alone. The treated group consisted of 80 (46.7 percent) male and 117 (58.3 percent) female patients. The sexual dysfunctions presented by these patients are summarized in Table 13–1.

Our group of male clients presented 36 erection problems (19 percent of the total group); 20 premature ejaculation problems (10 percent), 18 ejaculatory incompetence (9 percent), 4 male dyspareunia (2 percent) and 2 cases of alibidinismus (1 percent).

In the group of female patients we found 17 aversion problems (9 percent); 4 cases of alibidinismus; (2 percent); 16 arousal problems (8 percent); 18 (9 percent) orgasmic dysfunctions; 19 dyspareunia (10 percent) and 38 cases (20 percent) of vaginismus. The *ages* of these patients were: under 25: 51 (26.7 percent); between 26 and 30 years: 53 (28.8 percent); between 31 and 40: 63 (33 percent); between 41 and 50: 19 (9.9 percent); and 3 (1.6 percent) above 50 years.

The *duration of the problem* can be described as follows: in four patients the problem was present less than one year, in 110 between one and five years, in 47, between six and ten years. In 22 cases the problem existed more than ten years.

TABLE 13-1. Frequency of Sexual Dysfunctions (N = 192)

Sex	Dysfunction	Number	Percent
Male	alibin.	2	1
N = 80	erect. probl.		
41.7%	prim.	16	8
	sec/sit	20	11
	prim. ejacul.		
	prim.	20	10
	sec/sit	0	0
	anejaculation		
	prim.	11	6
	sec/sit	7	4
	dyspareunia	4	2
Female	aversion	17	9
N = 112	alibid.	4	2
58.3%	arousal probl.		
	prim.	4	2
	sec/sit	12	6
	orgasm.dysf.		
	prim.	15	8
	sec/sit	3	2
	dyspareunia	19	10
	vaginismus	38	20

As to the *motivation for therapy*: 103 patients came with a complaint about the sexual relationship itself; in 45 cases a wish for a child was the motivation. In 39 patients, a better general relationship was the motive for seeking sex therapy. The data concerning previous treatment were: 117 patients had no previous treatment, 33 received a somatic treatment, 32 psychotherapeutic help and 10 had a psychiatric hospitalization in their past.

Marital status: three patients were married for less than one year; 78 between one and five years, 44 between six and ten, 44 were married for more than eleven years. Thirteen lived together without marriage.

The *number of children* was: 127 patients had none; 15 had one and 29 had two children. Thirteen had three, and eight had four or more children. All patients were from

Flanders, most of them from a Roman Catholic upbringing. The group was a *real clinical group* referred to us by general practitioners, psychiatrists, gynecologists, and so on.

THERAPY

The therapy consisted of a Masters-and-Johnson type of sex therapy, influenced by Lobitz and LoPiccolo's [10] therapy and with the use of Rogerian therapy in the phases of resistance. In 33.5 percent of the cases, *cotherapy* was used. In 13 percent this cotherapy was done by two experienced therapists and in 20 percent by one experienced therapist and a cotherapist-in-training. The experienced therapist in 62.5 percent of the cases was a female psychologist. In the other 66 percent of the cases the therapy was carried out by one experienced therapist-psychologist or medical doctor. The experienced therapists were three females and three males, all about 30 years of age.

The *number of therapy sessions*: 23 patients had less than five sessions; 49 patients received six to ten sessions, 62 patients had eleven to fifteen sessions, 45 clients had sixteen to 20 sessions, and thirteen patients had 21 sessions or more. The duration of the session was one hour.

One group (50 percent) of the patients had an intensive residential therapy of three weeks every working day (Monday to Friday). The other half of the group received out-patient therapy (mostly one session a week).

GLOBAL EFFECT

The outcome can be summarized in four classes: worse, status quo, better and success. The results were: worse, 3.4 percent; status quo, 33.3 percent; better, 17.5 percent; and for 45.8 percent, therapy was successful. For 36.6 percent no therapeutic effect was found. (See Table 13–2.)

SOME CHI SQUARE ANALYSES

By means of a simple chi square test we found a lot of information about the dysfunctions, previous treatment, drop out, cotherapy, type of treatment, motivation, duration of the problem, social level of patients, age, and outcome of the therapy.

TABLE 13-2. Dysfunction and Therapeutic Effect

Dysf. Effect	-	sq.	+	Success
alibid. male		1		
Erect. probl. prim.	1	5	2	7
sec/sit		6	1	12
Prem. ejacul.	1	7	8	4
Anejaculat. prim.		4	1	6
sec/sit		4	1	1
Dyspareun. male			1	
Aversion	1	7	5	2
Alibidin. female		2	2	
Arousel dysf. female				
prim.		1	2	1
sec/sit	3	3	3	3
Anorgasm. prim.		4	2	6
sec/sit		2		
Dyspareunia fem.		2	1	15
Vaginismus		11	2	24
Tot. (N = 177)	6(3.4%)	59(33.3%)	31(17.5%)	81(45.8%)

No significant relation was found between *dysfunction* and drop out. However, a significant relation was found between the kind of dysfunction and the motivation, the duration of the problem, social level, the age and the number of children. No significant relation was found between dysfunction and previous treatment. *Previous treatment*: no relationship was found with the outcome. As to the *drop out,* no relationship was found neither with the duration of the problem, the social level, the fact of being married, no influence of the distance of the residence of clients to the center. A significant relationship was found between *drop out* and cotherapy (chi$_1^2$ = 4.71 (p < 0.05); C = 0.17). A significant relationship was found between *cotherapy* and outcome (chi$_1^2$ = 5.75 (p < 0.05); C = 0.19). No significant relationship was found between the duration of therapy and outcome. *Intensive therapy* was significantly related to cotherapy (chi$_1^2$ = 11.97 (p < 0.001) and to *outcome* (chi$_1^2$ = 3.41 (p < 0.05); C = 0.15).

The *motivation for treatment* was not significantly related to intensive or outpatient type of therapy. The *motivation for treatment* was significantly related to outcome. When the motivation of the patient was sexual functioning or wish for a child, there was a good therapy outcome in two of three cases. When the patient expected a more general improvement of the global relationship, only in less than half the cases a good outcome was found (chi$^2_2$ = 8.16; p < 0.05).

The *duration of the problem* was not significantly related to drop out, nor to type of treatment, or outcome.

The social level of the patient was not related to motivation, nor to outcome. *The age* was not related to motivation or outcome. The sex of therapist was not related to outcome.

DATA FROM THE ANALYSIS OF VARIANCE (ANOVA)

One of the statistical problems was that the number of patients in the different conditions was uneven. We used the "least squares" method instead of the "unweighted means solution." Some trends we already found, were now confirmed. A repeated measurement design (split-plot design SPF) was used with the following values: worse = one; status quo = two; better = three; and success = four. The base score before treatment was for all cases: two.

After treatment, when the therapist judged that there was no therapeutic effect, a two was given, and so on. The difference of the variance from zero was tested. This form of analysis is, in fact, very severe: the levels of significance are divided by the number of conditions.

The results can be summarized as follows: An overall effect of the therapy on the outcome was found. When only the main complaints were considered, therapy was found to be effective for erection problems, dyspareunia and vaginismus. When the same analysis was repeated for all complaints (main complaints, secondary problems of partner and patient) a significant effect was found for every dysfunction, excepted for aversion. For libido problems only a slight effect was found. Female dyspareunia and vaginismus were very successfully specially treated. Some further analyses were carried out with the variance of "dysfunction, outcome, cotherapy" and one with "type of treatment, outcome and motivation." (See Tables 13-3, 13-4, 13-5, and 13-6.)

Motivation for therapy and type of treatment were again significantly related to the outcome, while they were both

TABLE 13-3. Design 1

Dysfunction	Before	Measurement	After
1. Erection probl.		n = 34	
2. Ejaculatio praecox		n = 20	
3. Anejaculation		n = 17	
4. Aversion		n = 15	
5. Fem. Arousal probl.		n = 20	
6. Anorgasmia		n = 15	
7. Dyspareunia		n = 15	
8. Vaginismus		n = 37	
		N = 177	

TABLE 13-4A. ANOVA-Table 1a (Main Problems [only]/Main Effects: N = 177)

Source	SS	df	MS	F	sig
1. Between subj.	81.16	176	0.46		
2. Dysfunctions	11.55	7	1.65	4.02	p < 0.01
3. Subject within groups	69.61	169	0.41		
4. Within subj.	895.00	177	5.06		
5. Effect	99.84	1	99.84	21.52	p < 0.001
6. Dysf. x Eff.	11.55	7	1.65	0.36	n.s.
7. Eff. x Subject within groups	783.61	169	4.64		
8. Effect:					$(\alpha/8)$
a. erection probl.	23.53	1	23.53	5.07	p < 0.01
b. ejac. praec.	5.63	1	5.63	1.21	n.s.
c. anejaculation	7.53	1	7.53	1.62	n.s.
d. aversion	2.13	1	2.13	0.46	n.s.
e. Fem. Arousal Probl.	3.60	1	3.60	0.78	n.s.
f. anorgasmia	6.53	1	6.53	1.41	n.s.
g. dyspareunia	28.66	1	28.66	6.18	p < 0.01
h. vaginismus	33.78	1	33.78	7.28	p < 0.01
9. Total	976.16	353			

TABLE 13-4B. ANOVA-Table 1b (Dysfunctions/Outcome: N = 297)

Source	SS	df	MS	F	sig
1. Between subj.	134.97	296	0.46		
2. Dysfunctions	15.75	7	2.25	5.49	p < 0.01
3. Subject within groups	119.22	289	0.41		
4. Within subj.	279.50	297	0.94		
5. Effect	144.52	1	114.52	352.5	p < 0.001
6. Dysf. x Eff.	15.76	7	2.25	5.49	p < 0.01
7. Eff. x Subject within groups	119.22	289	0.41		
8. Effect bij:					$(\alpha\alpha/8)$
a. erection	28.76	1	28.76	70.15	p < 0.01
b. ejac. praec.	12.50	1	12.50	30.49	p < 0.01
c. anejaculation	13.52	1	13.52	32.98	p < 0.01
d. aversion	2.63	1	2.63	6.41	n.s.
e. Fem. Arousal Probl.	8.	1	8.	19.51	p < 0.05
f. anorgasmia	16.20	1	16.20	39.51	p < 0.01
g. dysparenuia	36.38	1	36.38	88.73	p < 0.01
h. vaginismus	42.28	1	42.28	103.12	p < 0.01
9. Total	414.47	593			

TABLE 13-5. Design 2--Type of Treatment/Outcome/Motivation

Treatment (A)	Motivation (C)	Measurement (B)	
		Before (b_1)	After (b_2)
Intensive	sexual (c_1)		n = 46
	child wish (c_2)		n = 25
(a_1)	relation (c_3)		n = 18
Out-patient	sexual (c_1)		n = 49
	child wish (c_2)		n = 18
(a_2)	relation (c_3)		n = 20
			N = 175

TABLE 13-6. ANOVA-Table 2: Type of Treatment/Outcome/Motivation

Source	SS	df	MS	F	sig
1. Between subj.	119.22	175	0.68		
2. A	1.36	1	1.36	2.06	n.s.
3. C	4.25	2	2.13	3.23	$p < 0.05$
4. AC	1.56	2	0.78	1.18	n.s.
5. Subject within group	112.04	170	0.66		
6. Within subj.	135.50	176	0.77		
7. B	98.28	1	98.28	546	$p < 0.001$
8. AB	1.36	1	1.36	7.56	$p < 0.01$
9. BC	4.25	2	2.13	11.83	$p < 0.01$
10. ABC	1.56	2	0.78	4.33	$p < 0.05$
11. B x Subject within group	30.04	170	0.18		

12. AB (error = MS_B x s.w.g.); $\alpha/2$

	SS	df	MS	F	sig
B at a_1	61.94	1	61.94	344.11	$p < 0.01$
B at a_2	37.71	1	37.71	209.50	$p < 0.01$

13. BC (error = MS_B x s.w.g.); $\alpha/3$

	SS	df	MS	F	sig
B at c_1	59.14	1	59.14	328.56	$p < 0.01$
B at c_2	35.17	1	35.17	195.39	$p < 0.01$
B at c_3	8.22	1	8.22	45.67	$p < 0.05$

14. ABC (error = MS_B x s.w.g.); $\alpha/6$

	SS	df	MS	F	sig
B at ac_{11}	39.13	1	39.13	217.39	$p < 0.01$
B at ac_{12}	16.82	1	16.82	93.44	$p < 0.01$
B at ac_{13}	7.11	1	7.11	39.50	$p < 0.05$
B at ac_{21}	21.59	1	21.59	119.94	$p < 0.01$
B at ac_{22}	18.78	1	18.78	104.33	$p < 0.01$
B at ac_{23}	2.02	1	2.02	11.22	n.s.

	SS	df			
15. Total	254.72	351			

unrelated to each other. Cotherapy was also significantly related to outcome. Intensive therapy proved to be more effective than outpatient therapy. Patients with a demand for sex therapy from a motivation about the general improvement of the relationship had lower outcome, in outpatient and in intensive treatment as well. All these data confirm the previous findings.

PROGNOSTIC EVALUATION:
MULTIPLE REGRESSION METHOD

Finally, with a multiple regression method a prognostic evaluation was made. By means of this analysis a set of predictors is given in a decreasing range of their unique support to the variance of the criterion. The main outcome is considered as the dependent variable and all other variables are the independent ones. Then we searched for the variables by which the correlation between both sets of variables is defined. In the first analysis only "drop-out" was found as a predictor. The important result, however, was that a large number of variables had no relation to the therapeutic effect: the duration of the problem, the number of sessions, the social level, the age, the number of children, had no prognostic value. Other variables (previous treatment, cotherapy, type of treatment, motivation) had a slight prognostic value. A second multiple regression as then carried out on these relevant variables. *Motivation* seemed to have the most prognostic value. Previous treatment was also important.

CONCLUSIONS AND COMMENTS

The intriguing results of this exploratory clinical outcome study can be summarized as follows. In our Clinic for Sexual Dysfunctions *cotherapy* is clearly more effective than therapy with one therapist: the drop-out rate is lower and the outcome is better. In our setting, *residential intensive* (three weeks) sex therapy is more effective than an outpatient once-a-week treatment. These results are in contradiction to the studies of Heiman and LoPiccolo [6], Clement and Schmidt [7]. Improving sexual functioning and child wish are two *motivations* that lead to more effective outcome. A demand for sex therapy with, as a goal, an improvement of the general relationship is followed by a successful outcome in only half of the cases. The most difficult sexual problem to treat is aversion.

Our results can be compared with the outcome of Masters and Johnson [1], Kolodny, Masters and Johnson [11], Arentewicz and Schmidt [2] and our own review of therapy outcome literature [9] (see Table 13–7).

It seems that the effectiveness of our clinic is much lower than the effectiveness of all other centers, except for anorgasmia. Our drop-out rate is very similar to the drop-out rate of the Hamburg group. The failure rate of one third is an accepted rate in the general psychotherapy outcome literature [12]. In another study [13],[14] at our Clinic the outcome rate for couples with a good relationship was very similar to the results of Masters and Johnson.

TABLE 13-7. Comparison of Failure Rates*

Dysfunction	M and J		K, M, and J		A and S		V, L and D		B
	%	N	%	N	%	N	%	N	
Inorgasmic dysf.	20.8	342	28.1	388	31	108	31	48	21
Vaginimus	0	29	1.9	54	22	27	29	37	11.5
Prim. Impot.	40.6	32	21.1	19	21	57	40	15	32.5
Sec. Impot.	30.9	213	14.6	288			33	18	
Prem. Ejacul.	2.7	186	4.9	246	16	31	30	20	10
Ejacul. Inc.	17.6	17	25.9	58			49	17	3
Total	20	790	7.7	1053	25	223	33.3	155	-
Drop out	3.2	(?)	?		19		22.9		-

*M. and J.: Masters and Johnson [1]
K., M. and J.: Kolodny, Masters and Johnson [11]
A. and S.: Arentewicz and Schmidt [2]
V., L. and D.: our results
B: our review of Billen [9]
%: Failure rate
N: number of treated patients

NOTES

1. Masters, W. H., and V. E. Johnson. *Human sexual inadequacy.* Boston: Little, Brown, 1970.

144 / A. Vansteenwegen et al.

2. Arentewicz, G., and G. Schmidt, eds. *Sexuell gestörte Beziehungen.* Berlin: Springer, 1980.

3. Luyens, M. Een kliniek voor seksuele dysfuncties: achtergronden en werking (A clinic for sexual dysfunctions). *Leuvense cahiers voor Seksuologie,* 46–54. Antwerpen: DNB, 1978.

4. Verhulst, J., and C. Bakker. Marital therapy in an educational group setting: The Communication Center in Leuven, Belgium. D. Upper, and S. Ross, eds., *Behavioral group therapy, 1980,* 105–23. Champaign: Research Press, 1980.

5. Vansteenwegen, A. Intensive psycho-educational couple therapy: therapeutic program and outcome research results. *Cahiers des Sciences Familiales et sexologiques,* 1982, 5:91–135.

6. Heiman, J., and J. LoPiccolo. Clinical outcome of sex therapy. *Arch. Gen. Psychiatry,* 1983, 40:443–49.

7. Clement, U., and G. Schmidt. The outcome of couple therapy for sexual dysfunctions using three different formats. *J. Sex. Marital Therapy,* 1983, 9:67–78.

8. Kolodny, C. R. Evaluating sex therapy: Process and outcome at the Masters and Johnson Institute. *The J. of Sex. Res.,* 1981, 17:301–18.

9. Billen, J. *De effectiviteit van therapie voor sexule dysfuncties.* Licentiaatsthesis, o.l.v. Alfons Vansteenwegen, K. U. Leuven, Louvain, 1982.

10. Lobitz, W. C., and J. LoPiccolo. New methods in the behavioral treatment of sexual dysfunctions. *J. Behav. Ther. Exp. Psychiatr.,* 1972, 3:265–71.

11. Kolodny, R. C., W. H. Masters, and V. E. Johnson. *Textbook of sexual medicine.* Boston: Little, Brown, 1979.

12. Garfield, S. L. Evaluating the psychotherapies. *Behav. Ther.,* 1981, 12:295–307.

13. Vansteenwegen, A., and J. Verhulst. Behandeling van seksuele dysfuncties met Masters-en Johnsontherapie. *Tijdschrift voor Geneeskunde,* 1974, 230–34.

14. Vansteenwegen, A., and J. Verhulst. Residential psycho-educational therapy III: Changes in sexual functioning and sexual satisfaction. Paper presented at the Fourth World Congress of Sexology, Mexico, 1979.

14

Psychosexual Dysfunction: Diagnostic Criteria and Prognosis in Short Sex Therapy

F. Manara and G. Cantoni

In recent years much progress has been made in the search for a reliable and objective method of discriminating between organic and psychic pathologies which underlie the sexual syndrome. Thus it has become increasingly rare that patients suffering from impotence of vascular etiology undergo useless psychotherapeutic treatments. However, it is still quite common that a patient with a sexual syndrome stemming from a complex psychopathological situation and tied to intrapsychic problems is recommended to follow short sex therapy. Naturally, in these cases the prognosis will be as bad if the patient's psychopathological condition is serious, or the level of hostility present in the relationship is high. It is just for this reason that so much effort has also been made in the area of clinical psychosexology, as it is this field which must confront the majority of sexual problems, to find a better way of defining the psychological events in play.

The contributions in this area have been directed at:

1. A better organization of the data emergent from psychodiagnosis referring in particular to the person with the symptom.
2. A more accurate investigation of the individual psychopathological problems of which the sexual syndrome is the, or one of the, somatic manifestations.
3. A more accurate study of the relational problems of the couple which lie at the root of the sexual dysfunction.

DISCUSSION OF THESE CONTRIBUTIONS

In 1979, in its periodic revision of the *Diagnostic and Statistic Manual of Mental Disorders* (DSM III), the American Psychiatric Association inserted, for the first time, sexual pathology among psychiatric disorders. The contribution thus brought to sexology is not only nosographic, but, more importantly, methodological. In fact, DSM III recommends a multiaxial evaluation that takes into consideration various classes of information.

Axis I   includes the entire classification of mental disorders. The clinical syndromes which are the basis of a particular symptom are recorded here. Besides, Axis I includes those conditions which cannot be attributed to mental disorders, but which make up the focus of the treatment.

Axis II   includes personality disorders and specific disorders of the evolutive development. Specific personality traits can also be indicated in this Axis when structured personality disorders are not present.

Axis III includes the disorders and physical conditions external to the mental disorder, but which can illuminate the etiology of the diagnosed disorder.

Axis IV   refers to the seriousness of the psychosocial stressors. This axis provides a code with which it is possible to formulate a prognosis. In fact, it serves to codify the importance of possible stressors which significantly contribute to the development or worsening of the existing disorder.

Axis V   refers to the way the patient has behaved during the year previous to the consultation. This information as well can have a prognostic significance.

To exemplify the use of DSM III, consider two examples in the following tables. They show a psychosexual dysfunction which will be treated by sex therapy (Table 14–1) and a psychosexual dysfunction depending on a psychiatric syndrome (Table 14–2).

The arrangement proposed by DSM III concerning psychosexual disorders should be considered for a moment. As far as concerns psychosexual dysfunction, the novelty of this proposal is that it tries to categorize in these five axes everything that relates to the psychological aspects of the disorder. Thus its major contribution is that of setting up

TABLE 14-1. Multiaxial Evaluation (DSM III)

Psychosexual Dysfunction: Premature Ejaculation

Axis I	300.02	Anxiety
	302.75	Premature ejaculation
		(Focus of treatment)
Axis II		Traits of dependent personality
Axis III		Hypertension
Axis IV		Psychosocial stressors: New career.
		Severity 4--Moderate
Axis V		Highest level of adaptative
		functioning past year: 3--Good

TABLE 14-2. Multiaxial Evaluation (DSM III)

Psychosexual Dysfunction: Inhibited Sexual Desire

Axis I	296.23	Major depression
Axis II	301.60	Dependent personality disorder
Axis III		None
Axis IV		Psychosocial stressors: 5 - Severe
Axis V		Highest level of adaptative
		functioning past year: 4 - Poor

---

a diagnostic prospective in which the symptom is studied in relation with any other psychiatric problems which might be present and affecting the situation. We have shown that with such guidelines, the margin of error in proposing a therapy would be greatly reduced. It thus offers the possibility, if correctly utilized, of differentiating those cases in which a sex therapy would be useful, from those where the elected therapy should be of a completely different kind: for example, psychoanalysis or psychopharmacological therapy.

DSM III seems to have another important advantage, that of being a serious and well-codified instrument for an epidemiological study of psychosexual disorders and in particular of psychosexual dysfunction, allowing us to determine to what extent the sexual symptoms are pure, and to what extent they are expressions of other psychiatric problems, as well as the incidence and diffusion of sexual pathology. This, being a relatively untouched field of research, will surely lead not only in a speculative direction, but moreover in an applicative direction, perhaps finally shedding light on an abused and hardly fertile terrain, namely that of those sterile queries into whether or not sex therapy be truly valid.

DSM III seems indeed to be a formidable instrument for defining that which lies within the realm of psychosexology and differentiating this from what belongs to psychiatry. Only in this way, can it be clearly shown whether psychosexual therapy has a vast, or a partial utility, or none at all.

To be able to correctly fill in the blanks of the five axes proposed in DSM III, it is necessary to use adequate guidelines which can provide the most precise indication of the incidence of the individual psychopathological elements, and of the relational problems of the couple which bring about sexual dysfunction. To do this we employ a system of measurement having three objectives: 1) to make a diagnosis or description of the problem; 2) to try to clarify the etiology of the problem; 3) to suggest adequate therapeutic strategies for solving that problem.

Our diagnostic program comes from a fusion of the conceptual vision of psychodynamics and several elements borrowed from the behaviorist and cognitivist methods. Assuming that any diagnostic program should be flexible in relation to the specific needs which arise, it can be postulated that the couple must be involved in the psychodiagnostic program so that all the pertinent material for a correct diagnosis either on the intrapsychic or on the relational level is available. For this purpose, we utilize a form composed of a hundred items that explore diverse areas concerning:

1. the patient or patient's birth and marriage data and their sociocultural status;
2. the patient(s)' remote pathological anamnesis;
3. the patient(s)' remote sexual anamnesis;
4. the data relating to the sexual education of the patient as well as his or her preceding sexual experiences;
5. the present relationship;
6. the couple's attitude towards their bodies;
7. the couple's sexual habits;
8. their knowledge of contraception; and

9. any treatment or medical tests which have been performed.

The advantage of this form consists in the fact that it not only allows the same data for both partners to be collected and clearly organized, but also that it facilitates the programming of this data on a computer. This form thus permits a quite efficient diagnostic evaluation, and is a "spontaneous" document relating to the symptom, which during any consequent sex therapy, gives the possibility of evaluating any possible modification or remission of the given symptom.

Through this first diagnostic approach it can be seen beforehand where resistance is apt to occur, and thus the prognosis will be nearer the truth, and consequently the therapeutic contract with the patients will be more precise.

In the case that the interviews indicate that an important psychopathology might be generating the sexual syndrome, traditional psychodiagnostic instruments are employed, such as the projective tests (Rorschach, Thematic Apperception Test), having the aim of uncovering certain aspects of the patient's inner world, or personality tests such as the Minnesota Multiphasic Personality Inventory (MMPI), which are meant to measure the general psychological functioning of the individual. Then, if the data gathered indicates the need for sex therapy, the couple is further studied using a questionnaire, specifically, the "Sexual Interaction Inventory" (SII) of LoPiccolo, Steger 1974. This questionnaire was principally designed to pinpoint the sexual behavior of the couple and the pleasure they derive from it. The SII questionnaire provides a description of the sexual relations of the couple (given separately by the two partners and later comparing the scores) in terms of the frequency and pleasure of a specific sexual activity, besides providing information relative to the type and level of communication between the partners concerning these activities.

Another questionnaire which we use with the couple, administered separately, is one which evaluates their attitudes towards masturbation. This questionnaire, designed by P. R. Abramson and D. A. Mosher in 1974, gives us an insight into three principal factors: 1) a positive or negative attitude towards masturbation; 2) false beliefs about the dangers of masturbation; 3) any negative effects personally felt by masturbating. This test, as is well known, begins with the hypotheses that a negative attitude concerning masturbation (which this test is designed to reveal) is correlated with a reduced pelvic vasocongestion when confronting erotic stimuli. As good pelvic vasocongestion obtained by erotic stimuli is a pre-requisite of a good sexual response, the data gathered by the answers to the 30 items of this test offer a valuable clue to the seriousness of the sexual dysfunction.

It should be stressed at this point, that none of the instruments which we have cited can provide, by them-selves, an adequate measurement, simply because sexual dysfunction is not something which exists on its own, independently, but rather, it is tied to the history of each partner, to his (or her) real sexual behavior in private, to attitudes and cognitive factors, to intrapsychical defenses, and above all to the network of interpersonal relations, not to mention psychiatric conditions and biological factors. Therefore, only in its totality, and adapted to the partic-ular situation, can this diagnostic method be useful for those who wish to utilize a multidimensional approach.

Following this diagnostic procedure, we have treated, in the last two years, 62 patients suffering from disorders which were certainly psychosexual in nature. To be pre-cise the data are reported in the following tables (Tables 14–3 and 14–4). In Table 14–4 we show the types of ther-apy to which we address the three groups.

The couples or patients belonging to the first group were treated with short sex therapy of a psychodynamic-behaviorist orientation, lasting from eight to twenty-two sessions, with an average of sixteen. The results were largely positive as far as the resolution of the symptoms was concerned. In fact, only two patients suffering from impotence, three from anorgasmia, and one from dyspareu-nia were not able to overcome the sexual symptom, but even in these cases an improvement in the intimacy and climate of the sexual relationship was obtained.

The couples of the second group were advised to follow a projectual therapy of the couple, therapy focused on relational problems (conflict, hostility, and so on). Six couples (three premature ejaculation, one impotence, one female orgasmic dysfunction [F.D.D.] one dyspareunia) did not follow this suggestion and in all six cases the choice was made by the dysfunctional partner. Of the remaining cases, three ended in separation (one premature ejaculation, one F.D.D., one dyspareunia). Three began the therapy but withdrew after several sessions (two Inhibited Sexual Disorder [I.S.D.] one impotence), hence without improving their conjugal problems. Seven (two premature ejaculation, three impotence, one F.D.D., two dyspareunia) could finally be treated with a "projectual therapy of the couple" which yielded, in five cases, a noticeable improvement in

TABLE 14-3. Patient Characteristics

Total No. of Cases (62)	Psychosexual Dysfunctions	Group 1 Light Related Problems and Neurotic Psychopathol. Traits	Group 2 Serious Related Problems	Group 3 Serious Psychopathology or Relevant Intrapsychical Conflicts
8	Inhibited Sexual Desire	3	2	3
14	Impotence	5	5	4
15	Premature Ejaculation	8	6	1
2	Inhibited Male Orgasm	0	0	2
11	Female Orgasmic Dysfunction	6	3	2
7	Dyspareunia	2	3	2
5	Vaginismus	3	0	2

TABLE 14-4. Therapy

Group 1 (27 cases)	Group 2 (19 cases)	Group 3 (16 cases)
Short Sex Therapy	Projectual Therapy of the Couple	Individual Psychotherapy and/or Psychopharmacological Therapy

the climate of relationship to the point of allowing, later on, a direct treatment of the sexual dysfunction.

Concerning the patients of the third group, advised to follow individual psychotherapeutic treatments or psychiatric treatments, we do not have complete and reliable data. This is due to the fact that the therapy, which 12 of the 16 patients to whom this was recommended, chose to follow, has a long duration. Also, these patients were sent to work with other psychiatrists and psychotherapists.

We can deduce from the above, the importance of a careful diagnostic screening in the field of psychosexology, to differentiate psychosexual disorders from different etio-pathogenesis and, above all, to differentiate therapeutic programs according to the prevailing problem. Just as a correct instrumental and laboratory diagnosis permits an adequate therapy to be chosen for organic disorders, with a correct psychodiagnosis, our patients can avoid undergoing short sex therapies when actually there is a psychiatric pathology at the root of their sexual syndrome, which must be treated as such. In the first place, this will be of great use to patients. Additionally, it will protect short sex therapy from the indiscriminate and sometimes unjustified criticism, which should instead be attributed to improper diagnostic standards.

BIBLIOGRAPHY

Abramson, P. R., and D. L. Mosher. "The development of a measure of negative attitudes toward masturbation." *J. Consult. Clin. Psychol.*, 1974, 43:485–90.
Bentler, P. M., and P. R. Abramson. "The science of sex research: Some methodological considerations." *Arch. of Sex. Behav.*, 1981, 10:225–51.

DSM III—Third Diagnostic and Statistical Manual of the American Psychiatric Association. Washington, D.C.: American Psychiatric Association, 1979.

Kaplan, H. "The new sex therapy." New York: Brunner/ Mazel, 1974.

Lo Piccolo, J., and J. C. Steger. "The sexual interaction inventory: A new instrument for assessment of sexual dysfunction." *Arch. of Sex. Behav.*, 1976, 3:585–95.

Manara, F. "Compendio di psicosessuologia." (ed.) SIRFS. In press.

Manara, F., and A. Tridenti. "Scheda epidemiologico-clinica per terapia sessuale." Third World Congress of Sexol., Roma, 1978.

Manara, F., and A. Tridenti. "Problemi metodologici nella diagnosi e nella terapia delle disfunzioni sessuali psicogene." In A. Ermentini, ed., *Psichiatria*. Brescia: Mattarollo-Cavinato, 1981.

Manara, F., and A. Tridenti. "Sex therapy and/or couple therapy." Fifth World Congress of Sexol., Jerusalem, 1981.

Masters, W., and V. Johnson. *Human Sexual Inadequacy*. New York: Little, Brown, 1971.

15

Panel Discussion:
Integrating the Disabled into Sex Therapy

M. E. Dunn, S. Kelley-Linton, and H. Rousso

INTRODUCTION

Rehabilitation agencies have always assumed the responsibility for the health care needs of disabled men and women. In recent years, in response to increasing demand, sex counseling and educational services have appeared in various rehabilitation settings. However, these services are rarely sufficient to meet the changing needs and expectations of the disabled population striving for integration in the community. It is, therefore, likely that disabled men and women will turn to the same kind of sexual health care services that are available for their non-disabled neighbors.

In the past few years, sex therapists have been seeing more people with a range of organically caused sexual dysfunctions. These problems are being increasingly recognized because of better diagnostic tools and increased research on conditions that can cause sexual problems. The dichotomy between apparently healthy people with psychogenic dysfunction and those with subtle medical problems appears to be far from clear-cut. Expanding services now to include the disabled, seems the next logical step.

We wish to offer, in this chapter: 1) a model for measuring sexual capacity that can benefit both disabled and able-bodied clients; 2) consideration of the clinical and countertransferential issues that complicate treatment of the disabled; and 3) one center's experience in integrating disabled clients into their treatment population.

A MODEL FOR MEASURING SEXUAL CAPACITY

While Masters and Johnson's sexual response cycle is a fine model for the assessment of function and dysfunction in genital response, its application to assessment and treatment of broader sexual concerns is limited. Therapists are now seeing greater numbers of clients who are concerned with the qualitative, subjective aspects of their sexual experience and who feel deficiencies in desire and/or satisfaction. Research corroborates what many of us have believed for a long time: what a person feels, believes, thinks, expects is a much more powerful influence on sexual experience than the way the body responds. Acceptance of this idea is vital in working with people whose limbs may move differently or whose genitals may respond differently.

The following model is designed to assess an individual's capacities to experience a pleasurable sexual life and may be particularly useful in work with disabled or chronically ill clients. The model looks at three capacities: 1) desire, or the individual's wish to engage in sexual activity; 2) the individual's capacity to experience pleasure; 3) the individual's capacity to give pleasure. The therapist can assess the ways that favorable or problematic physiological, psychological, or social factors enhance, detract, and interact with these capacities.

Capacities	Influences		
	Physiology	*Psychology*	*Social*
Desire			
Capacity to experience pleasure			
Capacity to give pleasure			

It is clear that physiological, psychological, and social (that is, scripting) variables all shape an individual's desire for sexual activity and capacity to give and receive pleasure. It is rarely obvious which factors in a person's life are the primary causative ones in a sexual problem. For example, a client with muscular dystrophy may have limited capacity for experiencing pleasure on the basis of his poor muscle tone, a "secondary" deficiency in social skills or, because of a narcissistic self-absorption that has flourished in the absence of opportunities for rewarding interpersonal experiences. Similarly, acute pain in a patient with chronic lumbar disc disease can directly limit physical activity, but may have a more profound impact through lowering the individual's self-esteem and thwarting social opportunities because of recurrent hospitalization.

The complex interweaving of these causal factors means that facile conclusions about the "cause" of the patient's sexual problem must be vigorously avoided. It is clearly missing the boat for a therapist to actively assist his spinal cord patient to master new and indeed physically more manageable sexual positions, when his motivation for sexual activities has been stunted by other more critical psychological and social factors.

This model is useful in organizing treatment planning for sexual dysfunctions in disabled and chronically ill individuals. Each of the "nine" cells in this matrix must be assessed to determine the degree to which the patient's sexual capacities can be favorably altered.

Simi Kelley-Linton

CLINICAL AND THEORETICAL ISSUES

Sex counselors, therapists, and other clinicians encountering physically disabled clients for the first time commonly report one of two reactions. They may assume that without specialized training, they will be unable to handle sexual issues with disabled clients. In this case, there will be an inclination to refer to a specialist, possibly in a rehabilitation facility. If no specialist is available, therapists will begin their work feeling overwhelmed and inadequate. Alternatively, clinicians may feel that there are no special issues facing disabled clients, that disability does not significantly impact sexuality, and that the treatment of disabled and non-disabled clients is identical. While the latter position may be closer to the truth—at least for some disabled clients, and in any case may be more functional in allowing the treatment process to begin—both of these polarized viewpoints represent partial truths. I suggest that they indicate particular countertransference reactions to disabled clients.

Disability affects sexuality in various ways. There are the physical effects: on the neurological, vascular, and hormonal systems or on the mobility and flexibility needed for sexual positioning. There are also the psychological effects: alterations in self-esteem and body image which inevitably influence a sense of sexual entitlement and, therefore, sexual performance. In addition, there are social effects that arise from negative societal attitudes toward the disabled person and pursuant limitations of social opportunity. For the clinician to deny the impact of these physical, psychological, social realities is indeed countertherapeutic.

On the other hand, the growing body of literature on sexuality and disability can provide the interested clinician with an orientation, sufficient to begin the treatment process with disabled clients. Specific disability-related issues may be researched as they emerge. Indeed, most of the treatment techniques already known to the well-trained therapist or counselor are equally applicable and particularly useful to disabled clients. In the face of negative societal stereotypes regarding the sexuality of disabled people, the therapist's capacity to be curious about all aspects of the disabled client's sexual interest and activity can be an important counterbalance facilitating a sense of sexual entitlement and providing reassurance that there are positive ways to think, feel and function sexually.

Unfortunately, therapists fail to appreciate the value of their own curiosity and creativity, and instead prefer to view work with disabled clients as a specialized field beyond their grasp because of the conscious and unconscious attitudes, feelings and anxieties which disability raises. Recognizing and working through these attitudes is the major prerequisite to successful work with disabled clients.

Research on attitudes of nondisabled people toward disabled people document the preponderance of negative attitudes. These socially prevalent attitudes include the notion that disability is contagious, that disability is punishment for sin, and that disabled people are helpless, dependent and inherently socially and economically inferior.

Throughout history, most cultures have put a high value on physical perfection; physical imperfection has been equated with moral and intellectual imperfection. Disabled people tend to be viewed as asexual, or sexual within narrowly defined limits and may not meet a narrow definition of sexuality also based on physical intactness and Madison Avenue standards of beauty. Therapists and counselors, having been socialized in this society, are in no way exempt from these attitudes. Such negative attitudes can be understood in part as the result of lack of exposure to disabled persons and realistic information about disability and may reflect the therapist's experiences with illness and temporary disability. It may be hard for nondisabled people to appreciate the process of adaptation which can occur over time with proper supports and opportunities when faced with a permanent disability.

However, we must also view such attitudes in terms of their unconscious meaning. Disability in others raises anxieties regarding one's own wholeness, perfection, impermanence, and fragility. Intrapsychic factors such as castration anxiety, fears about body integrity, fears about one's destructive impulses, and anxieties over lovability are easily stimulated by contact with disabled people.

Therapist's anxieties, fears, and attitudes toward disability can impede work with disabled clients in a variety of ways. Most importantly, it may prevent the therapist from achieving the optimal distance from the client, from getting close enough to empathize with the client's deepest thoughts, feelings, and experiences, while remaining separate enough to be impartial and objective. Sometimes, in an attempt to feel safe in the face of feelings evoked by the client's disability, the therapist may become too distant. The distance may be a psychological one—or a physical one, that is, referring the client to another facility. At the other extreme, the therapist, overwhelmed by feelings surrounding the disability, may over-identify with the disabled client's experiences, particularly his or her negative experiences and feelings. In such a case, the therapist's curiosity may be particularly impaired for in the face of the client's pessimism about his or her sexual future, the therapist may think (and possibly say), "Of course, I would feel the same way," as opposed to the more helpful response, "What makes you feel that way?" which suggests that there are options. We should also note that if the client is not that pessimistic while the therapist is, the therapist may misinterpret the the client's attitude as evidence of denial and fail to recognize his or her own countertransferential projective identification.

There are other typical countertransferential responses which may be interwoven with the therapist's failure to achieve optimal distance. One is overprotectiveness on the part of the therapist and a reluctance to encourage risk-taking and experimentation for fear that the client will fail and be devastated. Thus the therapist may hold back on offering certain suggestions or strategies unless there is a high likelihood of success, thereby limiting his or her own spontaneous, creative problem-solving process as well as the disabled client's right to make choices. Disabled people may be physically fragile but are not necessarily psychologically so; disability is not a psychiatric diagnosis. It is important to keep in mind that risk-taking and failing, particularly when there is support—the therapist's support—can be a source of considerable growth and learning. Clients and therapists alike need permission to fail some of the time.

Another common type of countertransference involves the able-bodied therapist's fear of the disabled client's anger. In particular, the therapist may be concerned that his or her very physical intactness may evoke in the client a feeling of, "How can you possibly understand my sexual problems?" and that a client may react with rage to suggestions which involve other than traditional forms of foreplay and lovemaking. While some clients may indeed respond angrily to the therapist's presence and suggestions, this is not necessarily the case; much depends on the client's own dynamics and transference responses. In addition, if anger is produced, it is not necessarily a bad thing, but rather an important part of the therapeutic process, to be worked through, like any other response. The therapist must address his or her own fear and possibly guilt at being non-disabled first, so that anger, if and when it arises, can be handled and fully utilized.

It should be noted that disabled therapists, while in some ways possibly more attuned to the issues of disabled clients, are by no means exempt from countertransferential issues. Disabled therapists, along with the able-bodied counterparts, have been socialized in the same society filled with negative stereotypes toward disability, which they most likely have internalized to some extent; they too will have conscious and unconscious attitudes toward disability in need of careful scrutiny. In addition they may have some unique countertransferential responses. For example, the therapist with a disability may be too quick to assume that he or she understands the disabled client's experience. Rather than respecting the client's uniqueness, this may lead to attempts to impose solutions on the client which have been useful in the therapist's own life. Or, the therapist may be impatient with the client's slow progress, insisting "If I could do it, you can and must too!"

This discussion is at best an introduction to the types of countertransferential issues which can emerge in work with disabled clients. Major emphasis is given to countertransference here because it is believed that this is often a more significant impediment to integrating disabled clients into sex therapy services rather than the therapist's lack of specific knowledge and training on disability issues. Knowledge is readily obtainable, but only by a receptive mind. As has been indicated, most therapists already possess two major tools for successful work with disabled clients; curiosity and creativity. Anxieties and fears often block full utilization of these tools. In addition, we should note that disabled clients are really clients who happen to have disability as one of their characteristics. Disability is one factor affecting their sexual functioning and sexuality, but not the only fact. One of the greatest challenges facing therapists as they begin to work with disabled clients is finding a way to put the disability in perspective—for themselves and their clients. When it comes to the sexual response cycle, there are more similarities than differences between disabled people and their nondisabled counterparts. As therapists, it is part of our professional responsibility to scrupulously examine the resistances within ourselves which prevent us from appreciating those similarities.

Harilyn Rousso

PROGRAM IMPLEMENTATION

For the past two years, disabled and chronically ill clients have been integrated into the general clinical population at the Center For Human Sexuality of the Downstate Medical Center. Prior to this time, we took it for granted that our traditionally trained sex therapists lacked the requisite expertise for this group of clients. We were quite surprised then when agencies for the disabled began requesting our services for their clients. We quickly learned that these specialized agencies did not have personnel with the training or skill to assist clients in their sexual functioning. I will briefly review the impact on our sex therapy staff, and on our training program, from this innovation in our service delivery program.

Perhaps the most unexpected and salutary effect of treating disabled clients has been a deepening in our understanding of some of the underlying tenets of sex therapy.

One of the key messages of the sexual therapy movement was to guide people away from goal-oriented sex into more pleasure-centered sexuality. We urged men and women to stop working towards arousal, erection, and orgasm, and to broaden their personal definition of sexuality. We asserted that pleasure, intimacy, and closeness were preferred goals that would result in an enhanced relaxed sexual response. This was the basic philosophical message that we inherited from Masters and Johnson: that performance-geared sexuality often resulted in disappointment, while relaxed, sensual, communicative sexual experiences most often resulted in greater pleasure. Yet at our clinics and in our practices as sex therapists, we often quietly screened out patients whose sexual response might be compromised by serious illness or disability.

Working with severely chronically ill and disabled clients, has forced us as therapists to examine what is important in sexual interaction and what ought to be enhanced, and valued. We have seen able-bodied couples who could function multiple-orgasmically, yet in a very detached, uncaring manner. And we have seen other couples, who because of physical limitations could not complete a Masters and Johnson standard sexual response cycle and yet who had achieved enviable sensuality and sexuality. Thus, working with disabled clients helped us confront our own bias and paradoxical messages about what sexuality really is. It has helped us to work more effectively with disabled and chronically ill clients but also shored up and strengthened our treatment of able-bodied clients as well.

But the integration of the disabled population had other, quite pragmatic benefits in terms of increasing, as well as broadening our client census, and strengthening our training program. Since we have a large and active training program, we as a center need a constant stream of patients to work with. Now, since we only reject cases for treatment where the major difficulty is in the marital relationship, or in deep-seated intrapsychic problems, we have a more dependable available case load. Our trainees are also experiencing a more realistically composed treatment population. In this age of medical marvels, many more people are living longer but are living with some kind of chronic illness, disability or are on a drug regime that may inhibit sexual functioning. We feel in training our students to be able to work with all kinds of patient groups, we are aiding them in their future practices by giving them flexibility and a broader knowledge base. We have also found that working with disabled clients usually results in the therapist needing to learn some new approaches, techniques, studying some new literature, dealing with consultants more actively, all of which keep the therapist from becoming bored or jaded. Therapist burn-out is an issue in any form of therapy. If the therapist is exposed to new clients with somewhat different difficulties requiring somewhat different approaches and solutions, it seems to enliven the therapist and revitalize his or her work.

We have been impressed, as have others, with the commonality of sexual issues shared by both able-bodied and disabled populations. However, certain new skills are initially required. We would like to review some of the modifications in technique that evolved from our work with the disabled.

A sex therapist needs a cadre of consultants available even when working with supposedly able-bodied clients. For our disabled clients we have, at times, also needed the consultive services of a physical therapist. We usually cannot judge whether clients will be able to position their bodies or thrust well enough to accomplish intercourse, for example. The disabled clients themselves, perhaps inexperienced or very anxious, may not be the best reporters of their physical abilities. We have been pleased to find that once the therapeutic alliance has been established, most disabled clients are comfortable allowing their therapist to make a home visit with a physical therapist for an evaluation. We assure the clients that we will not be asking to watch sexual activity but rather to see them dressed and work with them towards seeing what range of motion they are capable of. On one such visit, for example, we saw that a client with severe cerebral palsy had no hip movement and could not angle her body in any way so that her severely disabled husband could penetrate for intercourse. He had no lower body strength and poor upper body movement so penetration was impossible. As they had initially entered sex therapy, in part, because they wanted to be able to have intercourse, we would have worked with them towards that end if we had not seen with them *in vivo* that intercourse was not a possibility. The physical therapist was able to teach the clients, in that single home visit, how they could position themselves in their chairs for maximum cuddling and body contact, and what positions they could use combining bed and chair contact. He also showed the female how she could comfortably and safely roll from her bed to her husband's bed for full body contact when they wished it.

Disabled clients are often, unfortunately, inured to outsiders entering their personal life space. They are sometimes dependent on home health aides for personal care and home visits of nursing personnel. It is not usual for us as therapists to see our clients in bed or to as dramatically need to imagine how love-making might be achieved. It was a more personal intervention than even we, as experienced, verbal, listening therapists were used to. We developed comfort with this practice as with every other form of sexual learning. Our clients were accepting and forgiving of our initial lack of total ease.

We have found the major necessary quality for being able to work effectively with disabled and chronically ill clients is the therapist's willingness to learn. The therapist needs often to learn from the client what is possible. It is exciting work because the therapist has to be an even more creative problem-solver than when working with able-bodied clients. While the same important training in couple inter-action, the same concern with communication, with inhibi-tion, with anxiety, with sexual entitlement become relevant issues when working with disabled clients, newer approach-es come into play when the therapist is trying to figure out how to enhance contact and facilitate sexual pleasure. We have, therefore, become somewhat more knowledgeable about ways that people can give each other pleasure or orgasm that require little body strength or mobility.

The effect of working with visibly disabled clients on our staff has been interesting. Those of my colleagues who were not working with such clients seemed initially de-pressed by the presence of disabled persons at our center. The clients' problems appeared overwhelming. The thera-pists were made very aware of their own fears of body injury and loss. As these same staff members saw changes in the mood, interaction and persona of our clients, their negativism and anxiety diminished. In staff conferences they were enthusiastic about changes that therapists were reporting. They, themselves, were now willing to take on similar cases. A broadening definition of sexuality, away from a high performance model, needs reinforcing in sex therapists as well as in the general population. Case discussions on severely, chronically ill and disabled clients dramatically taught and retaught us that lesson. Adminis-trative and clerical personnel also experienced attitude changes and had a new awareness that people with disabil-ities were sexual people. In short, the very presence of disabled persons in our institution raised consciousness.

Defining success in sex therapy has always been prob-lematic. If a client had erectile difficulty with no known organic basis, a successful outcome would mean his ability to resume intercourse. Yet even able-bodied males told us that the greatest benefit for them was that they learned if they lost an erection it was not the end of the world, or the end—necessarily—of a sexual encounter. With disabled clients who may have more complicated problems to over-come, a successful outcome from the client's point of view, may be mastering some mechanical aspects of sex, or becom-ing assertive enough to feel entitled to construct their lives so that they have a sex life. For example, one of the couples we were working with were dependent on home health aides to put them to bed, to wash them, to dress them, and so on. The greatest asset of their brief sex therapy was that the couple began to feel entitled to sexual pleasure. This meant that they felt assertive enough to ask their reluctant and resistant aides to undress them and leave them alone in the room so that they might have sexual contact. Often too, a successful outcome can depend on some small yet significant change in the way that a disabled couple is able to be together. As was the case for one couple we were working with, learning how to roll towards one another so that they could have her head on his chest and cuddle was a major and significant accomplishment for them. This achievement was sweeter to them than the fact that they could now bring each other to orgasm. The glow that their faces took on when they told us about being able to cuddle was a significant moment in the treatment process. The measure of our success then, is, as always, in whether an individual or a couple feel successful, feels that they have learned, or grown. It is person-centered rather than mechanical- or technical-centered.

We have found that our work with persons with disabilities has benefitted us as clinicians and expanded our view of sexuality. We are pleased with this long-needed integration.

Marian E. Dunn

Our goal in this panel has been to offer methods of integrating people with disabilities into sex therapy services. We believe this integration is an important part of the full social and economic integration that people with disabilities are working toward.

It is, of course, not only sex therapy which should be integrated. Sex education at all levels must include accurate and sensitive treatment of the sexuality of people with disabilities. Proper training of sexual health care professionals must include preparation for this work.

We must recognize that disabled people do not comprise a homogeneous and discrete group. If the definition of sexuality on which we base our work is broad enough, sex therapy can be useful for all people.

16

Biofeedback and Erectile Dysfunction

K. B. Segraves and J. Schipke

In recent years, a variety of therapeutic modalities have been developed for the treatment of secondary psychological erectile dysfunction and many causal factors have been hypothesized (Reynolds 1977; Kilmann and Auerback 1979). A number of clinical studies have found anxiety to be an important etiological factor and several investigators have demonstrated the effectiveness of anxiety-reduction techniques in eliminating an erectile dysfunction Wolpe (1958). Wolpe and Lazarus (1966) and most prominantly Masters and Johnson (1979) have used in vivo desensitization as part of their successful treatments for erectile dysfunction.

Wolpe (1958) has also advocated the use of systematic desensitization to reduce anxiety associated with erectile dysfunction. Wolpe taught his clients Jacobson's relaxation exercises (1938). Once relaxation was mastered, they were instructed to imagine a series of sexual scenes while attempting to remain in a relaxed state. Wolpe maintains that as a result of the desensitization process, the client is conditioned to respond with relaxation to stimuli that previously elicited anxiety. Wolpe (1958), Glick (1975) and Lazarus (1965) have all used systematic desensitization successfully to treat erectile dysfunction.

Friedman (1968) combined systematic desensitization successfully with intravenous injections of metholextol sodium to facilitate muscular relaxation during scene presentation. He reported that eight out of ten clients treated, regained normal erectile functioning and maintained change at 12-month follow up. Systematic desensitization has also been applied to a group format by Lazarus (1969) and Auerback and Kilmann (1977). Finally, Auerback and Kilmann (1977) compared group systematic desensitization with an "attention" control group. After 15 sessions, they reported a 40 percent improvement in the erectile functioning of those men in the systematic desensitization group, while those in the control group only improved 3 percent. If *in vivo* desensitization and systematic desensitization are effective in treating erectile dysfunction, perhaps other anxiety reduction techniques such as relaxation training would be effective. The concern of this study is to assess the effectiveness of relaxation training in treating secondary psychological erectile dysfunction.

One indication that an individual is in a state of high arousal (anxious) is a decrease in skin temperature. Research combining electromyograph (EMG) and temperature feedback has shown that decreases in skin surface temperature are associated with conditions of anxiety or stress; increases in finger temperature are associated with relaxation (Taub 1977; Taub and Emurion 1976; Bandewyns 1976; Fahrion 1977).

Peripheral hand-temperature can be used to validate the relaxed state. The rationale behind this is that an increase in surface temperature in the hand is associated with an increase in blood flow. An increase in blood-flow, in turn, results from vasodilatation to the surface area of the hands, and is dependent only on the decrease in neural outflow in the sympathetic sector of the Autonomic Nervous System (ANS). Simply put: in order to warm the hands by voluntary control, it is necessary to "turn off" automatic sympathetic activation (Green et al. 1970, 1975). Several writers have conceptualized erectile dysfunction as a parasympathetic response that is inhibited by sympathetic components of anxiety.

During an anxiety response, there is a decrease in circulation of the capillary beds of the digits which results in a decrease in skin temperature. Once there is a cognitive association of surface temperature and changes in arousal, a local warming effect can be self-induced by learning to self-regulate the hand temperature. It seems reasonable that training to carry out this task could provide a useful therapeutic approach to anxiety. Such training would have the client behave with a new response that would be antagonistic to anxiety. For this skill to be effective, the person must become "aware of existing tensions." Discrimination of slight changes within the body is necessary. Before training, these changes exist below our level of awareness. By focusing one's attention on the body, these changes can be brought to consciousness.

This treatment was aimed at teaching the patient how to relax under "ideal" conditions; in the therapist's office (a quiet place, no interruptions, eyes closed, comfortable). Once relaxation is mastered in this environment, the patient practices this skill under less "ideal" conditions (such as in his bedroom, or wherever the patient is most likely to have sex). This will help to make the skill more applicable to the patient's situation. The patient is then taught to relax without biofeedback, simply by using the subjective experience of his hand temperature as a cue.

In summary, the experimental treatment, "Thermal Relaxation Training," is designed to teach the client to control anxiety by: (a) "conditioning" relaxation responses to discrete and internal physiological cues; (b) teaching the client to intervene and use the skill when needed; (c) lessen the experience and frequency of erectile dysfunction.

The patient was a black male, 33 years of age, of lower socio-economic status, employed part-time, had a high school diploma, and was involved in an on-going sexual relationship of some stability. He had at least a six-month history of the erectile dysfunction. A recent physical examination suggested no organic etiology, normal serum testosterone, and prolactin levels; pH nocturnal penile tumescence recordings indicated psychogenic impotence, and a diagnosis of secondary psychological erectile dysfunction from an independent rater was made. Self-report data was collected. The most important outcome measure for this study involves the change in the target problem as reported in the patient's data. To chart this, information was collected throughout the study.

The form in the appendix was used to get a detailed picture of the erectile dysfunction, to assess the relationship between anxiety and the dysfunction, and to assess the overall level of day-to-day stress. Each time the patient obtained an erection, he would rate its firmness and duration. If the erection was lost before the completion of the intercourse, he would note the antecedent of its loss. To make erection rating a less subjective experience for the patient, the Knopf Scale (1983) was used to standardize data collection. Two different apparatuses were used for thermal biofeedback training. For office practice, a sensor called a thermistor was used for measuring temperature changes. The thermistor was taped comfortably (so as not to restrict blood flow) to the middle finger of the patient's dominant hand. The thermistor transmits the surface temperature of the skin through a wire to the biofeedback machine, which then translates the signal from the thermistor into a digital readout of the skin temperature. With this instrument, the patient receives feedback on variations in skin temperature up to one-tenth of a degree.

For home practice, temperature was monitored via a small inexpensive cardboard-backed thermometer which the patient taped to the pad of the middle finger of the dominant hand. The scale of the thermometer was marked in increments of 2° F. Although much less accurate, this thermometer was sufficient to give the patient some sense of the effectiveness of home practice periods. The instrument given to the patient was tested for its accuracy and was found to contain an error factor of less than two degrees.

Biofeedback was the treatment choice because of its congruence with the needs of the patients: both in physiological conceptualization, and in the relatively short time required for mastery (two to four sessions). The treatment used in this study closely follows a strategy outlined by Noonberg and Olton (1980).

SESSION 1

Before beginning, the rationale of biofeedback was outlined and patient's questions were elicited. After discussing the rationale, we introduced the patient to the biofeedback equipment, exploring the way in which the general processes discussed in the rationale become operationalized in treatment. The thermistor was then attached to the patient's dorsal digit of his dominant hand. Our next step was to obtain a baseline psychophysiological profile of the patient when relaxed and stressed. This data provides a baseline against which future changes, as a result of biofeedback treatment, can be compared. To obtain the relaxed psychophysiological profile, the patient is asked to sit quietly for five minutes, without feedback of any kind, doing whatever he would normally do to relax. Once the reading had stabilized, the temperature was recorded. To obtain a psychophysiological profile when stressed the patient was asked to describe, in as much detail as possible, the last occasion on which he lost his erection due to anxiety. The patient was asked as he described this situation, to re-experience this situation as much as possible. The therapist received constant biological feedback, so that reactions to the requests could be seen. After five to ten minutes, when the temperature had stabilized, the stress reading was recorded.

When the profile was concluded, the patient was told to relax. If there were changes in skin temperature, the therapist took this opportunity to discuss physiological changes noted by the patient and highlighted temperature changes that occurred.

At this point, the patient was taught paced breathing and received continuous thermal feedback. During the practice session, the therapist reinforced the patient ver-bally for increases in skin temperature. This initial session lasted 15 minutes and questions or comments were elicited from the patient at the end of practice.

Next, the patient's stress logs and erectile function logs from the baseline period were reviewed and discussed. During each session the patient was retrained in data collection procedures.

Finally, home biofeedback practice and the home practice audio tapes were introduced. Home practice was considered an integral part of the intervention, giving the client an opportunity to develop the skill of voluntary control learned in the clinic and to generalize that skill to his natural environment. The procedures for home practice were: (a) patient records beginning practice room and hand tempera-ture; (b) patient practices biofeedback skill learned in clinic as outlined by audio tapes; (c) patient records end-ing hand temperature and completes practice session eval-uation form.

The patient practiced twice a day for 15 minutes. To standardize and structure home practice, each patient received an audio tape that guided the patient through the skills being practiced that week and reminded him to record the data appropriately.

SESSION 2

The second session, like the first, focused on helping the patient master the relaxation response. After reviewing the patient's self-report data, the patient was given autogenic training to be combined with paced breathing. Autogenic training (Schultz and Luthe 1959) produces relaxation by having the client concentrate on verbal cues which are repeated silently or aloud. The basic exercises are phrases that are repeated facilitating muscular relaxation and pe-ripheral blood flow, lowering the heart rate, decreasing respiration, relaxing the upper abdominal cavity, and creating general sedation and drowsiness. The patient focused only on the phrase that was designed to increase peripheral blood flow (Noonberg and Olton 1980). Following introduction of the phrases, the patient practiced autogenic training for 15 minutes. During the practice session, the patient received continuous skin temperature feedback, was reinforced verbally for increase in skin temperature, and was asked by the therapist to focus on the sensations in his hands as the temperature changed. Finally, the patient was retrained on data collection and given the second home practice tape. This tape included guided paced-breathing and autogenic phrases.

SESSIONS 3 AND 4

By the third session, the patient had mastered thermal relaxation training. The goals of these final two sessions were to help the patient shift from the external cues of the biofeedback to his own internal cues of subjective hand temperature. Ideally, the patient should develop the confidence so that the physiological control can be carried out without feedback. The patient should develop the ability to assess the outcome of thermal relaxation training without immediate feedback from the machine.

Practice without feedback was introduced by alternating periods of feedback with training, with periods of no feedback. At the end of these sessions that lacked feedback, the patient was asked to report how successful he was during the session and then given information about the progress of his skin temperature over the course of the session.

As the patient began to demonstrate more voluntary control, obtain a relaxed state more quickly, and correctly assess no-feedback practice sessions, less and less feedback was given, and the no-feedback training periods became longer. The patient's records were also an important part of these final sessions. These records were reviewed at the beginning of each session. Where appropriate, the patient was praised for successful practice sessions, questioned about his performance (when using his new skills in stressful situations) and offered suggestions for future practice and implementation. In terms of home practice, the audio tapes for sessions three and four were much less directive and mirror the content of office sessions.

SESSION 5

Session five was planned as the final assessment. Rest and stressed psychophysiological profiles were again obtained, and the final batch of self-report data was reviewed and assessed. A four-week follow-up appointment was scheduled. Ideally, there would be periodic sessions after the final assessment to help maintain change.

Results of office practice for the patient are presented in Figure 16–1 of the appendix. The data is presented in graphic form. The number of the session is plotted along the horizontal axis, and peripheral skin temperature is plotted along the vertical axis. The data demonstrates the increasing ability of the patient to raise hand temperature at will, a skill that he continued to use effectively even with the reduction of external biofeedback in sessions three and four (see Figure 16–1). Followup at three months indicates that the patient had a return of normal coital function.

Figure 16–1. Results of the office practice for the patient

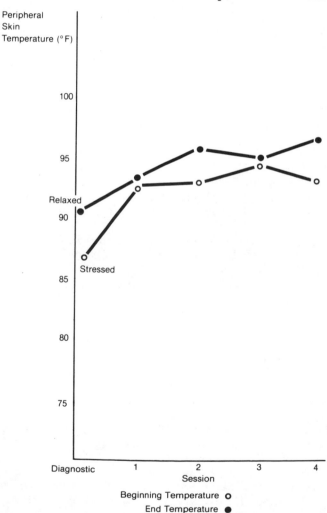

DISCUSSION

It is apparent from the available data on the patient that he was able to master thermal biofeedback training in the therapist's office. Subjective verbal reports by the patient suggest that he did experience some improvement in erectile functioning over the course of treatment, but the dubious reliability of such data prevents us from considering it as definitive.

The data from this single case study suggests that thermal biofeedback treatment merits further investigation as a treatment strategy for psychogenic erectile dysfunction. Our limited data does not allow a conclusion as to whether biofeedback or other variables were the primary effective treatment component.

NOTES

1. Auerback, R., and P. Kilman. The effects of group systematic desensitization of secondary erectile failure. *Behavior Therapy,* 1977, 8:78–83.

2. Bandewyns, P. A. A comparison of the effects of stress versus relaxation instructions on the finger temperature response. *Behavior Therapy,* 1976, 7:54–67.

3. Fahrion, S. L. Autogenic biofeedback treatment for migraine. *Mayo Clinic Proceedings,* 1977, 52:776–84.

4. Friedman, D. The treatment of impotence by brietal relaxation therapy. *Behavior Therapy,* 1968, 6:257–61.

5. Glick, B. Desensitization therapy in impotence and frigidity: review of the literature. *American Journal of Psychiatry,* 1975, 132:169–71.

6. Green, A. M., E. E. Green, and E. D. Walters. Psychophysiology for Inner Awareness. Paper presented at Association for Humanistic Society Conference, Miami, 1970.

7. Jacobson, E. *Progressive Relaxation: A Physical and Clinical Investigation of Muscular States and Their Significance,* 2nd ed. University of Chicago Press, 1938.

8. Kilmann, P., and R. Auerback. Treatments of premature ejaculation and psychogenic impotence. *Archives of Sexual Behavior,* 1979, 8:81–98.

9. Knopf, J. Knopf Erection Rating Scale, Unpublished, 1983, by Systematic Desensitization. *Journal of Abnormal and Social Psychology,* 1961, 63.

10. Lazarus, A. Group treatment for impotence and frigidity. *Sexology,* 1969, 36:22–25.

11. Lazarus, A. *Treatment of Sexually Inadequate Men, Case Studies in Behavior Modification.* New York:

Holt, Rinehart and Winston, 1965.

12. Lundgren, D. C., and M. R. Schwab. Perceived appraisals by others, self-esteem, and anxiety. *Journal of Psychology,* 1977, 97, 205–13.

13. Masters, W., and V. Johnson. *Human Sexual Inadequacy.* Boston: Little, Brown, and Company, 1970.

14. Noonberg, A., and D. Olton. *Biofeedback.* Englewood Cliffs, N.J.: Prentice-Hall, Inc., 1980.

15. Reynolds, B. Psychological treatment models and outcomes results for erectile dysfunction: a critical review. *Psychological Bulletin,* 1977, 84:1218–38.

16. Schultz, J. H., and W. Luthe. *A Psycho-physiologic Approach in Psychotherapy.* New York: Grune and Stratton, 1959.

17. Taub, E. Self-regulation of human tissue temperature. In G. E. Schwartz and J. Beatty (eds.), *Biofeedback: Theory and Research.* New York: Academic Press, 1977.

18. Taub, E., and C. S. Emurian. Feedback-aided self-regulation of skin temperature with a single feedback locus:i. Acquisition and reversal training. *Biofeedback and Self-Regulation,* 1976, 1(2):147–68.

19. Wolpe, J. *Psychotherapy by Reciprocal Inhibition.* Calif.: Stanford University Press, 1958.

20. Wolpe, J., and A. Lazarus. *Behavior Therapy Techniques.* Oxford: Pergamon Press, 1966.

17

Orgasmic Preferences Among 40 Female Partners of Males with Erectile Dysfunction

A. J. Wabrek

In the early 1950s, a 46-year-old women traveled a thousand miles to see a Chicago gynecologist. It appears, that after 25 years of marriage, she was planning to divorce her husband. Although she did not have anyone else in mind, she liked people and if the occasion presented itself she would remarry and if so, wanted to bring her new husband a tight vagina. The gynecologist asked her if she was looking for a young man 20, or perhaps even 30 years old—only to be told "Why, of course not!" Later the gynecologist stated "Nature has been wise: as the turgor of the phallus decreases, the commodiousness of the vagina increases. Man would be wise to leave well enough alone, at least until he is able to repair the shaft too." [1]

Devices for measuring penile rigidity are available [2,3] and "repairing the shaft"—for purposes of increasing rigidity—is now possible with penile implantation. Although diagnostic testing for erectile dysfunction has become more sophisticated and the range of therapeutic options has expanded, the role of the female partner in the evaluation and treatment has received varying degrees of emphasis. Gee [4] examined the female's motives and attitudes and stressed that physicians understand the importance of coitus for her. The female partner's acceptance—after implantation—has generally been quite favorable [5]. In one study [6], 74 percent of females were either fairly satisfied or very satisfied with their partner's implant. One disquieting finding—in the same study—was the 16 percent of female partners who were either fairly or very dissatisfied. In a more recent study [7], 25 percent of female partners were dissatisfied with implantation and most eventually admitted to general dissatisfaction with their partners. The authors rightfully acknowledged "This may have been elicited had they been interviewed prior to implantation."

A more disturbing finding [8] was the report that slightly less than 50 percent of female partners were seen—preoperatively—by the urologist. Renshaw [9], in an editorial comment, stated "Unless the genitourinary surgeon sees the sexual partner before and after implant, there will be a perceptual handicap for the physician that is as severe as seeing the world through a microscope."

The sexual response patterns among female partners of impotent males has not been previously reported; the purpose of the present investigation was to study this one aspect of the female partner.

METHODS AND MATERIALS

In the present series 40 males with erectile dysfunction were referred by their physicians to a hospital-based medical sexology program. As part of that evaluation, each female's ability to be orgasmic and her orgasmic preference were assessed by structured interview [10]. Questions were asked about each of the following behaviors: (a) intercourse, (b) manual manipulation of the female genital area by the partner, and (c) oral stimulation of the female genital area by the partner. Specifically, four questions were asked about each behavior: (1) is it acceptable? (2) have you experienced it? (3) is it arousing and (4) do you have a climax or orgasm that way?

Data were recorded on forms, as shown in Figure 17–1, using a seven point Likert type scale to differentiate orgasmic ability (top scale) and orgasmic preference (bottom scale) ranging between penetration (left side) and external genital stimulation (right side). No observation of sexual activity took place.

RESULTS

Fifteen percent of the females preferred being orgasmic by external stimulation of their genitals (Group I) and 42.5 percent preferred being orgasmic with internal or intravaginal stimulation (Group III). The remaining 42.5 percent of the females (Group II) was orgasmic with both external *and* intravaginal stimulation. Although the abilities

Figure 17–1. Form to Record Female Orgasmic Abilities and Preferences.

Female Response

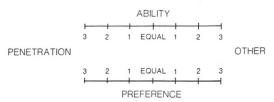

were equal, the preferences for being orgasmic were strongly in favor of intercourse. Those data are summarized in Figure 17–2.

Figure 17–2. Differences in Orgasmic Preferences Among Females with Equal Orgasmic Ability.

GROUP II – 42.5%

	EXTERNAL	INTRAVAGINAL
ABILITY	YES	YES
PREFERENCE	18%	82%

IMPLICATIONS FOR TREATMENT

A profile of the females who typically were orgasmic during intercourse and preferred coital behavior is as follows: a very clear distinction existed between "foreplay" and intercourse and oftentimes foreplay was quite brief (1–3 minutes) and consisted of "getting ready" for intercourse. With the onset of erectile dysfunction, sexual frequency decreased precipitously and a shift to noncoital sexual stimulation (to orgasm) would have been "difficult" or "impossible."

A profile of the females who typically were orgasmic with external genital stimulation includes a concept that intercourse is not a crucial aspect of sexual enjoyment. With the onset of erectile dysfunction, sexual frequency was much more likely to be maintained. Since the male was unable to have intercourse, sex play focused on holding, touching and caressing with genital stimulation and this represented for many of these females the best sexual experiences they have ever had.

Statistically, all females were wives of males with erectile dysfunction. Prognostically, they separate into different groups based on orgasmic preferences. Therapeutically, the females who preferred to be orgasmic with intravaginal stimulation were much more likely to opt for implantation if the males were found to have a nonreversible organic etiology of the impotence.

Hopefully, health care professionals assessing erectile dysfunction will routinely include the female partner. To do less, loses out on her very important contribution.

NOTES

1. DeCosta, E. J. Dance Me Loose. *Obstetrics and Gynecology,* 1955, 6:120.

2. Wabrek, A. J. Penile rigidity: concepts, measurements, and correlations. *Sexology,* Hoch, Z., and H. I. Lief, (eds.), Excerpta Medica Amsterdam, 1982.

3. Virag, R. Personal communication.

4. Gee, W. F., J. W. McRoberts, J. O. Raney, and J. S. Ansell. The impotent patient: surgical treatment with penile prosthesis and psychiatric evaluation. *Journal Urology,* 1974, 111:41–3.

5. Furlow, W. L. Inflatable penile prosthesis: Mayo Clinic experience with 175 patients. *Urology,* 1979, 13:166–70.

6. Gerstenberger, D. L., D. Osborne, and W. L. Furlow. *Urology,* 1979, 14:583–87.

7. Light, J. K., and F. B. Scott. Management of neurogenic impotence with inflatable penile prosthesis. *Urology,* 1981, 17:341–43.

8. Kramarsky-Binkhorst, S. Female partner perception of small-carrion implant. *Urology,* 1978, 12:545–48.

9. Renshaw, D. C. Inflatable penile prosthesis. *Journal American Medical Association,* 1979, 241:2637–638.

10. Wabrek, A. J., and C. J. Wabrek. History taking in sex counseling. *Clinical Obstetrics and Gynecology,* 1978, 21:183–90.

18

Rehabilitative Sex Therapy for Organic Impotence

M. A. Perelman

In our zest to pursue technological innovation in surgery and medicine, it is critical not to lose sight of the mind/body's ability to successfully compensate for its own deficits [1]. Our improved ability to diagnose organic pathology in impotence with the sophisticated assessment devices of nocturnal penile monitoring, penile blood flow and pressure monitoring, arteriography, corpus cavernosogram, evoked sacral potential, and hormonal assay has given rise to the view that the role of organicity in impotence was previously underestimated.

This view, when combined with the advancement of technique for surgery, has resulted in a dramatic increase in the number of men undergoing surgical prosthesis [2]. Additionally, there seems to be growing evidence that primary care physicians are becoming more reluctant to refer impotent cases for sex therapy [3]. This trend must be tempered by the recognition that sex therapy may still be the treatment of choice for some impotent men with documented organic deficits. This is feasible because of the omnipresent psychogenic component existing in any potency problem regardless of the degree of organicity. Clinical experience convinced me that anxiety can severely complicate the presenting picture of even a mild organic deficit, quickly escalating it into a complete and seemingly total dysfunction. Additionally, there is a growing body of evidence coming from other investigators that this is so. Blaivis at Harvard in 1980, discussed 100 patients of whom

50 percent had organic pathology—34 percent underwent sex therapy—which was effective for 62 percent of them [4]. Bullard, Mann and Caplan's 1978 article, went so far as to indicate all impotent men should first have sex therapy [5]. I question that, but want to present my experience in providing rehabilitative sex therapy to obtain your reactions to my approach. Our population's aging demographics make it likely that all of us will come to see an increasing number of cases with organic components, making such a dialogue between us a necessity.

There is a problem in defining this group of patients. All the men I am considering have at least one of the following: poor vascularization, diabetes, pharmaceutical reactions, hormonal insufficiencies. Yet, how do you define organic, when our current measures are still so inexact? How organic is it? How much do *you* trust equivocal, yet repeated nocturnal penile tumescence monitoring, Doppler or hormonal studies? Unfortunately, the more sophisticated we are, the more we seem to add to the tautological nature of our definitions. Nevertheless, I was particularly interested in cases where the organic element itself could not be completely corrected, but where sex could be improved. For instance, a switching of antihypertensive medication may improve the odds by producing some early morning swelling, but without a turgid erection, intercourse is still perceived as impossible. Something more than a change in medication is needed. Many men seen are borderline cases where erectile functioning is impaired, but not defunct. However, these same principles of enhancement to be discussed can be used with more severe cases.

Regardless of the organic deficit present, the range of capacity remaining varies extraordinarily. In terms of presenting symptomology, the cases I have seen are characterized by one or more of the following, independent of age: erections which are not reliable; erections which are not turgid; erections which do not last; latency for any tumescence is substantially greater than a previous period of functioning; lost "automatic functioning"; compulsive attempts at penetration or complete avoidance of sexual attempts; the level of stimulation required for erection produces an immediate ejaculation (this is especially likely to be seen in individuals with a previous history of premature ejaculation); and finally, no erection at all under any circumstance. You will, of course, notice how many of these common chief complaints parallel normal changes occurring in the aged male. All were saying to me, "it's not like it used to be." I believe the general theory in how to treat the majority of these people is the same. What will vary are the specific strategies suggested for each individual, depending on the particular nature of the organic and psychogenic factors.

Any of these organic deficits can make a man vulnerable to impotence by decreasing the probability he will reach the threshold of arousal necessary to obtain and maintain an erection. This threshold is like a point in space representing the sum total of all the vectors that are required to get "the darn thing to work." This reflects a sort of critical mass theory of potency. The greater the organic deficit in one or more spheres, the greater the need for compensatory thoughts and behaviors to bypass the deficit and reach the threshold necessary for erection. It becomes critical, therefore, to assess how the patient and his partner are handling the dysfunction. It appears that in all the cases I have seen, the patient's negative reaction to his diminished capacity (initially organically determined) exacerbated the problem into complete dysfunction. In other words, the degree of dysfunction consistently exceeds the degree of impairment in "organically impotent" men.

To treat this problem, I used a cognitive-behavioral sex therapy to develop new sexual scripts for the man and his partner(s), whereby psychic and physical stimulation were increased in order to compensate for the organic impairment [6]. Experimentation was encouraged, as well as redefinition of expectations, in order to produce an optimistic, but reality-based attitude. Patients were seen individually and/or conjointly with partners. I worked with single and married men, with treatment time varying from five sessions to 18 months—usually once per week.

A brief word about the spacing of sessions. Much more than working with other kinds of disorders, I find that after assessment and an introductory phase of treatment— allowing more time between sessions, is very helpful. Following eight sessions, one 56-year-old man with impotence secondary to circulatory problems, found one month between sessions ideal timing. This allowed him and his wife to find one to three comfortable times when they could successfully integrate a host of new suggestions simultaneously—which is what was necessary for him to function. If you want people to maximize all the positive conditions, they need more time to practice.

My general procedure to assess etiology is derived from Kaplan (1983), well described in her latest book—*Evaluation of Sexual Disorders* [7]. A comprehensive medical and problem-focused psychological work-up leads to an understanding of the physical, immediate, and remote psychological causes enabling a treatment plan to be developed.

Once alerted to the issue or organicity, a subtle shift must take place in analyzing your patient's responses and laboratory information. It is critical to assess the current parameters of sexual functioning and remaining capabilities. All must be analyzed in great detail in order to successfully formulate a precise individualized treatment strategy. Special emphasis is placed on finding any situation in which tumescence can be experienced. For instance, even partial nocturnal penile tumescence (NPT) erections may be extraordinarily encouraging to a diabetic man who has not seen one in three years and has avoided sex with his wife until the night before his visit with you. This immediately indicates a tentative level of potential success available—that awakened functioning becomes at least equal to that experienced during sleep.

The overlap of assessment and treatment is obvious, and this becomes clearest when carefully taking a "sexual status exam" [8]. Here is where a trained sex therapist can be the most helpful. A clear video picture of the sexual experience will tell you if there are any ways in which the couple is aggravating the problem unnecessarily. The following example illustrates how you might focus your questions. A 34-year-old diabetic with peripheral neuropathy tells you, "as soon as I penetrate, I lose my erection—that's it, Doc." Indeed, this information is consistent with his NPT erratic wave pattern. However, by asking specifically what happens at that moment of penetration, you find:

1. His change in position from oral sex to coitus takes 30 seconds.
2. This results in a mere softening of erection. However, this did not happen to him a few years ago.
3. He immediately starts obsessing about whether or not his penis will stay hard. This causes a rushed and awkward penetration attempt. His partner resents this and tenses up. He feels this and a complete negative feedback system is established.
4. He worries about disappointing her and anticipates a fight. He becomes enraged with her and himself.
5. Sex is aborted. Instead of a loving experience, they have another huge argument and he ends up sleeping on the couch.

Is this an organic problem requiring surgery? There is definite neuropathy and some diminished circulation, probably secondary to the diabetes. What is causing his impotence?

This particular couple had a successful intercourse experience after their seventh therapy session. Seemingly critical elements in their treatment involved redefining their expectations regarding the nature of stimulation required to maintain his erections. Specifically, they found female superior coitus with continuous stimulation until penetration an effective technique. This was combined with exercises to reduce performance anxiety and marital therapy. One year follow-up indicated a coital frequency of once per week, with the potency problem reoccurring approximately one time in ten. Previous to treatment, the patient was told he might never have intercourse again, and was offered a referral for a prosthesis. In ten years he may indeed require a prosthesis, but let us reevaluate the problem then.

The basic strategy in sex therapy is to modify the immediate causes of the impotence. This usually translates into exercises designed to reduce performance anxiety and improve communication. Naturally, with these individuals we often use the traditional exercises such as sensate focus with gradual progression to genital stimulation. However, there are subtle differences in treatment technique with this population. First, overcoming initial fears of failure can be more profound. For instance, requesting a man to intentionally lose whatever degree of erection he learned to have after weeks of practicing different stimulation techniques can elicit intense resistance. Men with organic deficits are more likely to lose erections periodically and more likely to have intermittent difficulty with potency, even with successful treatment. Therefore, reframing loss of tumescence as a "nonevent" is a critical process in their sex therapy.

Work with this population also requires greater than usual emphasis on developing new methods for increasing stimulation to further eroticize the sexual situation. Masturbatory experimentation is encouraged to discover what helps most, by varying frequency, intensity, location and type of stimulation. Many of these men are older and there is a reticence to engage in that kind of "kid stuff." Zilbergeld's *Male Sexuality* is helpful when the resistance is superficial [9]. This experimentation is often a critical stage in helping them gain the necessary confidence to function again.

Management of partner resistance plays a big role in helping these men learn to maximize their functioning. For instance, resentment of masturbation is common. Use of fantasy by the dysfunctional man is often critical to help reach his threshold for success. The fragility of their erectile system usually requires this extra push, yet a partner may initially resist this notion vehemently.

The man himself may resist using fantasy if it is perceived as forbidden. One 68-year-old hypertensive man was overwhelmed by guilt at wanting to fantasize about the prostitute "who could get me hard 50 percent of the time." It was the discovery of his infidelity with the prostitute which caused the huge marital argument that precipitated the referral in the first place. Therapy required considerable working through of his wife's rage and his guilt before they could accept his use of fantasy as a sexual aid. When he used the fantasy, while relaxed and rested he could get erections sufficient for coitus, although not hard. As an aside, it is important to teach that coitus does not require a raging "hard on," especially if your partner has been educated to help you penetrate. Helping her learn to be a more skilled sexual partner was an important part of treatment and a number of changes in attitude and technique were necessary. On follow-up, she stated, "I never thought I could accept massage, oral sex, or being the initiator." While eventually gratifying, many older passive women find it very difficult to learn to be more aggressive and initiate sexual experiences. Yet successful therapy often requires a change in script.

Sometimes the script change can be very dramatic. A 71-year-old man, with severe circulatory problems, had "forbidden fantasies" of a homosexual love affair of 40 years earlier. This was a fascinating case where the man "came out" at that late stage of life. His last sex experience prior to treatment was in a heterosexual marriage of convenience which ended 20 years before.

Erotic tapes viewed at home helped another couple achieve success, yet it was months before they were willing to try this. She was fearful of rejection and afraid of his response to young sexy women. Their situation was interesting because they first saw the tape late at night when he was fatigued. Both had been drinking and not surprisingly he had no response. The next session involved helping them to carefully orchestrate an experience where the tape was used and all his conditions for good sex were met—a modest intercourse was possible. If you are to maintain credibility, orchestration of the experience is critical. So often patients will tell you, "I tried this, I tried that—it didn't do a thing for me—nothing." Convincing them to suspend disbelief and systematically introduce changes one by one, knowing they are likely to work only when done cumulatively, can be difficult.

This type of cure could easily cause another problem. Such careful orchestration by the therapist can lead to the patient anticipating or experiencing sex as too mechanical or clinical. While a common resistance in sex therapy, it is exacerbated by the approach I am recommending. Striking the right balance between spontaneity and planning requires trust and motivation from the patient and considerable finesse and sensitivity by the clinician.

The emphasis on maximizing potential creates the additional risk of the patient becoming too erection-focused. The therapist must guard against creating iatrogenic performance demands. He must sufficiently reeducate the couple to the pleasures and importance of noncoital sexuality.

Finally, the clinician must be continuously aware of the dangers of creating false hope and subsequent depression. A consistent theme of reality-based expectation, experimentation, and reframing of experience must be maintained. It is, of course, emotionally risky when one is using multiple sexual enhancement techniques to merely achieve a modest level of performance. Especially, since such performance was once so taken for granted and may be no longer.

Before concluding, allow me a brief word about single men who lack a continuous partner. Three important additional considerations arise.

- You must work with them on who, what, where, when and how to tell a new woman in their life about their problem and what is needed to improve it.
- This usually requires more assertiveness training and role playing by the patient than working with couples.
- You must prepare them for the likely recurrent bouts of impotence they will have in the beginning of a new relationship. They can then utilize all they learned to function effectively again.

So will these techniques always work? *Of course not!* I do not have sufficient data collected to discuss success rates. Recently, one man who was able to have coitus with his girlfriend opted for an implant, because he correctly assessed his inability to achieve that level of functioning in his disharmonious marriage. He still wanted to have sex and his wife wanted to remain passive. Under such circumstances, his prognosis even with the implant is guarded.

In fact, some of you may accurately ask: "How do you know if these patients really had organic deficits that primarily caused the potency problem? How do you know that the results of assessment and physiological measures, and presumed disease and pharmacological reactions were not false positives; that these men were not merely the basic sex therapy case with one or two more interesting complications which were "red herrings"? The answer is that I do not know for sure, but neither would the surgeon implanting a prosthesis. I will however, have a good idea of their progress and prognosis within six sessions; using a nonintrusive, and fundamentally emotionally benign technique. At the end of three to six weeks, a surgeon will hopefully have a patient who is recovering nicely from a procedure, which had all the risks of the operating room and who still may need some sex counseling. What would you want for yourself, your father, your husband, or boyfriend?

I am not saying all cases should be treated with sex therapy first. However, this option should be discussed with every patient before he is sold a prosthesis. Perhaps, I am bringing coals to Newcastle in recommending this approach at a Congress of sexologists, but I feel this information must be disseminated and advocated by sex therapists like ourselves.

NOTES

1. Perelman, M. A. *Non-Surgical Interventions in Cases of Organic Impotence.* Paper presented at Fifth World Congress of Sexology. Jerusalem, 1981.

2. Wasserman, M. D., C. Pollack, A. Spielman, and E. Weitzman. The differential diagnosis of impotence. *JAMA,* 1980, 243:2038–42.

3. Rosen, R. C., and E. Gendel. Sexual problems: current approaches in primary care practice. *Postgraduate Medicine,* 1981, 6:127–34.

4. Blaivis, J. G. *Diagnosis and Treatment of Erectile Impotence.* Paper presented at the annual meeting of the Society for Sex Therapy and Research. Cambridge, 1980.

5. Bullard, D. G., J. Mann, H. Caplan, and J. M. Stoklosa. Sex counseling and the penile prosthesis. *Sexuality and Disability,* Fall 1978, 1–3.

6. Perelman, M. Premature ejaculation. Lieblum, S., and L. Pervin (eds.), *Principles and Practice of Sex Therapy.* New York: Guilford Press, 1980.

7. Kaplan, H. S. *The Evaluation of Sexual Disorders.* New York: Brennan/Mazel, 1983.

8. Ibid., Term suggested by Sharon Nathan, Ph.D.

9. Zilbergeld, B. *Male Sexuality.* Boston: Little Brown & Co., 1978.

19

Spontaneous Remission of Sexual Dysfunctions

S. G. Nathan

Although this chapter on spontaneous remission has been included in the section on "Psychotherapy of Sexual Dysfunction", I will discuss how people get better without it. And getting better without treatment is all that "spontaneous remission" implies. Even though the term would seem to connote that the improvement is somehow involuntary, unsolicited, chance, perhaps even inexplicable, we label it so only because we have not been able to identify the curative factors—not because the factors themselves do not exist. One of the main reasons why we have not identified the curative factors is that we have so little bothered to look.

The idea that people overcome sexual problems without benefit of professional ministrations makes many therapists uneasy, and this may in part account for why the remissions are so blithely dismissed as "spontaneous." But there is certainly no reason to believe that people with sexual problems exist in a state of suspended animation. As therapists, we often hear of our patients' unsuccessful pretreatment efforts to overcome their symptoms. It is therefore quite plausible that people who never come for treatment also attempt to improve their conditions—and that some of them succeed, thereby accomplishing what we call spontaneous remission. In order to learn more about such self-cures, I have been attempting to locate people who report having had an experience of this kind and to interview them about it. I will report some preliminary findings from this research below.

But first the question arises as to why we should study spontaneous remission at all. The classic reason for doing so has been to "discount" therapy outcome figures by netting out the number of people who would have gotten better even without treatment. If we cure 50 percent of patients with a particular complaint, but 25 percent would have had a cure without our help, then a somewhat more modest claim for the efficacy of our methods is probably in order. This reason for studying spontaneous remission leads to a quantitative approach to the subject.

There are also good reasons to study spontaneous remission *qualitatively*. Doing so can teach us something about the natural history—the untreated course—of the sexual dysfunctions, a subject about which very little is known. Other pathologic conditions suggest several possible models for the course of the sexual dysfunctions. Are they like the common cold—likely to get better on their own? Like a spinal cord transection, where the impairment is once and for all? Like pancreatic cancer with its progressive downward course? Like multiple sclerosis, involving alternating exacerbations and remissions? Which, if any, of these patterns best describes the course of untreated sexual dysfunctions is yet to be learned.

Another reason for examining spontaneous remission qualitatively is to benefit from the experience of people who have effected self-cures. Learning what conditions and methods facilitate improvement can help us in developing new therapeutic techniques and approaches—an endeavor that seems increasingly important as we encounter more and more sex-therapy-resistant dysfunctions.

In addition, knowledge about the characteristics and circumstances of people ripe for spontaneous remissions can be an aid in triage. Whether we employ this information to select the most promising or the most difficult cases for treatment, it is useful to know which is which.

But is there any evidence that spontaneous remission of sexual dysfunctions takes place at all? There is, although much of it is indirect.

In the first place, we know that a wide variety of other psychiatric complaints and conditions are subject to spontaneous remission. Although Eysenck's [1] contention that two-thirds of neurotic symptoms remit spontaneously is no longer generally subscribed to, most experts on the subject still place the rate at a not inconsiderable one-third to one-half [2,3]. And Stanley Schachter [4] has recently offered impressive evidence that the rates of self-cure for smoking and obesity far *exceed* the rates of cure achieved by professional therapists.

We encounter other indirect evidence of spontaneous remission in our clinical practices. Most therapists have had occasion to treat patients who present with partial spontaneous remissions—say, a formerly totally preorgasmic woman who learned to have masturbatory orgasms on her own but who seeks treatment when she cannot climax with her partner. Most therapists have also had experience with "minimal treatment cures," patients who need only one or two sessions of education or permission-giving to overcome their symptoms. It is only a small step to imagine this education and permission-giving coming from some source other than a professional therapist, and there we have a "no treatment cure" or spontaneous remission. (If that seems at all fantastic, remember that 15 years ago it would have seemed incredible that a serious problem like anorgasmia could succumb to 10 sessions of sex therapy rather than to five years of psychoanalysis.) One other line of clinical evidence relevant to spontaneous remission is our often-shared lament that "There are no easy patients anymore." One explanation for this is that the easier cases are taking advantage of the ubiquitous information about sex available today and using it to cure themselves.

In addition to these very suggestive lines of indirect evidence about the spontaneous remission of sexual dysfunction, we have a smattering of direct evidence as well. The first piece comes from Kinsey's [5] *Sexual Behavior of the Human Female,* in which data are reported on the percentage of married female respondents remaining anorgasmic at various times after marriage. The percentage declines precipitously in the first year of marriage—51 percent had not experienced orgasm after one month of marriage but only 25 percent were still anorgasmic after one year. The rate continues to diminish thereafter so that only 10 percent had not had an orgasm 15 years after they married. Since therapy for anorgasmia was seldom undertaken in the days when Kinsey collected his data, we are safe in considering virtually all of this remission spontaneous.

In a more recent study, Segraves and his colleagues [6] contacted 66 men referred, but not treated, for erectile impotence a year after their referrals. Almost 14 percent reported they were no longer symptomatic. How rates for these men—concerned enough to report their problems but disinclined to engage in sex therapy—compare with those for men never seeking treatment at all is not known (a limitation shared with other types of waiting list control studies), but it nonetheless provides more evidence that some sexual dysfunctions do indeed improve without treatment.

Ellen Frank and her colleagues [7] were able to follow up 73 of the original 100 "normal" couples they asked about sexual dysfunction in the mid-1970s [8]. Five years later, they found substantial movement out of (and into) symptomatic status (in other words, evidence of spontaneous incidence as well as of spontaneous remission). The remission rate varied from one dysfunction to another (premature ejaculation and anorgasmia showed the lowest rates of improvement, erection problems and reaching orgasm too quickly on the part of women, the greatest) but the overall remission rate was 33 percent—similar to what has been found for a variety of other psychiatric symptoms. Like Kinsey's respondents, Frank's were not patients, and this may be one reason why their reported remission rate is higher than Segraves' (another may be the longer time elapsing before follow-up); it may be that a person only presents as a patient when he has exhausted his avenues for self-cure.

It thus seems clear that sexual dysfunctions do at times remit spontaneously and that remissions may even take place in substantial numbers. But *who* is likely to remit *what* dysfunctions, and *how* is it done?

As for who is likely to remit, we know from studies [9,10] of the remission of other kinds of symptoms that remitters in general are more likely to be female, to be of higher socioeconomic status, to have greater self-esteem, and to be more likely to talk to others about their problems (all as compared with nonremitters). Segraves [6] found that his remitters of erectile impotence were more likely to be married and to be living with their spouses. In other words, spontaneous remitters tend to share many characteristics with those we label "good patients." This perhaps sheds some light on why such people are considered to be good patients in the first place; they may be primed for getting better whether we treat them or not!

What dysfunctions remit? As far as can be ascertained, all of them—although probably not all at the same rate. (Frank's [7] five-year remission rates ranged from 18 to 63 percent, depending on the dysfunction; Segraves [6] found that dysfunctions of short duration were more likely to remit than long-standing ones.) My own subjects have reported remission of even the most serious problems such as primary retarded ejaculation and long-entrenched desire disorder.

Perhaps the most interesting question of all about spontaneous remission is one of how they come about. In thinking about this question, I have kept in mind Helen Singer Kaplan's [11–13] model of the causes of sexual dysfunction. In this model, sexual dysfunctions are seen as invariably having immediate, here-and-now causes—causes like performance anxiety and inadequate stimulation—and as frequently having deeper causes as well. These deeper causes, which have their roots in the individual's relationship or in his psychodynamics, underlie the immediate causes and in fact *cause* the immediate causes that in turn cause the dysfunction itself. For example, take the case of a women whose problem is anorgasmia. The possible immediate causes are few and easily enumerated—spectatoring, inadequate stimulation, performance anxiety, inability to "let go"—but the underlying causes, themselves myriad, lead to dozens of possible combinations. For example, inadequate stimulation may stem from a woman's being with a withholding partner, or it may exist because her castration anxiety is so great that she cannot bring herself to touch her "mutilated" genitals.

From the reports of my subjects, it appears that spontaneous remissions can entail change at both immediate and deeper causal levels. Undoing only immediate causes was enough for symptomatic improvement in many cases. To accomplish this, many respondents reported invoking standard sex therapy techniques (masturbation combined with fantasy for female anorgasmia, for example), often learned from popular self-help books and articles. But others used techniques that were quite different from the ones we ordinarily recommend to our patients. For example, I interviewed a man who was able to overcome his longstanding erectile dysfunction by participating in group sex. The immediate cause of his symptom had been performance anxiety, and he found it much abated in a group sex situation because he knew that if he did not have an erection, someone else would. Knowing that someone could spell him if he faltered reduced his performance pressure and he achieved consistent erections, an accomplishment he was later able to transfer to a lone couple situation. In addition to subjects who reported success with methods we do not ordinarily recommend to our patients, a few reported success with methods we believe to be actually counterproductive, notably distraction techniques for premature ejaculation.

Of the deeper causes reported as worked through in order to bring about symptomatic improvement, the most common were relationship problems. Sometimes the curative factor was the chance meeting of a wonderful partner. But other respondents reported expending great effort to change their relationships—for example, a women who struggled to make the power balance in her marriage more equal, which she saw as necessary for achieving genuine sexual desire for her husband. At times, a remission was the unexpected consequence of a change sought for another reason. Take the case of one subject who vowed he would never again go to bed with a woman until he was comfortable enough with her to confide about his erection problems; by the time he achieved this level of trust and intimacy with a new partner, he found he was so at ease that he had no erection problem to report!

A few subjects reported remissions that involved change at the level of psychodynamics. For example, a formerly preorgasmic lesbian told of overcoming her dysfunction by allowing herself to use a fantasy of herself as a child being stimulated by an adult man, thereby accepting and integrating the excitement she had felt when she experienced incest with her father. After employing this fantasy to achieve her first orgasms, she was able to abandon it in favor of preferred fantasies of exciting sex with her actual loved female partner.

The one therapeutic process that was never reported as being involved in the remissions experienced by my subjects was insight. (What looks like insight in some of the cases vignettes reported above was the product of the interviews.) Although the subjects were able to report on the *circumstances* under which their remissions came about, they seemed to have no idea *why* this had been the case. This at first led me to suppose that insight was of no value to a person endeavoring to overcome a sexual symptom, and that the attempt we make to have our patients understand is perhaps more important for our own conception of what therapy ought to involve than it is for the patient's improvement. But then I began to think about why these subjects had volunteered to be interviewed in the first place and realized that almost all of them had come seeking some understanding of what had happened to them—that is, seeking insight. When, in the course of the interview, we were able to arrive at some formulation of what had brought about the subject's remissions, they seemed relieved, pleased, and very grateful. Evidently, there are at least some people with long-standing stable remissions who do not feel completely at rest until they know *why* they got better; until they do so, they appear to be left with a feeling that their progress might be snatched away as mysteriously as it seemed to them to arrive. It thus may be that a sense of intellectual mastery is one difference between a spontaneous and an in-treatment remission, and that to at least some people, it is a difference of great importance.

NOTES

1. Eysenck, H. J. The effects of psychotherapy: an evaluation. *Journal of Consulting Psychology,* 1952, 16:319–24.
2. Bergin, A. E. The evaluation of therapeutic outcomes. *Handbook of Psychotherapy and Behavior Change: An Empirical Analysis,* A. E. Bergin, and S. L. Garfield (eds.), New York: John Wiley & Sons, 1971.
3. Lambert, M. J. Spontaneous remission in adult neurotic disorders: a revision and summary. *Psychological Bulletin,* 1976, 83:107–19.
4. Schachter, S. Recidivism and self-cure in smoking and obesity. *American Psychologist,* 1982, 37:436–44.
5. Kinsey, A. C., W. B. Pomeroy, C. E. Martin et al. *Sexual Behavior in the Human Female.* Philadelphia: W. B. Saunders, 1953.
6. Segraves, R. T., J. Knopf, and P. Camic. Spontaneous remission in erectile impotence. *Behavior Research and Therapy,* 1982, 30:89–91.
7. Frank, E. Personal communication, 1983.
8. Frank, E., C. Anderson, and D. Rubinstein. Frequency of sexual dysfunction in "normal" couples. *New England Journal of Medicine,* 1978, 299:111–15.
9. Beiser, M. Personal and social factors associated with the remission of psychiatric symptoms. *Archives of General Psychiatry,* 1976, 33:941–45.
10. Endicott, N. A., and J. Endicott. "Improvement" in untreated psychiatric patients. *Archives of General Psychiatry,* 1963, 9:575–85.
11. Kaplan, H. S. *The New Sex Therapy.* New York: Brunner/Mazel, 1974.
12. Kaplan, H. S. *Disorders of Sexual Desire.* New York: Brunner/Mazel, 1979.
13. Kaplan, H. S. *The Evaluation of Sexual Disorders.* New York: Brunner/Mazel, 1983.

PART V

Surgical Interventions

Technical advances in surgical treatment of sexual problems have been remarkable. The development of an inflatable implantable penile prosthesis has restored sexual function for many men. Surgical techniques are available to create neovaginas. Perhaps the most remarkable surgical feat is the ability to change gender.

Unfortunately, our understanding of the psychological consequences of such surgery are less well understood. Considerable controversy still persists about the indications for transsexual surgery, and we possess minimal information concerning the impact of penile prosthesis surgery on marital relationships and self-esteem. It is similarly difficult to predict which individuals and marital units will have difficulty adapting to surgical interventions for birth control.

This is clearly an area requiring close collaboration between surgeons and mental health professionals. Human sexuality has profound personal meaning and significant interpersonal ramifications for most individuals. It is gratifying to observe early collaborations in this field of common interest.

20

The Retaining and Restoring of Sexual Functions by Means of Gynecologic Surgery

G. Vecchietti and F. Borruto

The recent growing awareness on the part of women of their own "sexual capability" has led to an increase in the number of reported cases of dyspareunia, anorgasmy, and psychogenic anxiety, the underlying causes of which may often be ascribable to psychosomatic factors, emotional disturbances or problems relating to the stress of everyday life and may occasionally be due to factors associated with hormone deficiencies or more specifically organic conditions.

The sexual difficulties of women are frequently attributed to subconscious states of inner conflict, neurotic disorders, somatization phenomena or to what may be broadly defined as problems of the couple, but, in those cases where anatomic disorders are at the root of sexual disturbances, there is no choice but to resort to surgical procedures in order to prevent the patient's awareness of her physical deficiency from triggering a guilt mechanism which might then lead to irreversible damage of a behavioral type, involving more than the strictly sexual sphere. Before labelling sexual difficulties as "psychosomatic disorders" or "emotional disturbances" of the relationship of the couple, there must necessarily be thorough clinical evaluation of patients complaining of dyspareunia, vaginismus or even complete inability to have sexual intercourse.

Poor knowledge of one's own body is more widespread than might first appear in the light of a superficial examination. In patients, ignorance of the human body is a decisive factor in sexual behavior, while, as regards the medical profession, it has repercussions in the form of superficial clinical investigations and a poorly thought-out, very often inadequate approach to the problem.

Sexual desire and satisfaction in women are often affected not only by biohormonal changes but also by the woman's perception of her own sexual potentiality during the various stages of her biological cycle.

The Rokitansky-Küster-Hauser syndrome is characterized by vaginal aplasia with total inability to have sexual intercourse; it is associated with a rudimentary uterus with normal fallopian tubes and ovaries. With the improved diagnostic procedures available today, it appears that this condition would appear to be much more frequent than has been reported in the past: one case out of every 5000 females born (Vecchietti and Ardillo 1970).

In the creation of a neovagina, one must take due account of those anatomo-functional considerations which make it possible to achieve the reconstruction of an organ with characteristics resembling as closely as possible those of a normal vagina. Care should be taken to avoid operations which not only fail to respect basic anatomic relationships but, on the contrary, have the effect of creating a vaginal canal, the characteristics of which prove radically different from those of a normal vagina. The creation of a neovagina with dermo-epidermal flaps and intestinal loops has notoriously not only failed to solve the patient's problem but may even aggravate it owing to the concomitant presence of unwanted side effects.

The operation proposed by Vecchietti respects basic anatomic conditions, in that the neovagina is created using the inter-urethro-vesico-rectal space, which is its natural site, and features the anatomic characteristics of a normal vagina.

The method has already been described in previous studies (Vecchietti 1970, 1980) and involves:

1. Pfannenstiel laparatomy.
2. Opening of the vesico-uterine fold.
3. Preparation of an inter-vesico-rectal tunnel.
4. Perforation of the pseudo-hymenal membrane by means of a suture holder to the end of which is attached an acrylic olive mounted on suture threads.
5. Subperitoneal passage of suture threads laterally in relation to the rectus muscles.
6. Traction of the suture threads using a spring appliance positioned on the patient's abdomen in the region of the laparatomy suture.

Figure 20—1. Opening of the vesico-uterine fold.

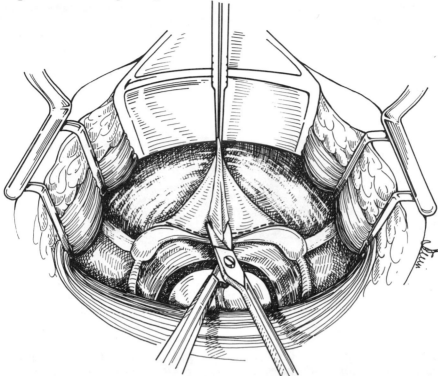

    After roughly one week, the progressive traction on the
olive will have had the effect of creating a vaginal canal
measuring from 8 to 10 cm. in length.
    The use of phantom falluses is confined to the first one
to two weeks after the operation and is discontinued on
commencement of sexual relations.
    Five hundred and twenty patients were operated on by
Vecchietti using this technique over the period 1962-1982.
The patient's ages ranged from a minimum of 15 years to a
maximum age of 39.
    All patients were followed up with the following control
percentages:

        after one month: 100% = 520
        after three months: 85% = 442
        after one year: 70% = 364
        after two years: 30% = 156

Long-term follow-up proved difficult as a result of the fact
that during the 20-year period Vecchietti operated in three
different cities (Padua, Turin, and Verona).

Figure 20–2. Perforation of the pseudo-hymenal membrane with a sutural holder at the end of which is attached an acrylic olive mounted on suture threads.

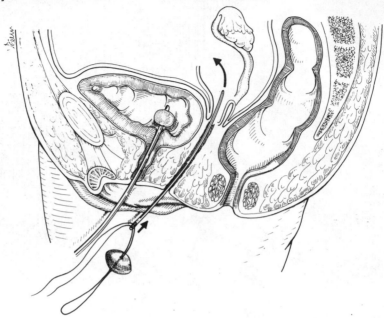

Figure 20–3. Subperitoneal passage of suture threads laterally in relation to the rectus muscle.

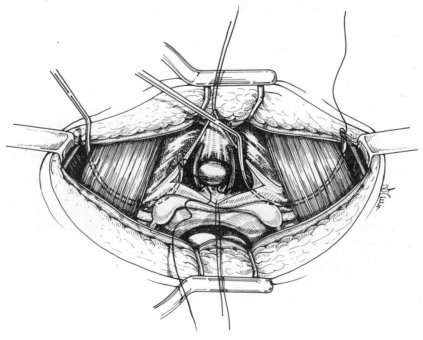

Figure 20–4.   Spring appliance positioned on the patient's abdomen.

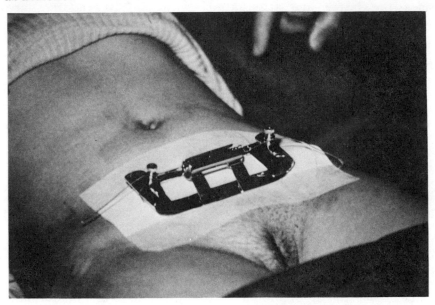

Twelve percent of the patients complained of dyspareunia at one month followups, but this had subsequently disappeared by the time the second followup was performed.

When examining the results of this surgical creation of a neovagina, we also investigated to what extent this type of patient was capable of having an orgasm.

Awareness of severe impairment of sexual capability will trigger what often proves to be an irreversible psychological disturbance mechanism, unless appropriate psychological assistance is given.

In a number of subjects, the creation of a neovagina would appear to afford the possibility of vaginal orgasm, despite the fact that, as we know, the female orgasm is an all-embracing phenomenon, which is by no means exclusively related to the specific area stimulated and is of entirely psychical origin.

The creation of a neovagina with anatomic characteristics corresponding as closely as possible to those of a normal vagina makes a decisive contribution towards restoring the psychological equilibrium of such patients, who, once treated, become perfectly normal apart from their reproductive capability.

Pregnancy has always been an event responsible for changes in the relationship of the couple, more often than not leading to a strengthening of the bond of affection between the partners. The state of pregnancy inevitably has repercussions on sexual relations and habits; in some cases the latter are attenuated, while in others they are experienced with greater intensity.

Normally, for both partners, pregnancy will involve substantial changes in sexual behavior: not infrequently, the relationship during pregnancy is characterized by less frequent sexual intercourse, lengthy intervals, a sense of repulsion, and concern on the man's part about harming the woman.

In the light of these considerations, we take the view that the surgical correction of a number of uterine or vaginal malformations (vaginal septa, cervico-isthmic incontinence, uterine malformations) not only makes successful pregnancy possible, but also helps to improve the quality of the sexual experience and the relationships between the partners.

In this case, too, we opt for procedures which respect basic anatomic conditions and remedy physical deficiencies in a manner which reflects as closely as possible normal physiological states and processes.

As regards the correction of cervico-isthmic incontinence, we have abandoned the practice of performing cerclage operations on the neck of the uterus at the level of the outer uterine orifice in favor of correction of incontinence at the level of the inner uterine orifice.

On the basis of our experience vaginal septa should always be removed, even in the absence of functional disorders, as they contribute towards creating an "imperfection syndrome" with all the above-mentioned associated psychological repercussions.

The same criterion also holds good for uterine malformations; once the diagnosis has been made and the woman is conscious of her condition, a uteroplasty procedure is advisable.

In conclusion, the surgical treatment of malformations justly deserves to take its place in the forefront of the new, fascinating science of sexology.

According to Descartes, pleasure consists in awareness of one's own perfection. Pleasure, including sexual pleasure, may, as we see it, take on a degree of intensity which elevates it above the purely biological sphere, but it is now a known fact that pleasure is generated by a whole series of delicate mechanisms, including sociocultural factors and, above all, the individual psychological make-up of the patient, who today more than ever before suffers as a result of her knowledge and awareness of her physical imperfection.

NOTES

1. Borruto, F. Sexualität nach operierter vaginal-aplasie. *Sexualmedizin,* 1982, 11:476–77.

2. Vecchietti, G. Die Neovagina beim Rokitansky-Küster-Hauser Syndrom. *Gynäkologe,* 1980, 13:112–15.

3. Vecchietti, G. Insufficienza cervico-istmica e cerchiaggio per via addominale. *Attual. Ost. Ginecol,* 1975, XVI–XXI:481–90.

4. Vecchietti, G. Istmectomia e fertilità. Atti 4° Simposio Italiano sulla sterilità – Varenna 28–29 maggio 1965. "Studi sulla sterilità" 1965 Coop. Tip. Modena.

5. Vecchietti, G. Neovagina nella sindrome di Rokitansky-Küster-Hauser. *Attual. Ost. Ginecol,* 1965, 11:131.

6. Vecchietti, G., L. Ardillo. La sindrome di Rokitansky-Küster-Hauser. SEU, Roma, 1970.

21

Genital Transformation
by Inverted Penis Skin Implantation Technique

W. Eicher

There are four techniques of the male-to-female conversion operation and each has modifications:

1. the neovagina by inverted penile skin implantation,
2. the neovagina by peno-scrotal flap implantation,
3. the neovagina by split-skin graft implantation,
4. the bowel-neovagina.

We perform the first technique: the genital transformation by inverted penis skin implantation.

THE PATIENTS

From 1975 to 1983 we have evaluated 210 transsexuals. There were 125 male-to-female and 85 female-to-male trans- sexuals. We performed surgery primarily on 65 male-to- female, 45 female-to-male transsexuals, and more than 50 corrections on patients who had surgery primarily else- where. It is now six months to eight years after surgery on the primarily operated male-to-female patients, with an average follow-up of two years.

Our patient selection has been strict and is based on the following criteria: psychiatric evaluation and consultation for more than one year. Other disturbances of gender identity, especially psychosis are excluded. The patient switched into the role of the desired sex. The hormone treatment has been effective for at least more than six months. If estrogen treatment does not result in an sufficient gynecomastia we implant inflatable silastic mammary protheses from a small auxiliary incision. These are the conditions for the genital transformation.

THE OPERATION TECHNIQUE

The patient is in the gynecological position—that is, in an exaggerated lithotomy position. We start with an incision dissecting the raphe of the scrotum beginning on the base of the penis downward to the perineum to four centimeters above the anus. The testes are removed after high ligation of both spermatic cords. In the midline under the urethral bulb we find the tendineous raphe, called *centrum tendineum*. On either side of it is the fossa perineum into which we can penetrate with a finger through the fossa ischiorectalis on either side and push the tissue, especially the levator muscle sidewards. The tendineous raphe and the rectourethralis muscle between urethra and rectum is cut and the cavity formed is lengthened now by dissecting the Denonvillier's fascia, so that the prostate gland can be separated from the rectum and the preperitoneal space is obtained. The length is now 14–15 centimeters and quite deep enough for the new vagina.

In the next step the shaft of penis is stripped from his skin. The urethra is separated from the corpora cavernosa and the corpora cavernosa are resected from the os pubis. The inverted penis skin is invaginated and sutured in the preperitoneal space. The urethra from which the corpus cavernosum urethrae is also dissected is shortened and explanted through the inverted penis skin under the symphysis in a female position.

Now the labia majora and minora are formed with some scrotum skin and the rest of the scrotum skin is resected. A clitoris-like aspect is attained by transplanting the top of the glans penis above the new urethra. A Foley catheter is placed into the urethra and a soft tamponade with polyvidon-iodine cream is inserted in the new vagina. A hard mold would cause necrosis of the implanted skin. After one week we give a hard prothesis or suggest a vibrator for dilatation.

RESULTS AND COMPLICATIONS

No one of the patients has regretted surgery. All of them stabilized psychologically following the operation. We have not seen any serious psychic complications because of the careful preparative selection. The implanted penis skin was taken in 50 percent not totally, but partially. Only in ten percent was there a total necrosis, which is not necessarily a failure for the new vagina. As a rule, there is a tendency to spontaneous epithelization, if the cavity is kept open. It is very important in general to use regularly a dilatator (prothesis or vibrator) to prevent shrinking until regular cohabitations are practiced. In eight cases we have seen a shortening or contracted vagina—too small for coitus—that is, in 15 percent. In five of these cases we have enlarged the cavum by additional surgery. In the three other cases the patients did not use the dilatator, had a difficult postoperative rehabilitation from lack of cooperation or were unreliable. We have had one rectovaginal fistula without incontinence, which we closed after five months without necessity of a colostomy. In five cases we have had bleeding around the resected urethra which did not recur since we removed the corpus cavernosum around the urethra. In five percent we observed a stenosis of the urethral meatus. It could be cured in all cases by repeated dilatation with Hegar dilators using a local anesthetic. For tenderness of the vaginal skin and for other reasons, sufficient estrogen substitution therapy is absolutely necessary. Problems with lubrication are frequent especially in the first half year, but in many cases forever. We recommend the use of a jelly for intercourse in these cases. Eighty percent reported orgasm during intercourse. All the operated patients had their identity legally changed after surgery.

NOTE

1. Eicher, W. *Transsexualismus, Möglichkeiten und Grenzen der Geschlechtsumwandlung.* Stuttgart: F. Fischer Verlag, 1983.

22

Vasectomy, Personality Factors, and Body Experience

R. Venturini, C. Simonelli, G. Pascale, and F. Maggiorano

Since vasectomy has become a contraceptive method in various countries, several researchers have attempted to enquire into the effects this technique can have at both the organic as well as the psychological level. As this fundamentally irreversible operation concerns the very delicate reproductive and sexual spheres, it is most important that both psychological and physical effects do not harm the balance of these functions or cause pathological consequences. The conclusions drawn by the various authors who have studied the problem are not entirely concordant. Some researchers emphasize the importance of family planning factors in the motivations which lead to the operation (Edey, Bernstein, and Ferber et al.); others indicate factors involving the couple: the value given to sexuality, difficulties in sexual identification or even psychiatric problems (Rodgers et al. 1965). Another motivation, which is not rare, is the sense of guilt towards the partner on the question of the responsibility for contraception and often there is a secret hope that vasectomy can solve sexual problems as well as those of the couple itself. As for the consequences on the psychological plane, some authors (Johnson) warn against the operation in patients suffering from serious psychological disorders or those suffering from problems of sexual identity, as well as in hypochondriacs

(Rodgers and Ziegler 1974), as the consequences can range from the development of neurotic disturbances to the onset of psychosis.

Normally, it is the sexual sphere which is most affected as some of the patients view the operation as a castration and doubt about sexual potency brings the sexual relationship under continual scrutiny, according to Rodgers and Ziegler (1968), to justify the increase in frequency of sexual intercourse recorded among those vasectomized. According to Ziegler, negative changes in sexual behavior develop in 33 percent of those vasectomized. Some authors maintain that the major consequences in sexual behavior occur at the level of libido, the postorgasmic state, and frequency in intercourse. Wolfers discovered sexual problems in 12 percent of the patients examined: alterations in the relationship of the couple are the consequence of these changes.

Other authors give very positive data on the sexual behavior of vasectomized subjects. According to Ferber, sexual intercourse is enlivened and occurs more often without particular pathological consequences. Dandekar, in research carried out on 1191 men, found that 92 percent had greater sexual satisfaction during intercourse, even though 35 percent experienced less desire. We should add that in the social group where vasectomy is contrary to explicit moral principles, there may be problems of self-acceptance and deviant or compensatory behavior. Given these kinds of results, the authors seem to agree on the need for a careful selection of the subjects who request the operation. On the other hand, differences in culture and sample groups can have important bearings on research results and the attitude of the researchers may also be influenced.

This research based on working experiences in a clinic of the Italian Association for Demographic Education, should be inserted into the above framework. We should remind readers that in Italy, voluntary vasectomy has only been available for a few years since the abrogation of a law on race conservation.

This is the first research in Italy on this subject and aimed above all at studying the possible effects that vasectomy may have on the personality and bodily experience of men who undergo it. As we have seen, various research projects on the subject have been carried out in various countries but our particular sociocultural conditions make a broadening of the survey interesting especially in view of giving an adequate structure to the counselling service offered to the applicants.

SUBJECTS AND METHODS

Those who wished to be vasectomized made an application at the clinic and, after a medical examination and several clinical tests, were invited for an interview with the consultant psychologist. During this talk the subject was asked a series of questions aimed at assessing: a) the motivation for the operation, previous contraceptive practices, and attitude to paternity; b) the attitude to the operation and possible doubts and fears about the consequences; c) the quality of the relationship of the couple; d) the process which had lead up to the decision for vasectomy; e) possible psychopathological precedents.

Following the interview, the subjects were selected on the basis of the following criteria: a) objective conditions: impossibility of using other contraceptive methods, risk of dangerous pregnancies for the partner, eugenic motives, serious economic factors; b) motivational factors: parity: age ratio, refusal and mistrust of other contraceptive methods, improvement of sexual life. The subjects were dissuaded who: a) were without any motivation regarding point a) above; b) showed obvious psychopathological signs; c) had serious disorders in sexual behavior; d) were in serious disagreement with their partner on the decision to take; e) had low or no parity with their partner and were very young; f) had serious doubts about the outcome of the operation from the point of view of their own mental health and the moral and cultural acceptability of vasectomy; g) were excessively afraid of others' judgment. The conversation had the aim of stimulating more attentive reflection in the applicant and a more profound, mature approach to the choice. Where necessary, the subject could return for further talks.

About 30 percent of the 200 who had applied for the operation followed the customary procedure, after the conversation, for obtaining the operation. The remaining 70 percent desisted for various reasons, but of these only 12 percent had been dissuaded during the preliminary interview.

The subjects in our sample (about 25 of the applicants chosen at random from the larger group of subjects who actually underwent the operation) were, before the operation, given a battery of tests which explored the dimensions of the personality and body experience, and a questionnaire on their sexual behavior. A year after the operation, the same subjects were given a retest. The subjects vasectomized at our clinic were also sent a questionnaire which included a series of questions on postoperative experiences, sexual behavior after the operation, the relationship within the couple, and possible pathological consequences.

The results of the first psychodiagnostic examination were compared with those of the second by studying the significant qualities of the differences in the values which emerged from the Student t test.

An analysis of the sociodemographic characteristics of the subjects enable us to make several observations:

1. The average age is around 38 years. These are fairly mature subjects who arrive at the choice for vasectomy after generally having experienced the principal sexual-affective experiences such as marriage and paternity.

2. There is a high scholastic level, working activity (professionals and white collar workers), and ideology which presumably places our subjects in a middle class open to new solutions and eager to accept them.

3. As for religious convictions, a high number of subjects declared they were of no religious persuasion while the majority declared they were nonpracticing Catholics.

4. An interesting datum is the comparison between the number of children in the family of origin which is higher than the number of children in the present family. This does not seem decisive as regards the choice of vasectomy since in 43 percent of the families of origin the average number of children was one to two, that is, an atypical number of children in an Italian family a few decades ago. We could put forward the hypothesis that the family structure helped to produce a responsible attitude toward contraception.

5. As regards the civil status, there is a generally low number of bachelors and particularly high number of separated men, which seems to bear out the hypothesis that these are people who are able to deal with various situations in life with a certain realism and maturity, act consequently, and take responsibility.

The battery of tests used for the research were:

Three Personality Tests

•   Thematic Apperception Test (TAT) tables 1, 2, 3, 4, 8, 10, 11, 12, 13, 17, 18; all the tables which could elicit useful information on the personality and specific sexual problems, using the Reuben Fine system for the scoring.

- Eysenck's Personality Questionnaire in the Italian version by Sanavio and Soresi.
- The Cattel Anxiety Scale in the Italian version.

Three Body Experience Tests:

- The Holtzmann Inkblot Technique from which the two Barrier and Penetration indices were extrapolated following the indications of Fisher and Cleveland.
- The Body Cathexis Scale of Jourard and Secord which explores the acceptance of the body.
- The Questionnaire on body distortion drawn up by Fisher which demonstrated possible distortions in perception of one's body associated with disturbances of contact with reality.

A Questionnaire on Sexual Behavior

It was drawn up by some of our team and included a series of questions on both behavior and present and progressive sexual attitudes to the education received on sexuality, the types of disconcertion encountered, and the way of dealing with them.

A Questionnaire with Closed *Ad Hoc* Questions

One year after the operation it was sent to a larger number of subjects who had availed themselves of the service. The questionnaire aimed at enquiring into the present attitude towards vasectomy, personal satisfaction about the operation, sexual behavior, social relations, present state of health, possible outcrop of various types of problems about work, those of an ethical nature, and so on.

RESULTS

The following considerations were obtained from the analysis of the TAT: the most frequent feelings in the experimental group in the first and second examination were, in descending order: depression, physical affection, anxiety, death, pain, pleasure. Some of these feelings were expressed the same number of times in the first and also the second examination, while other feelings such as frustration, pain, and pleasure occur consistently less often between the two examinations. Other feelings such as conflict and guilt decrease though to a lesser extent. The decrease in frequency of these feelings could lead one to think that there is a modification in profound experiences following vasectomy, as though certain unconscious complexes could have been somehow absorbed through the castration-expiation experience. When considering the results of the stories we did not find any differences between the examinations. No significant difference emerged from the analysis of the Eysenck Personality Questionnaire (EPQ) data, between the first and second examination, which are noticeably different from the Italian average with which they had been compared. In the case of Cattell Anxiety Scale (CAS), too, there was no significant difference between the two examinations.

The comparison made with the national averages showed that the experimental group had higher scores than the national average even though they were still within standard deviation.

The barrier and penetration scores obtained through the use of the Holtzmann Inkblot test also did not yield any significant difference between the two examinations. The comparison made with the Italian standardization gave an interesting datum. Our experimental group consists of subjects whose ratio between the scores differs from that discernible in the national average; this data could indicate that the subjects have a particularly open image of the limits of their own bodies, which is experienced as a mediating zone in relation to the surroundings, receptive to actions from the outside and also willing to undergo environmental influences without particular blocks or obstacles. This could explain the subjects' willingness to undergo an operation like vasectomy which is undoubtedly an obvious external manipulation, at least in terms of body experience as the operation is carried out under partial anesthesia and therefore with the subject fully conscious and involved. Unfortunately, this can only be considered a hypothesis because of the limits to the national sample even though there is an interesting confirmation of the particular qualities of the subjects who undergo vasectomy.

The body cathexis (BC) scale is a questionnaire which yields a score regarding acceptance of one's body. In the case of our experimental group we saw an increase in this acceptance of the body after the operation ($p = 0.02$). This data is not significant at a preselected probability level but at a higher level; it is, however, probably indicative of greater satisfaction concerning one's own body after the operation.

It would seem that vasectomy allows an improved experience of sexuality which leads to an increase in the acceptance of one's body. On the other hand, no particular attitude to particular organs or parts of the body emerged and therefore no other indication seems to confirm or contradict this hypothesis.

The data obtained from the Body Distortion Questionnaire are too scattered and have not been taken into consideration. The analysis of the replies to this questionnaire on sexual behavior produced some interesting indications of the typology of those who underwent vasectomy as a contraceptive method and also on their motivations. Some of the most significant data are:

1. On the attitude towards sexuality, 25.7 percent of the subjects gave "fundamental importance to sexuality" while 54.3 percent "great importance." On the motives concerning desire for sexual intercourse no less than 43.7 percent consider the search for pleasure important, while 31 percent attach importance to desire for human contact. According to 72.6 percent, men approaching old age do not lose interest in sexuality. This is a datum which confirms the importance that those vasectomized attach to sexuality and therefore the importance of the "sexual" motivation in the choice made for contraception.

2. Another section of the questionnaire covered the previous contraceptive practices of the subjects. All those interviewed declared that they had tried to avoid pregnancy and 80 percent were negatively conditioned by the problem regarding their own sexuality. The methods used were: oral estroprogestines by 6 percent; condoms 25 percent; coitus interruptus 24 percent; Ogino-Knaus method 14.8 percent; I.U.D. 4.6 percent; the diaphram 3.7 percent and basal temperature 1.8 percent. Almost all were dissatisfied with the contraceptives used and saw this problem as the cause for decrease in desire in their partners, less frequent intercourse, less satisfaction in intercourse, sexual functional disorders and other disturbances of a psychological nature. The average number of undesired children was 0.6 as against an average of 2.1 children desired. Of those interviewed, 41.8 percent admitted seeking abortions and the average number of abortions per subject was three.

3. Another section of the questionnaire dealt with the incidence of disorders in sexual functions. Eighty-eight percent of the subjects judged their own sexual potency satisfactory or normal, and 60.9 percent declared they have never had serious worries about

their genital apparatus. Forty-three percent declared that they had suffered occasionally from sexual complaints or dysfunctions, only 1.7 percent suffer from them often. Among the pathologies indicated were: premature ejaculation: 51.4 percent; no erection 17.1 percent; insufficient erection 14.3 percent; loss of erection at the moment of penetration 8.6 percent; no ejaculation 8.6 percent.

From the postoperative questionnaire we noted:

1. The first series of questions dealt with how the operation was experienced. The majority of those interviewed had no problems during the operation and where problems did arise they were only very slight.

2. On the question of how sexuality was experienced, 30 percent declared increased sexual desire while for the others interviewed, there was no change. Sexual pleasure increased in 52 percent of the subjects but was unchanged for 45 percent. For 35 percent of the subjects, desire increased in the partner, too, while in 61 percent of the cases desire was unchanged, 58 percent of the subjects maintained that the partner's sexual pleasure increased, while for 42 percent it remained unvaried. In 42 percent of the cases intercourse became more frequent while for 58 percent of the cases there was no change. This apparently enthusiastic picture seems to confirm the hopes of those vasectomized even though we must not overlook the compensatory and self-assertive factors which certainly, as is shown in other research, led to the exaltation of the choice made and saw all the consequences as positive, though overlooking possible future problems. We do not know whether a year is a long enough period between the operation and the questionnaire to obtain a correct assessment of the long-term effects of the operation, or whether the effect and need for self-assertion still play a decisive part.

3. The comments on the onset of postoperative sexual disorders are important. In nine percent of the subjects, occasional erection problems occurred and five percent had problems regarding ejaculation. It should be pointed out that the onset of sexual problems, especially if occasional, does not necessarily jeopardize the experience of sexuality or intercourse. If we are to speak about real pathological conditions we should wait for more than a year. Other non-

specifically sexual disorders such as insomnia, anxiety, tachycardia, tiredness generally appear only in the immediate postoperative period and only in 12.5 percent of the subjects, taking into account the nine percent of the subjects who had slight organic disorders after the operation. These data confirm therefore the overall positive experience as regards the operation together with the observations made in the first section of the questionnaire.

4. On the relationship of the couple, those interviewed declared that the harmony of the couple improved in 66 percent of the cases, whereas there was no change in 32 percent of the cases. Social relations and those in the work sphere saw no changes following the operation so that the reputed aggressive compensatory attitude which emerged from other research does not seem to appear in our sample. Only two of those interviewed had second thoughts over a question of morality, but they did not create dramatic situations.

On the whole, the data give a fairly positive picture of the postoperative experience and it is possible to state that in general the conscious experience of those vasectomized, which we dealt with, is one of satisfaction and an improvement in the conditions of the relationship which correspond to expectations in a positive and stimulating way.

DISCUSSION

There are not sufficient motives therefore to maintain that vasectomy has negative effects on the conscious, profound experience of those who undergo it. We must keep in mind, while stating this, the fact that our subjects were adequately selected; the conclusion is legitimate, therefore, only for those who fall into the categories observed. The interview probably acted as a good filter for avoiding and warning those who were neither deeply convinced nor able to deal with the postoperative situation. It would be interesting to go into the profound, motivational factors which underlie this choice and how they compensate the loss suffered. The fact should be taken into account that the time lapse between the operation and the retest was a year: probably too short a time for the profound experiences to change. We can offer the further hypothesis that the subjects were still enthusiastic about the operation so that a long-term control could give more valid information on this aspect.

Many subjects approached the operation with a sense of responsibility and openness towards their partner, demonstrating their awareness of the need to take their responsibilities regards family planning. Even though a sense of guilt towards the partner cannot be excluded, this attitude certainly demonstrates a profound change in the man-woman relationship within the family or the couple. If previously the onus of contraception fell entirely on the woman, an increasing number of men today are even willing to run risks, involving their virility, just to become coresponsible for contraception. Considering that all this occurs in a society like the one in Italy where up to a short time ago the virility myth was unquestioned, we cannot but underline the importance of this datum which emerged from the research and points to a profound transformation which has been taking place in Italian society over the last few years.

Vasectomy is obviously the extreme act of dissociation between sexuality and reproduction. The research data seem to offer the indication that the separation of the two functions does not, in sufficiently prepared subjects, bring any harm to sexuality. This confirms the enormous incidence of cultural factors in sexual experience, shows new functional possibilities for the human being and once again brings out the plasticity of behavior. If our results agree only partially with those obtained by other researchers it is probably due to the special conditions in which the research was carried out, the severity used in selection, and the willingness of the applicants to live through the operation and the new situations they discovered after the operation with a special sense of responsibility. The longitudinal control we have forecast is still being carried out and the results will be available shortly.

NOTES

Antonelli, F. Aspetti psicological della vasectomia. *Rivista di Sessuologia,* 1979, 3:215–28.

Barglow, P. Pseudocyesis and psychiatric sequelae of sterilization. *Arch. of General Psychiatry,* 1964, 11:571–79.

Bumpass, L. L., and H. B. Presser. Contraceptive sterilization in the U.S.: 1965 and 1970. *Demography,* 1972, 9:190–97.

Coviello, N. et al. *Il Problema della sterilizzazione volontaria,* Milano: Angeli, 1983.

Dandekar, K. After-effects of vasectomy. *ARTHA Vijana,* 1963, 5:212–224.

Edey , H. "Psychological Aspects of Vasectomy" presented at the First National Conference on Vasectomy, Chicago, Illinois, 1971.

Edey, H., and I. Bernsctein. "Psychologic and Psychiatric Aspects of Voluntary Sterilization." In M. E. Schima, I. Lubell, J. E. Davis, E. Connel, and D. W. K. Cotton (eds.), *Advances in Voluntary Sterilization* (Proceedings of the Second International Conference, Ginevra, Feb. 25–March. 1, 1973). New York: Eisevier Publishing Co., 1974, 277–82.

Ferber, L. et al. "Men With Vasectomies: A Study of Medical Sexual and Psychological Changes" *Psychosom. Med,* 1967, 29:354–66.

Johnson, M. H. Social and psychological effects of vasectomy. *American Jour. of Psychiatry,* 1964, 121:482–86.

Landis, J. T., and T. Poffenberger. The marital and sexual adjustment of 330 couples who chose vasectomy as a form of birth control. *Jour. of Marriage and the Family,* 1965, 27:57–8.

Mumford, S. D. The decision-making process that leads to vasectomy. *Diss. Abs. Intx.,* 37:3884–85, Feb. 1967.

Poffenberger, T. Two thousand voluntary vasectomies performed in California: background factors and comments" *Marr. Fam. Living,* 1963, 25:469–74.

Rodgers, D. A., and F. J. Ziegler. Changes in sexual behaviour consequent to use of noncoital procedures of contraception. *Psychosom. Med.,* 1968, 30:495–505.

Rodgers, D. A., and F. J. Ziegler. Psychological reactions to surgical contraception. *Psychological Perspectives on Population,* Fawcett (ed.), New York: Basic Books, 1974.

Rodgers, D. A., and F. J. Ziegler et al. A longitudinal study of the psychosocial effects of vasectomy" *Jour. of Marriage and the Family,* 1965, 27:59–64.

Simon Population Trust. Vasectomy, a follow-up of 1,000 cases. Letchworth and London: Garden City Press, 1969.

Wolfers, H. Psychological aspects of vasectomy. *British Med. Jour.,* 1970, 4:297–300.

Ziegler, F. J., D. A. Rodgers, and R. J. Prentiss. Psychosocial response to vasectomy. *Arch. of General Psychology,* 1969, 21:46–54.

Ziegler, F. J. Vasectomy and adverse psychological reactions. *Annals of Internal Medicine,* 1970, 73:853.

Ziegler, F. J., and D. A. Rodgers. Vasectomy, ovulation suppressors, and sexual behaviour. *Jour. Sex. Research,* 169–193, Aug 4, 1968.

23

To Inflate or Not to Inflate
. . . Is There a Rational Approach to Penile Prosthetic Implantation

D. J. Krauss

With only a few exceptions we consider that penile prosthetic implants are for men whose erectile dysfunction is primarily organic rather than emotional in origin. This is not as simple as it sounds. First of all, there is an emotional component, whether cause or effect, in every patient who complains of sexual dysfunction. Human sexual function and the emotions, as we surgeons must not forget, can not be separated.

Next, if we establish a diagnosis of a medical condition that can be associated with impotence, [1] diabetes, or medications for example, it does not automatically mean we have determined the reason for our patient's sexual disability. In a particular patient, the contributory medical factor may not be so disabling once the emotional aspects are treated. This helpful mnemonic lists the various categories of medical illness that must be considered in evaluating a man for erectile dysfunction: I-inflammatory and infectious (lower genitourinary tract); M-metabolic; P-postsurgical (for example, radical prostatectomy); 0-occlusive vascular; T-traumatic; E-endocrine; N-neurologic: C-chemical (drugs, toxins); E-endurance (cardiopulmonary disease, penile anomalies)[2]. These conditions are ruled in or out by our investigation.

Initially, our history includes many questions about the patient's presenting problems as well as his overall medical condition and sexual history. As it becomes indicated, especially if more intensive sexual- or psychotherapy is going to be necessary, we obtain a much more detailed psychological and past sexual history.

The physical examination is also directed toward evaluating the patient's general health, as well as his secondary sexual characteristics, looking for signs of any of the many conditions that may be associated with erectile problems. We routinely measure the penile/brachial blood pressure ratio also.

The laboratory investigation includes those specific tests that are indicated by our history and physical examination. We measure blood levels of testosterone, luteinizing hormone, and prolactin in all men. Additional studies, including hormone stimulation or suppression tests, computed tomography of the skull, nerve conduction velocity measurement, cystometrogram and others, are done only as necessary.

We have not been doing pelvic arteriograms to diagnose erectile dysfunction. We feel that although it is promising, the state of the art is such that the long term benefits of revascularization do not as yet outweigh the discomfort and risks of the study.

We do sleep erection monitoring on selected patients. The study should be done in a sleep laboratory where the entire polysomnogram can be performed by a qualified technician who also can awaken the patient and subjectively evaluate his erection.

We must remember that the phenomena of sleep and sleep erections are influenced by many factors, medications and depression for example. Thus, unless the erection tracing is completely normal, there is no way of beginning to determine the reason for an abnormality without measuring the other parameters: electroencephalogram, electromyogram, extra ocular movements, and electrocardiogram. While the sleep study is extremely helpful, it is far from infallible. It is only a part of the complete investigation of the man with erectile dysfunction. . . .

Once we determine that a patient is a potential surgical candidate, and before we discuss it with the patient, our psychologist does a screening interview in order to make sure that we have not missed any particular psychological factor which would contraindicate surgery. If we decide to offer the patient a penile prosthesis and he is interested, we then follow our detailed counseling process. This also serves as the informed consent. We must be sure that we cover all the possible negative points for psychological as well as medicolegal reasons.

Our first step is to meet with the patient's regular sexual partner, alone and also with the patient included. At this time we can evaluate the couple's feelings and desires as well as discuss our plans. We feel that if we do not include the partner in the decision-making and education process, the surgery may be doomed from the start [3]. The issue of the patient's and partner's expectations of the surgery is a critical factor. If either one expects a miraculous result, such as sudden resolution of their social or emotional problems, we advise them that they are being sadly unrealistic. An erect penis is all that we can provide. The intimacy, sensitivity, and feelings must come from the partners themselves.

Next, in order to explain the surgical results, we give the patient and his partner sample prostheses to examine. We stress that regardless of what they may have heard, the artificial erection, while excellent for intercourse, will not be "normal" compared to his previous natural one. Based on complaints from some patients we warn them that the artificial erection will not be as long, wide, or firm as they may remember his previous normal erection to be.

While cutaneous sensitivity will be undisturbed, the feeling of engorgement of the penis or "natural" feeling during sexual excitement will be lost because of the post-operative scarring within the erectile bodies (corpora cavernosa). Such scarring prevents blood from filling the corpora around the prostheses. Thus, however minimal his natural erection used to be, there probably was some tumescence sensation and after surgery he will no longer have that. In addition, some patients find that after prosthetic implantation their penises get very sensitive to cold and must be protected, especially in subfreezing weather. Orgasm and ejaculation, we explain, are unaffected and therefore unchanged by our surgery.

Successful use of the penile prosthesis depends on a gradual exploration and experimentation by the partners, in order to find out what is and is not possible and pleasurable. Since his erection is not the same as his natural one, we must not allow the patient to assume that his sexual activity will be the same as it was before. He and his partner must be prepared to adjust to a new situation. In the right frame of mind, the partners actually consider this quite a pleasurable adventure. We also try to allay the partner's fears of injuring themselves or each other—again we stress gentleness. The use of a water soluble lubricant, until the partners are accustomed to the prosthesis, is essential, especially if there is a problem with vaginal transudation.

In general, partner satisfaction is high. What is still needed is a large scale prospective study of patient and partner satisfaction.

Continuing the education process, the next issue with which we deal is frequency of intercourse. The partners must understand that once the novelty of the operation has worn off, their frequency of sexual activity should not be measured against some ideal or fantasy. Despite the "no fail" erection, they must realize that all the factors that governed their past sex life will continue to influence their new sex life. Sexual activity will still depend on their moods and desires; neither partner should feel obligated or expect the other to perform at any particular frequency which is markedly greater than they ever did before.

The risks of surgery are then explained to the couple. We tell them that in addition to the discomfort that accompanies any operation, some patients have persistent pain. We do not know the exact cause of this pain, but some believe it is due to the placement of too large a prosthesis. It may be neurologic in origin because some of these patients are cured by local anesthetic injections [4]. In some others the pain may have an emotional basis.

Infection has been reported in anywhere from one to ten percent of cases with diabetics having the highest incidence. An infected implant must be removed and later reinsertion, while not impossible, is much more difficult because of dense scarring.

Mechanical failures, if the inflatable prosthesis is used, must be discussed. Considering all instrument failures, and tubing kinks, there is almost a 30 percent incidence of reoperation for some problem with the inflatable prosthesis, in addition to the complications that it has in common with the other types of prostheses.

Perforation into the urethra is not common but it can happen and must be mentioned. If it occurs, it is usually at the time of surgery during the preparation of the erectile bodies to receive the prostheses. In like manner, excessive surgical trauma can also cause gangrene of the glans penis. The general or spinal anesthesia itself has its own risks and these are mentioned. Details of the anesthesia are left for the anesthesiologist to discuss. In the higher risk patients, with heart and lung disease we have been using local anesthesia. The entire operation can be done simply by making the penis numb. Emotional problems immediately after surgery are rare but can occur.

Complications that may occur several months after surgery may again include pain. As before, this symptom also may have an organic or emotional etiology. If attempts at controlling the pain are unsuccessful, the prosthesis may have to be replaced with a smaller size or even removed. If there is no perforation at the time of surgery, but the tunica albuginea around the erectile bodies is injured, or too big a prosthesis is used, it may lead to erosion of the prosthesis into the urethra or out through the skin.

Mechanical problems again may occur with the inflatable prosthesis. The malleable prosthesis, containing silver wires, has not been in use long enough to know its exact life span.

Emotional complications in either the patient or his partner have been reported. Hopefully these can be avoided by a careful counseling process.

The last question with which we deal is the choice of which prosthesis to implant. I wish I could say that I know the secret of a completely objective, unbiased method of counseling on this subject but I do not. The public has just about been saturated with information with which it has been provided by both biased and unbiased sources. Patients have spent a great deal of money in order to obtain the most expensive device, thinking that it will make them normal again; this is simply not realistic. All the prostheses provide good usable erections but none is "normal" or "natural." The inflatable prosthesis is extremely popular and is an example of both engineering and marketing genius. When counseled properly, patients accept and function excellently with the less expensive malleable or semirigid devices.

The counseling process does not end with the surgery. We see the patients at two weeks postoperatively to check their wound and then at the four-week point in order to reinforce all the above information, prior to beginning to use the artificial erection. In many patients, sex therapy techniques and exercises are very helpful in rehabilitating the couple and enabling them to use the prosthetic erection successfully, especially if many years have passed since their last intercourse.

In summary, we feel that complete evaluation of the cause of the patient's erectile dysfunction is essential. Once surgery is decided upon we must be satisfied that the partners are well informed and understand the information which we give them. In addition we must be confident that the partners' expectations are realistic and that they have been honest with us in their conversations. After this long counseling session we make sure that we provide support to both partners during the peri- and postoperative periods.

NOTES

1. Krauss, D. J.   The physiologic basis of male sexual dysfunction, *Hosp. Pract.,* 1983, 18:193.
2. Smith, A. D.   Causes of partial erection, *Med. Aspects Hum. Sexual,* 1980, 14:10.
3. Krauss, D. J. et al.   The failed penile prosthetic implantation despite technical success, *J. Urol.* in press.
4. Krauss, D. J.   The elimination of pain caused by the small-carrion penile prosthesis, *Urology,* 1983, 19:82.

24

Preoperative Evaluation of Candidates for Conversion Surgery

J. Wålinder and B. Lundström

During the fifties and sixties the endeavors towards effective help for transsexuals have been concentrated more and more on the aim of achieving harmony between on the one hand the patient's conviction of belonging to the opposite sex, and on the other, the physical appearance and socio-legal status. This has called for a combination of hormonal, surgical, and legal measures. Whether in the longer term these measures really have a positive effect has sometimes been questioned. During recent years the authors of a number of follow-up studies have claimed that the treatment has been of great help to the majority of those who have undergone it (for review see Lundström [1]). The reported approximately 80 percent success rate for sex reassignment must, however, according to Lothstein [2] be viewed cautiously, because there are not a sufficient number of long-term studies that lend themselves to correct statistical interpretations.

The following presentation aims to throw light on the routines for evaluation of candidates for sex reassignment developed and employed at the Department of Psychiatry and Neurochemistry, St. Jörgen's Hospital, University of Göteborg (former Psychiatric Research Centre, St. Jörgen's Hospital) since the mid-1960s.

DIAGNOSTIC CRITERIA

The diagnosis of transsexualism has been based on the following criteria, now widely adopted internationally. The person in question:

- has experienced, usually since childhood, a firm conviction of belonging to the opposite sex;
- experiences aversion for own sex characters;
- wishes to be regarded by others as belonging to the opposite sex;
- insistently seeks to undergo hormonal and surgical treatment to acquire physical characteristics more in accordance with the experienced gender identity and to obtain the socio-legal status corresponding to this sex.

INDICATION FOR SEX REASSIGNMENT

Over the last ten years, the main features for inclusion in the operative program have been as follows:

- The diagnosis must have been clearly established over preferably two years' observation by doctors well acquainted with the condition. Onset, development, and symptoms must be typical. Investigation must provide for close psychiatric observation and must also include somatic study to exclude physical disease as a cause for the symptoms. Investigation should be supplemented by psychological tests evaluating the dimension of femininity-masculinity and should preferably include a period of observation in hospital.
- The patient should for at least a year have lived and behaved in the contrary sex role and thereby have shown suitability and capacity for coping with a life in this role. (All experience shows that the genuine transsexual, despite many social difficulties, manages to become established in the aspired sex role quite early in life.)
- The personality endowment should be such that it will ensure effective resistance to the difficulties which the person will always meet in the new role. There must be no signs of psychotic reaction.
- Features such as physical build, voice, hair growth, and so on should be such that in the new role the transsexual will not appear too conspicuous.
- Close study of all the details of symptoms and personality must have produced a firm conviction that any other form of treatment either is not possible or has no prospect of success. In some cases social position or other circumstances may be such that one must advise great restraint towards active measures.
- Before medical and legal measures are undertaken,

the social situation should be under best possible control. Interest must be taken in working life, the attitude of relatives, and so on.

• Close and continuous contact with treatment team must be ensured during evaluation period and not least after active measures have been taken.

One of the most important research problems now facing workers in the field of transsexualism is the search for factors which predict outcome of sex reassignment. There has been increasing recognition of certain contraindications to sex reassignment and among others Hoenig et al. [3] have discussed the importance of these factors (for example, complicating psychosis, dementia and allied disorders, abuse of alcohol and drugs, repeated criminal acts. In a follow-up study of 24 sex-reassigned transsexuals, Wålinder and Thuwe [4] found that the following factors appeared prognostically unfavorable: unstable personality, excessive geographical distance between patient and treatment team, and long interruptions of hormone treatment. In a more recent study Wålinder et al. [5], when comparing five cases who regretted sex reassignment with nine successful cases, found that out of 12 conceivably unfavorable prognostic factors the following indicated poor outcome: criminality, inadequate support from family, physical build inappropriate to new sex role, and mature age at the time of request for intervention. The results suggest that the more of such factors there are present in a particular case the stronger are the reasons for restraint in embarking upon a course of active intervention. An extended series confirmed on the whole the results. Lundström [1] when reviewing the literature found that the following factors indicated poor outcome after sex reassignment: poor result of surgery, personal and social instability, diagnosis other than genuine transsexualism, and mature age (more than 30 years) at first medical contact for gender dysphoria.

Another issue of interest is that up to the present time, not a great deal of interest has been shown in studying the development of the situation of those patients with gender dysphoria [6,7] who have not been considered suitable for sex reassignment. In his study of 1981 Lundström tried to gain information on the way in which such patients managed to adapt themselves in their subsequent life. If the life of this group of patients is found to be generally free from problems this might be thought to justify some stringency when considering the indications for sex reassignment. If, on the other hand, the adjustment of these patients is found to be consistently very poor, then this might be taken as a reason for relaxing the stringency of these indications. Since it is to be expected that a group of patients who do not receive approval for sex reassignment may include patients with atypical conditions, it is of great interest to determine whether there is any difference between the various diagnostic subgroups in their ability to adjust in the biological sex role. Information on this could be important for the attitude to be taken to indications for sex reassignment when dealing with gender dysphoria conditions which border on homosexuality or transvestism. It would also be useful for prognostic assessment when sex reassignment is under consideration to determine whether there are other features common to patients who find it easy to adjust to their biological sex role and, conversely, to those who find difficulty in making this adjustment. Similarly, it is of interest to inquire whether there are any differences in adjustment between the male and the female patients in the group with gender dysphoria who have not received approval for sex reassignment. In patients who have undergone sex reassignment it has previously been claimed that the postoperative adjustment of the women is better than that of the men.

Lundström concluded after a personal investigation of 17 men and four women who were not accepted for sex reassignment that more men than women seek help with a wish to live permanently in the opposite sex role. This predominance of males may at least in part be explained by the fact that the male group contains more cases which are atypical for transsexualism, while in this respect the female group is more homogenous. He also found that of the patients originally diagnosed as genuine transsexuals, very few have given up their wish for sex reassignment.

Up to the present time, a number of factors have been found important to take into account when sex reassignment is under consideration (see above). Lundström concluded that the following factors should also be added, namely:

- Cross-dressing behavior of compulsive type is a symptom which reinforces the indications for sex reassignment, provided the other requirements for this are met.
- In the group of biological women who wish to undergo sex reassignment the risk of encountering unsuitable applicants appears to be considerably less than in the group of biological men.
- Psycho-social functional capacity seems in general to be independent of whether measures for sex reassignment are taken or not. In considering the indications

for sex reassignment, assessment of psycho-social stability is therefore of interest only by virtue of the fact that very poor psycho-social function makes it more difficult to sustain the stresses almost always associated with the change to the opposite gender role.

In summary, we think it is fair to state that our knowledge has considerably increased when it comes to identifying persons suitable or not for sex reassignment (see Table 24–1). However, more research is certainly needed. More methodologically sophisticated follow-up studies must be performed. In these respects we agree with Lothstein's [2] points of view. We think, however, that his opinion about the present state of affairs is too pessimistic and cannot find that he has put forward conclusive evidence for the statement that most gender dysphoric patients are secondary transsexuals, who will not benefit from sex reassignment. Recent reviews of pertinent findings [1, 8] corroborate our point of view.

TABLE 24-1. Sex Reassignment Consideration Factors

Poor outcome of sex reassignment is associated with:

• Poor result of surgery

• Personal instability

• Diagnosis other than genuine transsexualism (that is, transvestism or effeminate homosexuality)

• Inadequate support from family

• Physical build inappropriate to new sex role

• Mature age (more than 30 years) at first medical contact for gender dysphoria

---

NOTES

1. Lundström, B. *Gender Dysphoria,* A Social-Psychiatric Follow-Up Study of 31 Cases Not Accepted for Sex Reassignment. University of Göteborg, Sweden, ISBN 91-7222-426-6, 1981.

2. Lothstein, L. M. Sex reassignment surgery: historical, bioethical, and theoretical issues. *Am. J. Psychiatry,* 1982, 139:417–26.

3. Hoenig, J., J. C. Kenna, and A. Youd. Surgical treatment for transsexualism. *Acta Psychiatr. Scand.,* 1971, 47:106–33.

4. Wålinder, J., and I. Thuwe. A social-psychiatric follow-up study of 24 sex-reassigned transsexuals. *Scandinavian University Books,* Akademiförlaget, Göteborg, Sweden, 1975.

5. Walinder, J., B. Lundstrom, and I. Thuew. Prognostic factors in the assessment of male transsexuals for Sex Reassignment. *Br. J. Psychiatry,* 1978, 132:16–20.

6. Fisk, N. Gender Dysphoria Syndrome. In: D. R. Laub and P. Gandy (eds.), *Proc. of the Second Interdisciplinary Symposium on Gender Dysphoria Syndrome,* 7–14. Stanford University Medical Center, Stanford, California, 1974.

7. Fisk, N. Gender Dysphoria Syndrome—The conceptualization that liberalizes indications for total gender reorientation and implies a broadly based multi-dimensional rehabilitative regimen. *West. J. Med.,* 1974, 120:386–91.

8. Pauly, I. Outcome of sex reassignment surgery for transsexuals. *Australian New Zealand Journal Psychiatry,* 1981, 15:45–51.

PART VI

Physiological Substrates of Sexual Behavior

Our knowledge of the physiological substrates of sexual behavior are minimal. In this regard, the pioneering work of Graber and his associates at the University of Nebraska and the contribution by Marrama and his colleagues at the Universities of Modena and Parma are especially appreciated. Graber and his coworkers report a pilot investigation of the effects of naloxone (an opiate blocker) on sexual performance. Their results suggest that endogenous opiate-like peptides may play a role in modulating sexual performance. This study is especially valuable as a beginning effort to map the neurochemical pathways involved in sexual behavior. This work is complemented by the study of Marrama. Only comparatively recently have clinicians become aware that some patients with pituitary tumors may present to physicians with a sole complaint of diminished erectile function. Although the frequency of pituitary adenomas in any series of impotent men is quite low, the history may be suggestive of a psychogenic etiology. For example, many men with pituitary adenomas may report situational and episotic erectile failure. Most often, these men also will report diminished libido. It is not uncommon for the physical examination, and even a careful neurological examination, to produce no signs of physical disease. It is still unclear whether the main effect of adenomas is diminished libido or whether the erectile mechanism itself is impaired. The mechanism by which pituitary adenomas influence sexual function is also unclear. Some investigators have suggested that the hyperprolactinemia and diminished sexual function may both be the result of increased activity in the tubero-infundibular-dopamine axis whereas others have suggested that the sexual impairment is due primarily to high circulating levels of prolactin. The paper by Marrama is especially welcomed. Using sound methodology, they investigated the effects of bromocriptine therapy on prolactin levels, testosterone levels, sexual libido, sexual function, and nocturnal penile tumescence. Their work is definitely complemented by the work of Grafeille and associates from Bordeaux.

25

Gonadal Function: Sexual Behavior in Bromocriptine -Treated Men with Prolactinoma

P. Marrama, C. Carani, V. Montamini,
G. F. Baraghini, A. Tridenti,
R. M. Pederzini, M. F. Celani,
and D. Zini

INTRODUCTION

The side-by-side occurrence of hypogonadism and impotency is a well-known, common clinical finding in the hyperprolactinemic syndromes of pituitary adenoma [1]. There are many mechanisms which cause this and which have not yet been clarified from the viewpoint of the endocrine modifications which accompany the syndrome.

As premises, however, two fundamental questions suggest themselves. Firstly, can the hypotestosteronemia observed in such a syndrome be attributed to a primary action of prolactin (PRL) at the testes, given that specific receptors for PRL are present at the testicular level; or is the testosterone deficit secondary to a prolactin-induced dysfunction of the hypothalamus pituitary axis (HP) [2,4]? Secondly, it should be established if sexual impotence is correlated with either a primary or secondary decrease in testosterone (T), or with the action of PRL at the level of the central nervous system (CNS) [5]; or are hyperprolactinemia, impotence, and the depressive state associated with these, traceable to a single piece of neurogenic damage [1,6,7]?

The data in the literature relating to hypothalamus pituitary gonadotropic (HPG) patterns during hyperprolactinemia of pituitary adenomas appear to be in contrast. Regarding the pituitary gonadotropins and luteinizing hormone (LH) in particular, basal levels sometimes appear to be diminished [3], often unaltered [1] and at other times even increased [8]. Analogously, after stimulus with luteinizing hormone-releasing hormone (LH-RH) the gonadotropinic pituitary reserve sometimes appears to be normal or increased, or at other times to be in deficit [8,9]. Finally, Thorner and his coauthors (1974), came across a diminution in the response to Clomiphene [7]. Such data do not, therefore, allow us to draw unequivocal conclusions regarding the dysfunctional levels of the Hypothalamus Pituitary Gonad Axis (HPG) during hyperprolactinemia.

When studying the genesis of impotency, it should be emphasized that the relationship between levels of testosterone (T) and sexual inadequacy does not appear to be constantly codifiable. Recently, however, studies in both men and animals have shown that a threshold limit for T does exist, below which the libido and erection are compromised, even though this limit appears to vary from one individual to another and often low levels of T are compatible with a picture of seemingly normal sexual functioning [9,10]. It has even been suggested that the decrease in serum dihydrotestosterone (DHT), a peripheral metabolosis of T, found during hyperprolactinemia by Magrini and his coauthors (1976) could contribute to the genesis (or to "the causing of" impotency) [11].

The importance of PRL in sexology derives from the observation that sexual functioning in hyperprolactinemics seems, on the other hand, rather to be correlated to pituitary hormonal levels: in fact, therapy with Bromocriptine (CB) is generally, in almost all cases, able to improve the sexual functioning of patients affected with PRL-secreting adenomas [1,7,12,13].

On the basis of these premises we studied, in patients with PRL-secreting adenomas, the functioning of the hypothalamus pituitary gonad axis (HPG) paying particular attention to the biorhythm of T before and during therapy with CB. We simultaneously evaluated sexual functioning by means of both guided interviews and nocturnal penile tumescence monitoring (NPTM).

MATERIALS AND METHODS

The study was carried out on ten male subjects (18–64 yrs) with hyperprolactinemia: five had unoperated microprolactinemia and five had residual hyperprolactinemia after surgical removal of the tumour. Pituitary microadenomas were diagnosed by computer tornography scan. The results were compared with those of 12 adult male controls (21–59 yrs) who did not have any endocrine pathology or any alterations in the sexual sphere.

All the subjects were hospitalized. The functioning of the hypothalamus pituitary gonadal axis (HPG) was evaluated from a hormonal viewpoint before and during treatment with 2 α Bromocriptine. This was administered in doses of between 5 and 15 mg/day orally for a period varying from three to eight months. To determine T levels in both groups of men, blood samples were taken at 7:45, 8:00 and 8:15 a.m. and at 7:45, 8:00 and 8:45 p.m. Each T value in this report is the average measurement of the three samples in the morning and the three samples in the evening.

Serum T was measured by a charcoal dextran radio-immune assay (RIA) method using an antibody against T-3 oxime supplied by Dr. Borelli of Bologna, Italy. RIA was preceded by a chromographic step on a celite column. For each hormone all samples were run in triplicate and all samples for the same man were run in the same assay. Variability in inter-assay and intra-assay was 13.2 percent and 6.3 percent respectively.

Serum PRL was measured by a commercial kit using a double antibody RIA method with MRC - 222/71 (Medical Research Council, London) as a standard. The sensitivity was 1.5 ng/ml. For low-dose control serum the variability in intra- and inter-assay was 5.3 percent and 8.3 percent respectively, and for the high-dose the variability was 9.4 percent and 11 percent respectively.

The gonadotropins were assessed in basal conditions and after stimulus with LH-RH (100 ucg, intravenous, sampled at 0', 15', 30', 45', 60', 90', and 120'). Both LH and FSH were measured by a double antibody radioimmunoassay technique. The sensitivity, the intra-assay, and the inter-assay coefficients of variation were respectively 5.3 percent and 9.8 percent for LH, and 6.5 percent and 15.3 percent for FSH.

The T rhythm was studied by means of samples taken at 7:45, 8:00, 8:15 a.m. and at 5:45, 6:00, and 6:45 p.m. The morning and evening samples were averaged.

Sexual adequacy was evaluated before and during CB therapy by means of guided interviews with individual patients and by the completion of a sexological record for each patient showing the details of any alterations in behaviour with particular reference to libido, erection and orgasm. Any personality disorders which occurred during the illness were also studied. Nocturnal Penile Tumescence (NPT) was monitored in 8 out of 12 of the normal subjects and in 9 out of 10 hyperprolactinemic patients. NPTM was

performed according to the method of Karacan et al. (1972)·
[14]. NPT was studied in the sleep laboratory for three
nights. Patients arrived at the laboratory at approximately
10:30 p.m. and were allowed to sleep from 11:30 p.m. to
7:00 a.m. Sleep was monitored poligraphically. Penile
tumescence was recorded by means of two strain gauge
loops, one placed around the penis about one inch from the
base and the other just behind the corona of the glans.
This method has been validated and is able to record minute
degrees of tumescence. During the night preceding the
first blood-sampling night, visual checks were also carried
out to ascertain the degree of rigidity in relation to the
recorded increase in penile circumference. This was done
by awakening the subject during erection and having both
the subject and the investigator evaluate the degree on a
scale of one to ten. We calibrated the strain gauge with a
graduated cone. We made sure that movements of the
subject did not significantly affect the baseline. We considered "T max" or complete tumescence and "T p" or
partial tumescence in relation to an 80 percent and 20
percent variation of the baseline.

STATISTICS

All the results are expressed as the mean ± SE. The
responses of LH and FSH to LH-RH administration were
analysed by calculating, for each subject, the peak level
attained and the integrated area under the response curve
corrected for basal levels (Delta area).
   In order to evaluate the differences between control
values and values shown in hyperprolactinemic patients, the
unpaired student's 't' test was used; the paired student's
't' test was employed to study CB effects in hyperprolactinemic patients, as well as testosterone rhythm.

RESULTS

Prolactin

In controls sero-PRL was 8.6 ± 0.9 ng/ml. In hyperprolactinemic patients CB treatment induced a significant reduction of PRL levels (from 366.6 ± 120.7 ng/ml to 45.8 ± 18.0
ng/ml) p < 0.05.

Gonadotropin

Both basal levels and those after stimulus with LH-RH
showed non-significant modifications both before and during

therapy with CB as did the peak of the response (maximum attained level), the integrated area under the response curve and the incremental ratio (if we exclude a tendency to delay in the peak of the response of LH to LH-RH). In 8.3 percent of controls the peak was attained at 30 minutes whereas in the hyperprolactinemics, before therapy, 20 percent of cases peaked at 30 minutes and 50 percent of cases at 45 minutes. During therapy with CB 60 percent of the patients peaked at 30 minutes.

Testosterone

T was severely limited during hyperprolactinemia, with a complete loss of the morning/evening rhythm. Therapy with CB, together with a decrease in PRL levels, induced a significant increase in T with restoration of the circadian biorhythm (Table 25-1). It should, however, be emphasized that a statistically significant inverse correlation between T levels and PRL did not emerge.

Sexual Pathology and Psychopathology

In the period preceding drug therapy, all the patients interviewed reported a progressive drop in desire leading, in the majority of cases, to impotency. The younger pa-

TABLE 25-1. Testosterone Circadian Rhythm in Normal Male Subjects and in Hyperprolactinemic Patients before and During Bromocriptine (CB) Treatment

Subjects	Testosterone (ng/dl)		p*
	8 a.m.	6 p.m.	
Normal men (n = 12)	607 ± 45	472 ± 32	0.001
Hyperprolactinemic males before CB (n = 10)	207 ± 25	201 ± 17	NS
Hyperprolactinemic males during CB (n = 10)	488 ± 58	369 ± 46	0.001

*paired Student's t test (Means ± SE).

tients, although they complained of a slight drop in desire and a decrease in sexual drive, never arrived at real impotency. Older patients, on the other hand, reported a more marked decline in desire which led to difficulties in erection and reached actual impotency.

Together with this sexual pathology, all patients complained of asthenia, lack of motivation in social life, a desire to be alone, irritability, difficulty in socializing and the genuine beginnings of a depressive state. During therapy with CB, practically all patients reported that they had overcome the sexual problems and at the same time experienced an improvement in mood and overcome the depressive state (Tables 25–2, 25–3).

TABLE 25-2. Sexual Behavior in Hyperprolactinaemic Patients before and during Bromocriptine Treatment

PATIENT	AGE	LIBIDO		ERECTION		ORGASM	
		*	**	*	**	*	**
T.G.	64 ys.	+-	++	-	++	-	++
B.I.	25 ys.	+-	++	++	++	++	++
A.M.	26 ys.	-	++	-	++	-	++
C.I.	45 ys.	+-	++	+-	++	++	++
B.R.	62 ys.	+-	+-	-	+-	+-	+-
S.G.	18 ys.	-	+-	-	+-	-	+-
M.C.	37 ys.	+-	++	+-	++	+-	++
L.M.	34 ys.	+-	++	+-	++	+-	++
M.G.	39 ys.	+-	++	+-	++	+-	++
G.P.	22 ys.	+-	++	++	++	++	++

Notes:
* before treatment; ** during treatment
++ normal; +- reduced
- absent

TABLE 25-3. Nocturnal Penile Tumescence (NPT) in Hyperprolactinemic
Patients before and during Bromocriptine Treatment

	Controls (n = 8)	Hyperprolactinaemic Subjects (n = 9)	
		Before CB	During CB
PRL Levels** (ng/ml)	8.6 ± 0.9	367 ± 121	46 ± 18
FREQUENCY** (no. of NPT episodes)			
tmax + tp	4.5 ± 0.4	2.3 ± 0.8(a)	4.6 ± 0.7(b)
tmax	2.9 ± 0.4	1.2 ± 0.5(a)	2.9 ± 0.7(b)
tp	1.6 ± 0.4	1.1 ± 0.4	1.7 ± 0.4
WHOLE DURATION** (minutes)			
tmax + tp	109.0 ± 24.1	42.1 ± 22.8	93.6 ± 70.5(b)
tmax	86.6 ± 10.2	30.9 ± 20.1(a)	67.9 ± 17(b)
tp	28.6 ± 15.3	11.2 ± 4.3	25.7 ± 9.3

Notes:
CB = Bromocriptine treatment (5-15 mg/day per os)
**MEANS ± SE
(a) Hyperprolactinaemic subjects before CB vs controls ($p < 0.05$)
(b) Hyperprolactinaemic subjects before vs during CB ($p < 0.01$)
tmax = maximum tumescence
tp   = partial tumescence

Nocturnal Penile Tumescence Monitoring (NPTM)

The study showed clearly that before treatment this activity
was in deficit in all patients. In particular, when compared
with controls, there was a significant decrease in the
duration ($p < 0.01$) and number ($p < 0.05$) of T max/night;

the total duration of T max/night ($p < 0.01$); and finally in the total duration of T max plus T p/night ($p < 0.01$).

The treatment with CB normalized the pattern in six patients, while four subjects who did not have any episodes in T max/night before treatment, showed at least one episode during treatment. On the whole, significant improvements were documented for the total ($p < 0.05$) and for the total duration ($p < 0.01$) of T max plus T p/night (Table 25–4).

DISCUSSION

Our data confirm that in hyperprolactinemia, modifications in the HPG system exist side by side with sexual inadequacy. As far as the first aspect of the problem is con-

TABLE 25-4. Improvement of Depressive Syndrome in Hyperprolactinemic Patients during Bromocriptine Treatment

Patient	Age	Before CB	During CB
T.G.	64 ys.	++	-
B.I.	25 ys.	+-	-
A.M.	26 ys.	++	+-
C.I.	45 ys.	+-	+-
B.R.	62 ys.	++	+-
S.G.	18 ys.	+-	-
M.C.	37 ys.	-	-
L.M.	34 ys.	+-	-
M.G.	39 ys.	++	+-
G.P.	22 ys.	+-	-

++ marked
+- light
 - absent

cerned, our case study shows that hyperprolactinemia is constantly associated with a decrease in T levels. Furthermore, it is rather singular that such a finding is associated with normal basal levels of LH and FSH and also with a normal gonadotropinemic response to stimulus with LH-RH (if a delay in the LH peak is excluded).

Such a situation is difficult to interpret. It is known that hyperprolactinemia can induce a reduction in Leydig receptors for LH [15]. In the case where one considers hypotestosteronemia to be a phenomenon that has been induced directly and primarily by an increase in prolactinemic impregnation, the testosteronic deficit should in turn determine an increased secretion of LH. Moreover, Nakagawa et al. (1982) [4] have recently shown how complex the problem is. Treating six normal men with specific drugs, these authors observed variable results due to gonadotropin and T, with a frequent dissociation suggesting a direct action of PRL on the testes. In particular Bromocriptine induced, together with a marked suppression of serum PRL, a significant increase in T correlated negatively with the modifications in PRL itself. CB also induced a transitory modification of LH, where with Metoclopramide, PRL levels increased, those of T decreased inversely and LH and FSH remained unmodified. Sulphiride evoked an increase of LH and FSH but not of T.

Such data, although they confirm the existence of hypotestosteronemia in the presence of normal levels of LH, do not explain the mechanism which brings about such a situation. A possible explanation could be provided by the theory that PRL, simultaneously with an action on the testes, also has effects on the CNS, altering the hypothalamic sensitivity threshold to sexual steroids in general and T in particular. This has been suggested by the recent observations of MacNeilly et al. (1983) [3]. They in fact observed that in castrated rats, the increase in gonadotropins was secondary to negative feedback and prevented substitution therapy with both, on the one hand, adequate quantities of T, and on the other hand, small quantities with experimentally induced hyperprolactinemia. In subjects with PRL-secreting adenomas, the modifications to the central threshold could explain the varying results concerning the hypothalamic content of LH-RH, the pituitary content of gonadotropin and the responsiveness of the latter to Clomiphene and LH-RH.

It is in this context that our results from hyperprolactinemic patients are interesting. The normality of gonadotropin basal levels in the presence of hypotestosteronemia should be emphasized together with the delay in the LH peak response to LH-RH corrected with CB therapy. However, if on the one hand, T levels are lowered with an increase in PRL, and are raised during therapy with a hypoprolactinemicizing drug, a statistically significant inverse correlation between levels of T and those of PRL does not, on the other hand, exist. This further suggests that PRL can interfere in the functioning of the HPG Axis at various levels.

Interesting from another aspect, is the important fact we observed that in hyperprolactinemia not only is hypotestos-teronemia verifiable, but a loss in the biorhythm of T can also be documented, as we ourselves have already observed in elderly men (1982) [16]. In the majority of cases CB therapy is not only capable of restoring normal levels of T but also enables a recovery of a normal morning/afternoon rhythm for T. The loss of T biorhythm confirms clinically the data of Rubin et al. (1975, 1976, and 1978) [17,18,19] which were collected in the course of experimentally induced hyperprolactinemia. These authors treated five adult males with high doses of Haloperidol, a powerful drug which blocks Dopamine at the level of the CNS. These research-ers observed the loss of T biorhythm parallel to an increase in serum PRL. The loss of T rhythm could be as much due to an altered peripheral neuroendocrino-vascular function as to a modification of the central neuroendocrine profile.

Finally, it should be pointed out how therapy with CB not only improved the endocrinological profile of our pa-tients but also improved sexual activity, nocturnal erectile activity and depressive states when present. Following the indications of what has been said so far, this improvement could be determined by the effects of the drug at various levels.

From a psychoneuroendocrinological viewpoint, the pos-sible concomitance during hyperprolactinemia of hormonal changes with modifications of neuro-transmitters and neuro-modulators at a hypothalamic and supra-hypothalamic level should be emphasized. This concomitance could contribute to explaining sexual inadequacy, which is not always corre-lated with hypotestosteronemia [10,11].

The inter-relationships between prolactinemic and neuro-transmitter modifications, Dopamine in particular at the dopaminergic tubero-infundibular level, but also Norepine-phrine, 5-hydroxide triptine and Gamma-hydroxide butirate acid are complex, of course [20,24]. On the one hand, a diminution in dopaminergic tone can constitute a *primum mobiles* for the beginning of hyperprolactinemic situations. On the other hand, however, hyperprolactinemia could condition a secondary hyperactive tubero-infundibular-dopamine axis (TIDA) with a short feedback mechanism, a short loop, intensively increasing the dopaminergic turnover with obvious compensatory significance. The alteration of dopaminergic tone could be responsible for secondary alterations in the HPG axis through collaterals which inhibit LH-RH neurons. These collaterals have for some time already been considered in the pathogenesis of amenorrhea in female hyperprolactinemia [24].

Furthermore, we should not forget the findings of Carter et al. (1978) and Ambrosi et al. (1977) [1,5]. They suggested a direct action of PRL at the limbic and hypothalamic system level. These systems play a fundamental role in the realization of satisfactory sexual activity, the limbic lobe being a trigger point for NPT [25].

From a clinical pharmacological viewpoint it should also be pointed out that impotency in hyperprolactinemic hypogonadics is frequently corrected by substitution therapy which not only involves administration of T alone, but can also involve therapy with T and CB together, or even CB alone with the lowering of PRL concomitant with a raising of T.

Impotence can, moreover, be corrected with modification of the levels of T and PRL, even in patients with neither hypotestosteronemia nor hyperprolactinemia [1,8,12,13]. Significant neuro-endocrine alterations during psychiatric pathology are also known. These could be considered as epiphenomena in the clinical picture, or they could be taken as psychosomatic. One might think that emotional disorders existing at the basis of the illness determine more or less rapidly, by means of influence on the limbic system and on the hypothalamus, functional and somatic modifications of which endocrine alterations represent but one aspect. Such modifications, because of the formation of a vicious circle, could contribute in varying ways to the worsening or self-maintenance of the primary illness [26].

A particularly interesting picture is presented by depression, which is frequent both during impotence and hyperprolactinemia. In depression, a diminution in the tone of Norepinephrine, 5-hydroxide triptomine, and Dopamine occur alongside the following modifications in the prolactinemic profile: an increase in basal levels, an altered pattern of secretion—PRL sometimes shows an evening peak rather than an early morning one—major fluctuations in secretion, and varying response to specific stimuli, in particular to insulinic hypoglycemia, L-Dopa, thyroid releasing hormone (TRH) [27]. These data could be interpreted as a dopaminergic depression due to the illness itself. It is in this context that the behavioral and psychopathological aspects found in our patients with hyper-prolactinemia are most interesting.

From a strictly psychosexological viewpoint, the most important data established by the interviews carried out was that modifications in sexual behavior are constantly linked with modifications in mood tone. However, the data were obtained from a sample which was not sufficiently large enough to allow a precise judgment on the significance of this relationship. The data have not yet been evaluated with the rating scales for depression.

Analagous considerations regarding the relationship between sexual behaviour and mood tone have also emerged in another type of endocrinopathy associated with sexual inadequacy; here we are referring in particular to our previous research carried out on acromegalic males (1981) [28].

Concerning the relationship between sexual disorders and a mood state, it can be observed that the depressive state could, psychogenically, be secondary to the state of the recognized illness or to a decline in sexual performance and sensibility. However, a close anamnestic appraisal of the case histories excludes this hypothesis and shows rather the importance of how variations in mood in many subjects appear before the first sexual symptoms and therefore appear obviously before any objective recognition of the illness. This leads one to assume that the same mechanisms, which we hypothesized could be responsible for alterations in sexual behavior, could in some way be a causal factor in the eziopathogenesis of the correlated syndrome.

Such an evaluation leads one to hypothesize a relationship, much closer than one would have thought, between symptoms of sexual inadequacy, hypersecretion of PRL, and variations in mood tone. One could, moreover, put forward another hypothesis given that the inverse correlation between the depression syndrome and sexual inadequacy has for some time been accepted in psychiatric practice. In this case one can put forward the hypothesis that whatever the starting point for medical observation, be it organic or psychogenic, a somato-psychic or psycho-somatic mechanism closely linking sexual behavior and mood state could exist when looked at from a psychoneuroendo-crinological viewpoint.

NOTES

1. Carter J. N., J. E. Tyson, G. Tolis, S. Vauliet, C. Faiman, and H. G. Friessen. Prolactin-secreting tumors

and hypogonadism in 22 men. *New Engl. J. Med.,* 1978, 299:847–52.

2. Hochberg Z., T. Amit, M. B. H. Youdim, and J. A. Bar-Maor. Prolactin by testes of unilaterally cryptorchid rats: the effect of HCG, testosterone, prolactin and orchiopexy. *Acta Endocrinol.,* 1983, 102:144–49.

3. McNeilly A. S., R. M. Sharpe, and H. M. Fraser. Increased sensitivity to the negative effect of testosterone induced by hyperprolactinemia in the adult male rat. *Endocrinology,* 1983, 112:22–28.

4. Nakagawa, K., T. Obara, M. Matsubara, and M. Kubo. Relationship of changes in serum concentrations of prolactin and testosterone during dopaminergic modulation in males. *Clin. Endocrinol.,* 1982, 17:345–52.

5. Ambrosi, B., R. Bara, P. Travaglini, G. Weber, P. Beck Peccoz, M. Rondena, R. Elli, and G. Faglia. Study of the effects of Bromocriptine on sexual impotence. *Clin. Endocrinol.,* 1977, 7:417–21.

6. Thorner, M. O., A. D. Rogol, W. S. Evans, W. C. Nunley, and R. M. MacLeod. The effect of prolactin on gonodal function in man. In *Central and peripheral regulation of prolactin function,* 271–86. R. M. MacLeod and U. Scapagnini, eds. New York: Raven Press, 1980.

7. Thorner, M. O., A. S. McNeilly, C. Hagan, and G. M. Besser. Long term treatment of galactorrhoea and hypogonadism with Bromocriptine. *Brit. Med. J.,* 1974, 2: 419–22.

8. Laufuenti, G., P. M. Risi, A. M. DiBlasio, A. Pipan, and G. B. Serra. Effetto della Bromocriptina sulla responsività ipofisaria a stress acuto con LHRH. *Endocrinol. Invest.,* 1981, 4(Suppl. 1):107–10.

9. Damassa, D. A., E. R. Smith, B. Tennent, and J. M. Davidson. The relationship between circulating testosterone levels and male sexual behavior in rats. *Horm. Behav.,* 1977, 8:275–86.

10. Schwartz, M. F., R. C. Kolodny, and W. H. Masters. Plasma testosterone levels of sexually functional and dysfunctional men. *Arch. Sex. Behav.,* 1980, 9:355–66.

11. Magrini, G., M. Pellaton, and J. P. Felber. Prolactin induced modifications of testosterone metabolism in man. *Acta Endocrinol.,* 1977, 85:212, 143.

12. Nagulesparen, M., V. Ang, and J. S. Jenkins. Bromocriptine treatment of males with pituitary tumours, hyperprolactinemia and hypogonadism. *Clin. Endocrinol.,* 1978, 9:73–79.

13. Della Casa, L., P. Marrama, C. Carani, M. Grandi, G. Mariani, V. Montanini, F. Pignatti Morano, P. Riva, and

B. Bonati. Prolactin in male psychogenic impotence. Third World Congress of Sex., 1978.

14. Karacan, I., C. J. Hursch, R. L. Wiliams, and J. I. Thornby. Some characteristics of nocturnal Penile tumescence in young adults. *Arch. Gen. Psychiatr.,* 1972, 26: 351–56.

15. Morris, P. L., and B. B. Saxena. Dose and age-dependent effects of prolactin on luteinizing hormone and PRL-binding sites in rat Leydig cell homogenates. *Endocrinol.,* 1980, 107:1639–45.

16. Marrama, P., C. Carani, G. F. Baraghini, A. Volpe, D. Zini, M. F. Celani, and V. Montanini. Circadian rhythm of testosterone and prolactin in the ageing. *Maturitas,* 1982, 4:131–38.

17. Rubin, R. T., P. R. Gouin, A. Lubin, R. E. Poland, and K. M. Pirke. Nocturnal increase of plasma testosterone in men:relation to gonadotropins and prolactin. *J. Clin. Endocrinol. Metab.,* 1975, 40:1027–33.

18. Rubin, R. T., R. E. Poland, and B. B. Tower. Prolactin-related testosterone secretion in normal adult men. *J. Clin. Endocrinol. Metabol.,* 1976, 42:112–16.

19. Rubin, R. T., R. E. Poland, J. R. Sowers, and J. M. Hershman. Influence of methyl-TRH induced prolactin increase on serum testosterone levels in normal adult men. *J. Clin. Endocrinol. Metabol.,* 1978, 46:830–33.

20. Ben-Jonathan, N., and J. C. Porther. A sensitive radioenzymatic assay for dopamine, norepinephrine and epinephrine in plasma and tissue. *Endocrinology,* 1976, 98: 1947–52.

21. Lachelin, G. C. L., H. Leblanc, and S. S. C. Yen. The inhibitory effect of dopamine agonists on LH release in women. *J. Clin. Endocrinol. Metabol.,* 1977, 44:728–32.

22. Cronin, M. J., C. Y. Cheung, J. E. Beach, N. Faure, P. C. Goldsmith, and R. I. Weiner. Dopamine receptors on prolactin secreting cells. In *Central and peripheral regulation of prolactin secretion.* R. M. MacLeod and U. Scapagnini, eds. New York: Raven Press, 1980.

23. Grandison, L., and A. Guidotti. Gamma-amminobutyric acid receptor function in rat anterior pituitary: evidence for control of prolactin release. *Endocrinology,* 1979, 105:754–59.

24. Scapagnini, U., P. L. Canonico, and N. Ferrara. Regolazione degli assi neuroendocrini. In *Psiconeuro endocrinologia,* 57–74. U. Scapagnini, P. L. Canonico, and N. Ferrara, eds. Padova: Liviana Press, 1982.

25. Sawyer, C. H. Physiological studies on some interactions between brain and pituitary gonad axis in rabbit.

Endocrinology, 1959, 75:614–18.

26. Servais, J. F., C. H. Mormont, J. J. Legros. L'impuissance: aspects diagnostique et thérapeutique. *Rev. Méd. Psychosom. et Psychol. Médic.,* 1975, 17:263–70.

27. Halbreich, U., L. Grunhaus, and M. Ben-David. Twenty-four hour rhythm of prolactin in depressive patients. *Archiv. Gen. Psychiat.,* 1979, 36:1183–86.

28. Marrama, P., C. Carani, A. Tridenti, and R. Pederzini. Acromegalie, handicap et sexualité. Second Congr. Int., "Handicap et sexualité," Paris, 1981, 56, Abs.

26

The Effects of Opiate Receptor Blockage
on Male Sexual Response

B. Graber, C. Blake,
J. Gartner, and J. E. Wilson

The study of the effects of Naloxone, an opiate antagonist, on male sexual physiology was undertaken because of the following:

1. Chronic opiate addiction had been found to be associated with a significant level of sexual dysfunction [3, 4,20,22,24] while withdrawal from opiates has been reported to be initially associated with episodes of spontaneous erections and emissions and eventually a return of function to preaddiction levels [4,22,24].
2. Animal experimentation with either systemic administration of exogenous opiate compounds [12,17,23,24, 27,31] or intraventricular administration [18,27] of endogenous or endogenous-like opiate compounds, in lower doses partially inhibited, and in larger doses completely suppressed, male copulatory behavior while leaving general motor activity unimpaired.
3. Animal experimentation with Naloxone (or Naltrexone) given prior to the administration of an opiate compound usually prevented the suppressant effects of the opiate and when either given prior to an opiate agent or when given alone usually demonstrated facilitation of male copulatory variables to above baseline levels [6,12,17,18,24-28].

Only one experiment has been reported in which Naloxone was given to human males during actual sexual functioning [8]. Although the authors of that single subject pilot study reported no effects, other interpretations have been made of their data [25]. The following two experiments were undertaken in an effort to reexamine the effects of endogenous opiates in human male masturbation.

EXPERIMENT 1: ADMINISTRATION OF NALOXONE TO HUMAN MALE VOLUNTEERS IMMEDIATELY PRIOR TO MASTURBATION

Methods

In a double-blind random order design, males received either 20mg/2cc saline or 2cc/saline administered at 0.2cc/minute. After a ten minute baseline period, the investigators in the next room indicated via intercom to the subject to initiate masturbation and to signal the onset and termination of orgasm. Simultaneous measurements included wrist excursions (accelerometer taped to wrist) and sphincter activity.

Results

The effects of the Naloxone on anal contractions are shown in Figure 26–1. Naloxone produced a significant increase in anal contractions. Naloxone as seen in Figure 26–2 also produced an increase in "ejaculatory latency." This was a time period measured from the signal to commence masturbation until the first recorded anal contraction during ejaculation.

EXPERIMENT 2: MEASUREMENT OF PLASMA B-ENDORPHIN AND PLASMA CORTISOL DURING HUMAN MALE MASTURBATION

Methods

Males in random order design underwent four experimental trials:

 a) Attachment of physiological monitoring equipment, and placement of intravenous indwelling catheter, followed by no activity for experimental session duration (20 minutes).
 b) Attachment of physiological monitoring equipment, and placement of intravenous indwelling catheter, plus a ten minute period of wrist excursion on a plastic penis model attached to a board at subject's side.

Figure 26-1. Anal Contractions

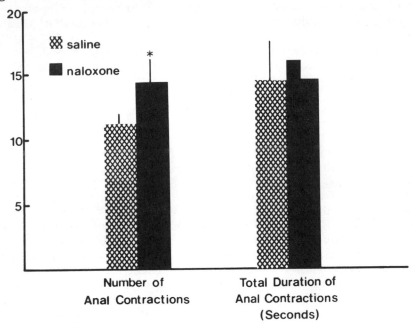

Figure 26-2. Ejaculatory latency

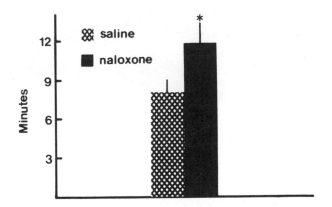

c) Attachment of physiological monitoring equipment, and placement of intravenous catheter, plus masturbation up to, but not including, ejaculation for 10 minutes.

d) Attachment of physiological monitoring equipment, and placement of intravenous indwelling catheter, plus masturbation continuing through ejaculation.

Blood samples were withdrawn from an adjacent room through approximately three feet of heparinized polyvinyl tubing. Samples were centrifuged and plasma separated and stored.

Assay for B-endorphin and cortisols were run blind by one of the authors who had not been present during experimental sessions (C.B.)

Results

B-endorphin results for the trial including masturbation are plotted in Figure 26–3 and plasma cortisol levels for all conditions are plotted in Figure 26–4. The results for both parallel each other quite closely in that neither the order or content of the trial (including ejaculation) produced any significant change in either plasma B-endorphin and plasma cortisol. For all conditions the sample at 70 minutes, which was taken after 60 minutes rest postcompletion of experimental trial, showed significant decreases in both B-endorphin and cortisol from baseline levels suggesting the initial "hook-up" procedures, and other factors may have produced an elevation at baseline above "resting" levels.

Figure 26–3. Plasma Beta Endorphin (pg/ml)

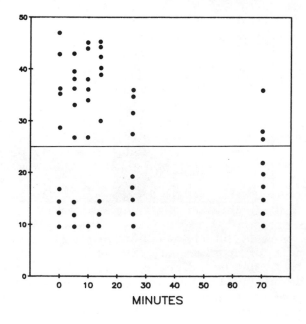

MINUTES

Figure 26–4. Plasma Cortisol Levels

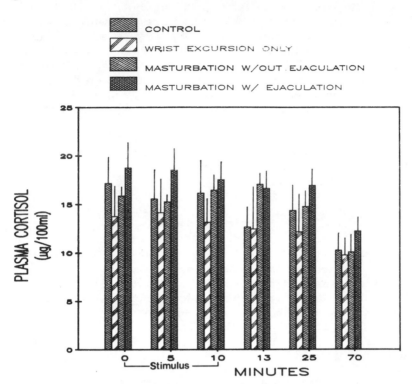

DISCUSSION

In a pilot experiment using one subject, Goldstein and Hansteen [8] reported no significant effect of five or ten mg of Naloxone. However, it has been pointed out [25] that their tabular data suggests that the time to full erection took almost twice as long with the higher Naloxone dose while time from erection to ejaculation was 50 percent that for saline, thus demonstrating initial inhibition and later facilitation.

Animal experiments as cited above have also shown both inhibition and facilitation by Naloxone although there has been a predominance of the latter. Specific facilitation shown has included: increased numbers (or percent) animals copulating [6,12,25]; decreased mount [17,25] or intromission; [17,25] latencies; decreased inter-intromission interval [17,25]; increased intromission rate [17,25]; decreased ejaculatory latency [17,25,26,28] decreased mount [17,25] or intromission [25,26,28] frequency. Specific inhibition has included: increased inter-intromission interval [28] and increased post-ejaculatory interval [26,29,30].

Elevation of B-endorphin in hamsters following their fifth ejaculation was reported by Murphy at the World Congress of Sexology in Jerusalem [24].

Due to time limitations, the possible explanations for these results cannot be discussed but include multiple opiate receptor sites [19], multiple endogenous opiates with different sensitivities to Naloxone [14,21], facilitation of spinal reflexes [7], simultaneous release of adrenocor-ticotropic hormone (ACTH), opioid-like peptides [5], differ-ential effects of opiates on vas deferens in different species [9-11,13-16,19,21,32] and variable effects of different dosages of Naloxone [2].

NOTES

1. Bohlen, J., J. Held, and M. Sanderson. The male orgasm: pelvic contractions measured by anal probe. *Archives of Sexual Behavior,* 1980, 9(6):503–21.

2. Cohen, M., R. Cohen, D. Pickar et al. Physio-logical Effects of High Dose Naloxone to Normal Adults. *Life Science,* 1982, 30:(23):2025–31.

3. Crowley, T., and R. Simpson. Methadone Dose and Human Sexual Behavior. *The International Journal of the Addictions,* 1978, 13(2):285–95.

4. Delean, G., and H. Wexler. Heroin addiction: its relation to sexual behavior and sexual experience. *Journal of Abnormal Psychiatry,* 1973, 81:36–8.

5. Fratta, W., Z. Rossetti, R. Poggioli, and G. Gessa. Reciprocal antagonism between $ACTH_{1-24}$ and B-endorphin in rats. *Neuroscience Letters,* 1981, 24:71–4.

6. Gessa, G., E. Paglietti, and B. Pellegrini-Quaran-totti. Induction of copulatory behavior in sexually inactive rats by Naloxone. *Science,* 1979, 204:203–205.

7. Goldfarb, J., and J. Hu. Enhancement of reflexes by Naloxone in spinal cats. *Neuropharmacology,* 15:785–792, 1976.

8. Goldstein, A. and Hansteen, R. Evidence against involvement of endorphins in sexual arousal and orgasm in man. *Archives of General Psychiatry,* 34:1179–1180, 1977.

9. Graham, J., Katib, H. and Spriggs, T. The isolat-ed hypogastric nerve-vas deferens preparation of the rat. *British Journal of Pharma (Chemother),* 32:34–45, 1968.

10. Huidobro-Toro, J. and Way, E. Comparative study on the effect of morphine and the opioid-like peptides in the vas deferens of rodents: species and strain differences,

evidence for multiple opiate receptors. *Life Science,* 28(12):1331–1336, 1981.

11. Henderson, G., Hughes, J. and Kosterlitz, H. A new example of a morphine-sensitive neuro-effector junction: adrenergic transmission in the mouse vas deferens. *British Journal of Pharmacology,* 46:764–766, 1972.

12. Hetta, J. Effects of morphine and naltrexone on sexual behavior of the male rat. *Acta Pharmac Tox,* 41(4):53, 1977.

13. Hughes, J., Kosterlitz, H. and Leslie, F. Effects of morphine on adrenergic transmission in the mouse vas deferens. Assessment of agonist and antagonist potencies of narcotic analgesics. *British Journal of Pharmacology,* 53:371–381, 1975

14. Jacquet, Y. Excitatory and inhibitory effects of opiates in the rat vas deferens: A dual mechanism of opiate action. *Science,* 210:95–97, 1980.

15. Lemaire, S., Magnan, J. and Regoli, D. Rat vas deferens: a specific bio-assay for endogenous opioid peptides. *British Journal of Pharmacology,* 64:327–329, 1978.

16. Macht, D. Action of opium alkaloids on the ducts of the testis. *Journal Pharmac Exp Ther* 9:121–127, 1917.

17. McIntosh, T., Vallano, M. and Barfield, R. Effects of morphine, B-endorphin and Naloxone on catecholamine levels and sexual behavior in the male rat. *Pharmacol Biochem & Behavior* 13:435–444, 1980.

18. Meyerson, B. and Terenius, L. B-Endorphin and male sexual behavior. *Euro J of Pharmacology,* 42:191–192, 1977.

19. Miller, R. Multiple opiate receptors for multiple opioid peptides. *Medical Biology,* 60:1–6, 1982.

20. Mintz, J., O'Hare, K., O'Brien, C., and Goldschmidt, J. Sexual problems of heroin addicts. *Archives of General Psychiatry,* 31:700–703, 1974.

21. Miranda, H., Huidobro, F., and Huidobro-Toro, J. Evidence for morphine and morphine-like alkaloid responses resistant to Naloxone blockade in the rat vas deferens. *Life Science,* 24(16):1511–1518, 1979.

22. Mirin, S., Meyer, R., Mendelson, J., and Ellingboe, J. Opiate use and sexual function. *American Journal of Psychiatry,* 137(8):909–915, 1980.

23. Murphy, M., Bowie D. and Pert, C. Copulation elevates plasma B-endorphin in the male hamster. *Soc. Neuroscience Abstracts,* 5:470, 1979.

24. Murphy, M. Methadone reduces sexual performance and sexual motivation in the male Syrian golden hamster. *Pharmacol. Biochem. & Behavior,* 14:561–567, 1981.

25. Myers, B. and Baum, M. Facilitation by opiate antagonists of sexual performance in the male rat. *Pharmacol Biochem & Behavior,* 10:615–618, 1979.

26. Myers, B. and Baum, M. Facilitation of copulatory performance of male rats by Naloxone: effects of hypophysectomy [17], Q-estradio-luteinizing hormone releasing hormone. *Pharmacol Biochem & Behavior,* 12:365-370, 1980.

27. Pellegrini-Quarantotti, B., Corda, M., Pagleitti, E. et al. Inhibition of copulatory behavior in male rats by D-ALA²-Met-ENKE-Phalinamide. *Life Sciences,* 23:673– 678, 1978.

28. Pellegrini-Quarantotti, B., Paglietti, E. et al. Naloxone shortens ejaculation latency in male rats. *Experientia,* 35:524–525, 1979.

29. Sachs, B., Valcourt, R., Flagg, H. Copulatory behavior and sexual reflexes of male rats treated with Naloxone. *Pharmacol Biochem & Behavior,* 14:251–253, 1980.

30. Szechtman, H., Simantov, R., Hershkowitz, M. Effects of Naloxone on copulation in rats and the role of endogenous opiates in a spontaneous rewarding behavior. *Soc Neurosci Abstracts,* 5:541, 1979.

31. Tokunaga, Y., Muraki, T. and Hosoya, E. Effects of repeated morphine administration on copulation and on the hypothalamic-pituitary-gonadal axis of male rats. *Japanese Journal of Pharmacology,* 27:65–70, 1977.

32. Waddell, J. The parmacology of the vas deferens. *Journal of Pharmacology and Experimental Therapeutics,* 8:551–559, 1916.

27

Plasma Prolactin Levels in 300 Cases of Sexual Disorders

N. Grafeille, J. C. Joutard, and A. Ruffie

Blood prolactin (PRL) levels were checked in patients with sexual disorders in which organic pathology could be diagnosed. Three hundred case records were thus selected.

We looked for a possible correlation existing between pathological levels of prolactin in the blood and the symptoms exhibited by the patients. Prolactin levels outside the range between minimum and maximum levels provided by laboratories were considered pathological.

MATERIALS AND METHODS

This study is based on data from 149 women (49.66 percent) and 151 men (50.33 percent). We attempted to draw a correlation between the PRL level and:

1. Disturbances in sexual drive: each patient was checked for disturbances in sexual drive
2. Disturbances in mood: (depression, normal mood, hypomania)
3. Sexual disorders

(I) Impotence: the impossibility for the man to engage in coital intercourse
(Er) Erectile dysfunction: the disturbance of erection, whatever the means (masturbation, spontaneous erection)

(PE) Premature ejaculation: involuntary ejaculation, occurring in a wakeful state
(A) Anejaculation and late ejaculation were grouped under the same heading
(F) Frigidity: the absence of sexual drive, coupled with a disturbance in, or absence of orgasm
(Ao) Anorgasm: the incapacity to achieve orgasm
(Do) Dysorgasm: possible but disturbed (vague, difficult, specific)
(V) Vaginismus: the tetanization of the vaginal constrictor muscles, preventing penetration of any kind
(Dp) Dyspareunia: painful sensation during penetration

BLOOD SAMPLES

Blood samples taken for the purpose of radioimmunoassay of prolactin levels were systematically carried out at times of low prolactin release, that is, between the hours of 10 a.m. and noon, and after a 15 to 20 minute period of imposed inactivity.

Fluctuations in prolactin level are thus minimal and this practice over many years has shown us that one venous blood sample is sufficient under these conditions.

Prolactin Radioimmunoassay Techniques

We used the kit that is found on the market from CEA-ORIS (PROL-RIA).

Normal Prolactin Levels

Normal values are established by each laboratory according to the following criteria: the origin and characteristics of the kit used; the physiological variations of the patients (age, period of cycle and their sex; the number of radioimmunoassays performed, allowing a more precise establishment of the range of normal values. We classified our test results into five groups:

Group 1: PRL levels less than 2.5 ng/ml = low basal serum prolactin concentrations.
Group 2: PRL levels between 2.5 ng/ml and the minimum normal value provided by the laboratory = moderately low basal serum prolactin concentrations.

Group 3: Normal PRL level (within the normal range defined by the laboratory) = normoprolactinaemia.

Group 4: PRL levels higher than the normal level provided by the laboratory, but less than or equal to 30 ng/ml = moderately high basal serum prolactin concentrations.

Group 5: PRL levels higher than 30 ng/ml = high basal serum prolactin concentrations.

RESULTS

We used Pearson's χ^2 test, a statistical method generally accepted and which can be easily applied to establish correlations between these data. We studied a number of different criteria, but we will refer only to those which are directly concerned with prolactin levels.

The normal level was the most frequently encountered (53.33 percent), but one out of two patients showed abnormal PRL levels, 27.33 percent with decreased levels and 19.33 percent with elevated levels.

Correlations Between Sex and Prolactin Level

There were significant relationships between the different criteria studied (see Table 27–1). One notes that the patients with normal prolactin levels constituted the largest group (PRL 3) in both populations; but whereas this groups includes 65.10 percent of the female population, it represents only 41.72 percent of the male population.

TABLE 27-1. Correlations Between Sex and Serum PRL

PRL	1	2	3	4	5	TOTAL
Men	24	33	63	29	2	151
Women	10	15	97	10	17	149
Total	34	48	160	39	19	300

In the male population, the moderate hyperprolactinaemia cases (PRL 4) were far more numerous (19.20 percent) than the cases of severe hyperprolactinaemia of group 5 (1.32 percent).

In the female population we found the opposite situation to prevail: moderate hyperprolactinaemia cases represented 6.71 percent of the population, whereas severe hyperprolactinaemia cases included only 11.40 percent.

The hypoprolactinaemia cases were distributed, for both sexes, in the following way: severe hypoprolactinaemia cases (PRL 1) represented 15.89 percent of the male population, compared to 6.7 percent of the female population. Moderate hypoprolactinaemia cases (PRL 2) represented 21.85 percent of the male population and 10.06 percent of the female population. Thus:

- Hypoprolactinaemia cases (PRL 1 and 2) represented 37.74 percent of the male population and 16.77 percent of the female population.
- Hyperprolactinaemia cases (PRL 4 and 5) included 20 percent of the male population and 18.12 percent of the female population.
- Severe hyperprolactinaemia cases (PRL 5) were more frequent for women than for men.
- The distribution of blood prolactin levels in the male population forms a bell curve, whereas the female population shows a prevailing peak at the normoprolactinaemia level.

Correlations Between Sex and Age

There is a significant relationship between sex and age in our sample. The female population is much younger (m = 29.9 years) than the male population (m = 42.5 years).

- 151 men ranging from 19 to 61 years of age, with an average age of 42.57 years.
- 149 women ranging from 17 to 55 years of age, with an average age of 29.94 years.

Correlations Between Mood and Prolactin Levels

There is no positive correlation between mood and prolactin levels (χ^2 well below significance).

Notice the rates of normal mood at extreme values of blood prolactin: 58 percent of men in group 1 and 70.5 percent of women in group 5.

TABLE 27-2. Average Age of Each PRL Group--Men

	m	number of cases
PRL 1	43.46 years	24
PRL 2	42.90 years	33
PRL 3	41.38 years	63
PRL 4	44.89 years	29
PRL 5	30.00 years	2

TABLE 27-3. Average Age of Each PRL Group--Women

	m	number of cases
PRL 1	29.1 years	10
PRL 2	29.5 years	15
PRL 3	29.85 years	97
PRL 4	32.9 years	10
PRL 5	29.59 years	17

Correlations Between Prolactin Levels and Sexual Disorders

The predominant symptom in men is a disturbance of erection. These disorders increase with prolactin levels. Rates of impotence are slightly higher with extreme variations in prolactin levels. There are no clear variations in premature ejaculation cases. Incidence of anejaculation is high in moderate hyperprolactinaemia.

Predominant symptoms in women are: frigidity (25 cases) and disturbances in orgasm (24 cases of anorgasm, 20 cases of dysorgasm).

Roles of frigidity seem to rise with prolactin levels (42 percent for PRL 4, 40 percent for PRL 5, 20 percent for PRL 1). Rates of dyspareunia are higher with extreme prolactin level variations.

Absence of orgasm is more frequent in cases of hypoprolactinaemia and orgasmic dysfunction is more frequent with average PRL levels. Disturbances in the female orgasm, in general, seem to be most strongly represented by cases of

hypoprolactinaemia. We did not find any orgasmic dysfunction in group 5, not did we find any case of vaginismus
in group 4 or frigidity in group 2.

Correlations Between Mood
and Disturbances in Sexual Drive

The χ^2 test confirms the association between mood and
disturbance of the sexual drive in men, but no correlation
can be drawn in women. Men seem to show disturbances in
sexual drive when not depressed or only slightly so,
whereas women exhibit a disturbance in sexual drive irre-
spective of mood.

Correlations Between PRL Level
and Disturbances in Sexual Drive

If there are substantially more women (70 to 80 percent)
than men (11 to 21 percent) that express a disturbance in
sexual drive, there is no positive correlation between sexual
drive disturbances and prolactin levels (see Table 27-4).

TABLE 27-4. Correlations Between Serum PRL and Sexual Drive

Men	PRL 1	PRL 2	PRL 3	PRL 4	PRL 5	TOTAL
Presence of disturb-ance in sexual drive	3	7	7	5	0	22
Absence	21	26	56	24	2	129
Women						
Presence of disturb-ance in sexual drive	8	12	68	7	13	108
Absence	2	3	29	3	4	41

DISCUSSION

The sample (300 cases) of sexual disorders on which this study was conducted showed a blood prolactin level distribution of:

- normal: 53.33 percent
- low: 27.33 percent
- high: 19.33 percent

Cases of Hypoprolactinaemia

In our study, 27.33 percent of the population showed low blood prolactin levels.

It was not possible in this work to systematically apply thyroid releasing hormone (TRH) stimulation test in all cases of hypoprolactinaemia in groups 1 and 2 as the study was performed on most of the patients *a posteriori*.

We noticed as early as 1975, in a previous study dealing with secondary amenorrhea in young women, that low prolactin levels in the blood could be found. Indeed, these levels were either at the threshold of radioimmunoassay detection (4 mg/ml group 2 like) or undetectable (group 1). Depending on the case, they were accompanied by highly variable levels of follicle stimulating hormone (FSH) and LH in a static state or in response to an injection of LH-RH.

We had at that time performed i.v. injection of 200 to 250 µg of TRH. In certain instances, a response of zero or an insufficient response led us to envisage the existence, until then contested, of hypoprolactinaemia.

Cases of Hyperprolactinaemia

According to our findings, 58 patients showed prolactin levels higher than the normal rates provided by the laboratories in which the blood samples were taken. Of these 58 patients:

- 39 are included in group 4: 10 women and 29 men
- 19 are included in group 5: 17 women and 2 men

Bromocriptine Study on Patients of Group 4

Of the 35 patients making up this group, 14 received bromocriptine (see Table 27–5).

Hormonal analysis and sella turcica examination of all the subjects were normal.

TABLE 27-5.   Treatment of Type 4 Hyperprolactinaemia With Parlodel

Sex	Serum PRL ng/ml	Normal rates	Sexual disorders	Duration of Treatment in Months	Clinical Improvement
M	30		Erectile dysfunction	3	0
	24		" "	1	+
	25	4	" "	2	0
	22		" "	1	+
	20		" "	1	+
	23		" "	1	+
	20		Anejaculation	3	+
	29		Premature ejaculation	2	0
F	30		Sexual drive disturbance	3	+
	27		"	3	+
	30	5	"	3	+
	29		Frigidity	3	±
	26		"	3	±
	30		Anorgasm	3	+

After one to three months of treatment (according to the case and the results):

In men: disturbances in erection ameliorated in more than half of the cases, as did anejaculation, which disappeared. The instance of premature ejaculation remained unchanged
In women: sex drive disturbances as well as anorgasm disappeared on the eighth day of treatment. The 14 patients expressed an improvement in sexuality. No intolerance or aggravation was indicated.

Bromocriptine Study on Patients of Group 5

In this group, levels of PRL range from 31 ng/ml to 224 ng/ml. In each of the cases, an X-ray and tomography of the sella turcica were performed and three cases were examined by scanner to complete the study (see Table 27–6).
We had only three cases of prolactin adenoma, which confirms the view that hyperprolactinaemia does not indicate

TABLE 27-6. Treatment of Group 5 Hyperprolactinaemia with Parlodel

SEX	SERUM PRL ng/ml	N	SEXUAL DISORDERS	SELLA TURCICA	DURATION OF TREATMENT IN MONTHS	CLINICAL IMPROVEMENT
F	33		Sexual drive disturbances--Vaginismus	Abnormal	6	In each case: After the
	52		Sexual drive disturbances--Frigidity--Amenorrhoea	Abnormal	8	7th day of therapy
	224		Anorgasm	Abnormal	6	
	36				3	
	80				4	
	51	5	Sexual drive disturbances	Normal	4	
	71	20			6	
	72				4	
	35		Sexual drive disturbances + Anorgasm	Normal	3	
	46				3	
	72				4	
	31		Sexual drive disturbances + Exhibitionism	Normal	3- Relapse 2	
	133		Sexual drive disturbances + Dyspareunia	Normal	3- Relapse 6- Relapse	
	160		Secondary Fridigity + Sexual drive disturbances	Normal	6	
	160		Secondary Frigidity + Vaginismus	Normal	6- Relapse	
	54		Secondary Frigidity + Vaginismus	Normal	4	
	32		Dysthymy	Normal	2	
M	59	4	Erectile dysfunction	Normal	4	+
	57			Normal	4	+

an adenoma. However, when we did this study, we did not systematically examine by scanner. Our experience has recently shown that certain adenomas could escape tomography detection. For this reason, we recommend that examination by scanner be performed every time prolactin levels are greater than 130 ng/ml.

The three cases of prolactin adenoma in our series were three women: the first consulted us for a disturbance in sex drive with secondary vaginismus and sterility, serum PRL = 33 ng/ml; the second patient consulted us for amenorrhea and secondary frigidity. She had been receiving anti-thyroidal and antidepressant drugs for six months, serum PRL = 52 ng/ml; the third patient showed an inability to achieve orgasm, serum PRL = 224 ng/ ml.

All 19 patients (2 men and 17 women) received bromocriptine.

Dosage: 1/2 tablet the first day,
1 tablet the second day (2.5 mg),
2 tablets per day thereafter.

The treatment lasted a minimum of two months and a maximum of several six-month periods. Indeed, we received one female patient who consulted us after an abrupt appearance of secondary frigidity, accompanied by a state of depression, without any other clinical signs (regular cycles, no presence of galactorrhea, no presence of ocular disturbance). The couple emphasized the sudden character of the condition.

This woman's first prolactin level was 133 ng/ml. X-rays and tomograms of the sella turcica were normal. Bromocriptine treatment, two tablets per day, was prescribed. After eight days, there was a clear improvement in mood, and sexual interactions were resumed after 15 days. A PRL analysis after three months showed a serum level of 20 ng/ml. Treatment was stopped. She experienced a relapse a month later. The same therapeutic approach was resumed. Parlodel was taken for six months as the woman refused to discontinue this medication. Seen again following this period of time, she declared that her sexuality was satisfactory. The treatment was discontinued. The patient did not come back for further help, but her primary physician indicated to us that "she had put herself back on Parlodel."

The other 18 patients treated with bromocriptine showed a rapid improvement of mood (six to eight days) with an improvement in sexual dysfunction, also (15 to 21 days). There were three cases of relapse after discontinuation of treatment. The results of the treatment are the following:

· sex drive: improvement in 100 percent of the cases

- the 2 men recovered the capacity to achieve satisfactory erection
- secondary vaginismus did not cease, but there was an overall improvement in mood
- anorgasm: 50 percent improvement
- no aggravation
- nausea at the start of treatment: three cases
- lypothymia at the beginning of treatment: one case (despite adherence to the progressive dosage).

We treated, with bromocriptine, *a total* of 33 patients (10 men, 23 women) who showed moderate or severe hyperprolactinaemia.

The results concerning mood are excellent, and concerning sexual disorders are good. Sex drive disorders and erectile disturbances dissipated rapidly. Anorgasm disappeared in approximately one of two cases. We saw no improvement in cases of vaginismus or premature ejaculation. No aggravation whatsoever was indicated. This confirmed the prolactin-decreasing effect of bromocriptine.

We feel that bromocriptine has a place in the treatment of sexual disorders *provided the disorders are associated with a moderate or severe hyperprolactinaemia*. It is for this reason we think it would be worthwhile to check the blood prolactin level when confronted with sexual disorders.

Additional Data

Other findings of this study demonstrated that there are correlations between age and sex, between sex and PRL levels, and between sex and the expression of disturbances in sexual drive. For example, in women, although not in men, there is a correlation between mood, sexual disorders and sexual drive disturbances.

There is, therefore, a difference between the two sexes, a difference in expression as well as in manifestation of sexual disorders. Men showed one symptom (184 sexual symptoms expressed by 151 men)—they rarely expressed a sexual drive or a lack of sexual drive. Women showed disorders, these disorders being much broader than in men (31 sexual symptoms expressed by 149 women), and women speak more readily of sexual drive disturbances (108 women whereas only 22 men expressed these disturbances).

This is undoubtedly due to a condition of our society, in which one readily accepts that a woman is unable to derive pleasure or experience desire, whereas a man is supposed to experience desire and therefore must be able to demonstrate it, at the present time, a time of acceptance of certain masculine sexual deficiencies, it is more readily accepted to speak of erectile dysfunction or impotence than of a lack of sexual drive. Virility has its cost . . . . One is therefore better off expressing what is thought to be a somatic symptom rather than admit one's lack of interest or absence of sexual drive.

Women express disorders at different ages and with different symptoms. Vaginismus is only encountered between the ages of 20 and 39 years. Between the ages of 20 and 29 years, the greatest number of cases concern orgasmic dysfunction (55 percent); between 30 and 39 years of age, the most frequent symptom is frigidity (43.7 percent). Are we dealing here with a difference in disorders due to the patient's age and to the length of time spent with her partner or, to a generation difference? Each society and each period has its trends. Was frigidity more common 10 or 20 years ago? Is the quest for "the orgasm at any cost" imposed by a media which caters to the female public? In other words, could not the cases of female anorgasm today be the cases of frigidity 10 or 20 years ago?

The same could hold true for men, where disturbances of erection constitute the symptom the most frequently expressed. In men under the age of 29, this disorder is clearly surpassed by instances of impotence.

It seems, in both sexes, that the distribution of disturbances in sexual drive is independent of age and prolactin levels.

Our findings reveal that, for sexual disorders:

- Hypoprolactinaemia (PRL 1 and 2) represents 37.74 percent of the male population and only 16.77 percent of the female population.
- Examination for erectile dysfunction in the male population and for frigidity in the female population were more frequent in cases of hyperprolactinaemia.
- Rates of impotence among men and anorgasm among women are higher for extreme PRL levels (PRL 1 and PRL 5).
- Percentages of ejaculatory dysfunction (PE and A) were nearly constant (between 26 and 29 percent), regardless of the serum PRL concentration.

Although disturbances in mood are independent of sex, age and PRL levels, they are nevertheless most frequently encountered in the severe hypoprolactinaemia group (PRL 1) (42 percent of the men and 70 percent of the women).

CONCLUSIONS

It is evident that hypoprolactinaemia does exist and that hyperprolactinaemia is definitely implicated in certain sexual disorders (which can be improved with bromocriptine).

It is difficult to quantify mood or sexual-drive disturbances. These disorders are often only expressed through their symptoms, this being the sole indication of depression or of bad verbal communication between the couple. The sexual symptom may also constitute a means of expression between two beings who, more often than not, dare not speak of their preoccupations or of themselves. It was, therefore, difficult to attempt to find possible correlations existing between such suggestive notions and a biological parameter. It appears, however, that the serum PRL level influences, as well as depends on, the psychic state.

NOTES

1. Bataille, D., and J. N. Talbot. The effects of vasoactive intestinal peptide (VIP) on prolactin secretion in man. *C.R. Acad. Sci., serie III; Sciences de La Vie,* 1981, 282, no. 7:511–14.

2. Board, J. A., and R. J. Fierro. Effects of cyproheptadine on chlorpromazine stimulation of prolactin in women. *Am. J. Obstet. Gynecol.,* 1981, 139, no. 2:160–63.

3. Boucher, D., and J. Hermabessiere. Amélioration de la spermatogénèse et améliorations hormonales après traitement par la bromoergocriptine. *Rev. Franc. Endocr. Clin.,* 1977, 18 , no. 2:158–59.

4. Brown, W. A., and T. Laughren. Low serum prolactin an early relapse following neuroleptic withdrawal. *The Am. J. Psychiatry,* 1981, 138, no. 2:237–39.

5. Buvat, J., M. Buvat-Herbaut, A. Racadot, and P. Fossati. Exploration neuroendocrinienne dans 68 cas de troubles de l'éjaculation idiopathique. Ejaculations prématurées et anéjaculations. *Cahiers Sex Clin.,* 1979, 28: 368–79.

6. Buvat, J., P. Fossati, M. Asfour, and J. J. Boutemy. La fonction prolactinique dans l'impuissance érectile idiopathique. *Probl. Actuel Endocrinol. Nutr.,* 1977, 21:165–83.

7. Empcraire, J. C., and A. Ruffie. Les dosages hormonaux chez la femme en dehors de la grossesse in ORGANON. *Service de Documentation Médicale,* 1983, 8–10. La Prolactine.

8. Feek, C. M., and J. S. A. Sawyers. The effects of thyroid hormone status upon the dopaminergic control of

thyrotrophin (TSH) and prolactin (PRL) secretion by anterior pituitary in men. *Scottish Med. J.*, 1981, 26, no. 1:87.

9. Fossati, P., J. Buvat, M. L'Hermite, J. P. Cappoen, J. C. Grenier, and M. Linquette. Etude de la fonction prolactique dans 14 cas de galactorrhée avec hypogonadisme et microdéformation de la selle turcique. *Ann. d'Endocrin*, (Paris), 1976, 37:157–69.

10. Caufriez, A., M. L'Hermite, A. Stevenaert, G. Copinschi, and C. Rubyn. Succès thérapeutique de la bromocriptine chez trois patientes prolactinémiques après adénéostomie trans-shpénoïdale. *Rev. Franc. Endocr. Clin.*, 1977, 18, no. 2:159.

11. Grafeille, N., and J. C. Joutard. Prolactine et sexualité. *Bordeaux-Médical*, 1981, 14:511–19.

12. Grizard, G., D. Boucher, and J. Hermabessiere. La sécrétion de prolactine chez l'homme stérile. *Gynécologie*, 1977, 28:421–28.

13. Hermanns, U., and E. S. E. Hafez. Prolactin and male reproduction. *Archives of Andrology*, 1981, 6, no. 2: 95–126.

14. Jaffiol, C., M. Robin, J. Mirouze, and A. Orsetti. Les hormones gonadotropes et la prolactine au cours des gynécomasties. Etude de l'action de la dibromoergocriptine. *Ann. Endocrin.*, (Paris), 1976, 37:469–70.

15. Kerbrat-Broard, C. La prolactinémie chez les déprimés et leur traitement par la bromocriptine. *Mémoire pour le CES de psychiatrie*, ROUEN, 1980.

16. Legros, J. J., C. Mormont, and J. Servais. Aspect neuro-endocrinien de l'impuissance érectile. *Bruxelles Méd.*, 1978, 58:155–65.

17. Leroith, D., and Y. Liel. The prolactin response to thyrotropin-releasing hormone is intact in the human male castrate. *Acta Endocrinologica*, 1981, 96, no. 2:163–67.

18. Lester, E., F. S. Woodroffe, and R. L. Smith. Prolactin and impotence in diabetes mellitus. *Annals of Clin. Biochem.*, 1981, 18, part 1:6–8.

19. Merceron, R. E., J. P. Raymond, J. P. Courreges, and H. P. Klotz. La sexualité chez les hyperprolactinémiques. *Probl. Actual Endocrin. Nutr.*, 1977, 21:184.

20. Nicolette, I., and P. Filipponi. Restoration of prolactin response to metoclopramide by chronic bromocriptine treatment in patients with prolactin secreting pituitary microadenoma. *IRCS Med. Sci. Biochem.*, 1981, 9, no. 4:375.

21. Reuter, A. M., P. Franchimont, and Y. Gevaert. Radioimmunoassay of prolactin in health and disease. *International Review Endocrinology*, 1976 e. (1976).

22. Roulier, R., A. Mattei, Reuter, A., and P. Franchimont. Etude de la prolactine dans les stérilités et les hypogonadismes masculins. *Ann. Endocrinol.*, (Paris), 1976, 37:286–86.

23. Spitz, I. M., U. Almaliach, E. Rosen, W. Polishuk, and D. Rabinowitz. Dissociation of prolactin responsiveness to TRH and chlorpromazine in women with isolated gonadotropin deficiency. *Journal Clinical Endocrinology and Metabolism,* 1977, 45, no. 6.

24. Tordjamn, G. Traitement des dysfonctions sexuelles masculines par le CB 154. *Probl. Actu. Endocrinol. Nutr.,* 1977, 21:191–195.

PART VII

Transcultural Studies

The influence of cultural standards on sexual functioning has been recognized by psychotherapists for years. Similarly, there is evidence of change in sexual standards and behavior in the United States and other countries. Sexual therapists with an international patient population are well aware of the need to modify their therapeutic approaches in accordance with the patient's cultural background. Even within the United States, a therapist's approach often requires change dependent upon the ethnic, social, economic, and regional background of patients.

This section includes four papers related to sexual attitudes and behavior in different cultures. The paper by Dr. Khattab on female circumcision was included for several reasons. This paper clearly documents the extreme extent to which cultural variables can influence sexual behavior. This paper was also included to mobilize public support of Dr. Khattab's efforts to prevent such surgery from continuing to be performed. The World Association of Sexology passed a resolution to express its concern over this procedure to the World Health Organization at its meeting in Washington during the Sixth World Congress.

28

Sexual Behavior of Japanese Students: Comparison Between 1974 and 1981 Surveys

S. Miyahara

AIM AND PURPOSE OF THE SURVEY

"Survey on the Sexual Consciousness of Youth" conducted in 1971 by the prime minister's office was the first nation-wide survey concerning sex in Japan. The results made it clear that young people of today are more aggressive and open towards sex and are becoming sexually aware at an age earlier than that of their parents' generation.

The second survey on the sexual consciousness of youth was conducted by the Japanese Association for Sex Education (JASE) at the request of the prime minister's office in 1974 [1]. For the first time in Japan it clarified the actual state of sex physiology, psychological growth, and development of sexual activity of young people on a nationwide scale. As a result, the following was learned: (1) the percentage of boys and girls who have experienced ejaculation, menstruation, masturbation, dating, kissing, petting, and sexual intercourse at different ages; and (2) the difference between boys and girls in the above items.

The social and cultural elements that promote and stimulate the activation and earlier age of sexual consciousness and sexual activity of young people, which were revealed in the 1970s, still exist in the 1980s and are becoming more multifold and complicated.

The first purpose of this survey was to clarify trends in changes of sexual growth and sexual activity by resurveying them on the same scale and with the same questionnaire used for the survey of 1974. The second purpose was to reveal the relationship between sexual growth, activity, family background, circumstances, and social and cultural elements. As for the second purpose, some data are now being analyzed and investigated; however, this report [2] deals only with the results of simple totals and comparison between the cumulative percentages of this survey with those of the previous survey.

METHOD OF SURVEY

The best way to conduct a social survey like this one is to hold an individual interview with a respondent chosen at random, but this method cannot be easily applied to a topic such as sex, which is influenced by strong social pressure. First of all, it has been, in our experience, extremely difficult to persuade selected people to be respondents. Because of the small number of our staff available, we had to entrust the role of persuader to school teachers. The next great difficulty is to obtain reliable answers. It is especially hard to imagine that respondents will tell of their sexual consciousness and activity honestly to an interviewer whom they see for the first time. However, if the interviewer is someone the respondent knows, it is very likely that other considerations will apply and that they will prevent the respondent from giving honest answers. Therefore, we decided reliability would be higher if we had the answer form filled out by the respondent himself. For these reasons, we decided to use a group answering method, adopting a school or a class as a homogeneous group. Taking problems of regional distribution into consideration, we set up seven definite cities (Sapporo, Akita, Tokyo, Nagoya, Kyoto, Matsue, Kumamoto) as objective study districts in this survey. Then, considering the number of students and the kind and scale of schools, we picked 75 schools. Finally, we chose some classes (all classes in some cases) from each of these schools as groups of respondents.

The survey was conducted utilizing all the members of the groups chosen in the way mentioned above. The respondents were not required to write their names. Needless to say, we paid great attention to the reliability of the respondents. For example, the sentences and arrangements of the questions were carefully studied in order to avoid fabricated answers. We prohibited them from communicating with each other and prohibited supervisors (teachers or association staff) from giving any advice to them when writing their answers.

This survey was conducted between May 1 and June 30 of 1981.

DESCRIPTION OF RESPONDENTS

In the end, 21,255 completed questionnaire forms were collected. But as mentioned above, the districts in which respondents lived were limited and the way of choosing groups of respondents was far from an ideal way. However, the results of this survey, which was conducted utilizing a large number of respondents (21,255), is believed to be a source for learning the actual state of sexual activity and consciousness of today's young people. After investigating the distribution of schools and grades of the respondents, we found that it was quite different from that of schools and grades in Japan today as a whole. Therefore, by allocating a certain number to each district, type of school, grade, and sex of the respondents, we extracted at random 4,990 answer sheets (boys 2,505 and girls 2,485) out of 21,255 and analyzed only these 4,990 answer sheets as the objects of this survey. There are, however, some points to be taken into consideration. The age of the respondents ranges from around 15 to 23 years old and those who were over 24 are included in a group labelled "over 23" together with those of age 23. But because of the sparsity of the number of those aged 23 compared with other ages, they were excluded in some cases. As for the distribution of area, a little less than 90 percent of the respondents live in cities, reflecting the fact that the survey was conducted mostly in cities. This must also be taken into consideration.

CALCULATION METHOD OF CUMULATIVE
PERCENTAGE OF THE EXPERIENCED

In order to show the process of growth of sexual consciousness and sexual activity, a "cumulative percentage of the experienced" for different ages, that is, the percentage of those who have experienced a specific consciousness or an act by the time they reach a certain age, was calculated by the following method. This method is similar to the one which A. Kinsey adopted in his report published in 1956 and exactly the same method used in the previous survey in 1974. For instance, taking the experience of ejaculation for boys 11 years old and under as an example, the number of boys who clearly answered "experienced" or "not experienced yet" is 2,374 (2,267 + 107); among these 2,374, the number of boys whose age at the time of their first experience was under eleven years is 173. Meanwhile, among the boys who answered "experienced," there are 543 boys who did not indicate the age of their first experience. Since these boys cannot be included as the objects of this calculation, it is also necessary to subtract a number calculated by the same ratio (543/2267) from the number of the inexperienced. This makes the number of the inexperienced 81. By dividing the above mentioned 173 by 1,805, which is the total of 81 and the number of boys who clearly answered the age of their first experience (1,724), 9.6 percent is obtained as the cumulative percentage of the experienced at the age of eleven. For the cumulative percentage of the experienced at the age of 15 or over, only the boys of an age equal to or over the respective age are included as respondents, and then the same calculation mentioned above was used. As a result, there are some points where the cumulative percentage decreases, although the rate is small.

PHYSIOLOGICAL SEXUAL GROWTH

Experience of Ejaculation (Seminal Emission)

To the question "Have you ever experienced ejaculation (seminal emission)?" 2,267 out of 2,374 definite answers were "yes." This is 95.5 percent, while it was 96.2 percent in the previous survey. The age of boys who experienced ejaculation for the first time ranges almost ten years, with boys of 13 at the top and most of them from twelve to 14. The cumulative percentage of the experienced (a total percentage of youth who have experienced the act by the respective age) is shown on Tables 28-1 and 28-2.

Comparing the results of this survey with those of the similar survey conducted on a nationwide scale by JASE seven years ago, almost the same trend is observed in the case of boys' ejaculation. In short, as far as ejaculation is regarded as an indication of boys' physiological sexual maturity, a trend of age decrease and promotion of sexual maturity is not clearly observed over the last seven years. The number of those who first experienced ejaculation by masturbation has increased (50.0 percent, compared with 42.5 percent in 1974) and those by nocturnal emission has decreased (42.0 percent, compared with 48.9 percent in 1974). This shows a trend toward active experience.

TABLE 28-1. Cumulative Rates of Experience in 1974 (In Percent)

Age		<10	11	12	13	14	15	16	17	18	19	20	21 yrs
Ejaculation	Male	6.5	12.5	34.4	53.8	76.7	89.1	93.7	94.4	95.6	96.4	96.6	95.4
Menstruation	Female	2.3	16.0	54.2	81.0	95.2	99.2	99.5	99.6	99.5	99.5	99.2	98.0
Sexual Interest	Male	14.9	23.0	44.0	59.4	75.2	87.2	92.4	94.8	96.8	97.2	97.2	96.8
Interest	Female	4.1	6.9	23.0	37.3	57.5	76.4	84.2	87.9	88.0	88.5	91.7	92.3
Desire for	Male	13.0	20.2	33.4	49.3	63.2	79.1	84.7	89.4	93.2	94.5	94.4	94.7
Body Contact	Female	0.9	1.7	5.4	8.3	14.4	25.7	30.9	34.8	39.2	41.7	46.0	50.0
Sexual	Male	10.9	17.1	35.3	49.7	65.1	77.9	84.5	88.0	89.9	93.5	95.4	96.6
Excitement	Female	2.0	3.0	7.6	11.9	19.2	29.1	38.9	45.4	48.4	58.6	66.7	67.7
Desire	Male	7.6	9.8	20.9	29.6	42.1	57.5	65.5	71.3	77.0	81.3	83.6	84.2
to Kiss	Female	0.5	1.1	4.9	9.1	16.8	30.7	39.8	44.7	50.1	54.0	56.7	61.0
Masturbation	Male	7.6	13.2	28.4	45.5	65.1	80.8	87.2	90.0	92.0	92.4	92.6	92.0
	Female	2.3	3.9	7.2	9.3	12.7	18.1	20.6	23.2	24.0	26.1	30.0	30.0
Dating	Male	1.8	3.0	6.3	10.3	20.0	34.3	45.3	57.2	65.0	73.1	75.0	73.3
	Female	1.0	1.7	4.1	10.5	20.0	39.0	51.0	58.4	66.3	73.5	81.0	84.2
Have	Male	2.3	2.6	3.5	5.1	8.6	15.0	19.4	28.0	36.7	43.6	47.2	49.7
Kissed	Female	1.0	1.3	1.5	2.3	3.4	7.8	13.3	19.6	25.7	32.3	42.9	45.7
Petting	Male	0.8	1.1	1.4	1.9	3.2	7.3	10.1	14.7	19.9	26.1	33.5	35.4
	Female	0.1	0.2	0.5	0.5	1.2	2.6	4.2	8.0	11.1	14.4	21.4	25.0
Coitus	Male	0.2	0.2	0.3	0.6	1.5	3.3	6.3	9.2	14.2	20.6	26.8	28.1
	Female	0.3	0.3	0.6	0.6	0.9	1.8	2.4	4.6	6.7	6.8	11.2	15.9

TABLE 28-2. Cumulative Rates of Experience in 1981 (In Percent)

Age		<10	11	12	13	14	15	16	17	18	19	20	21	22 yrs
Ejaculation	Male	4.1	9.6	31.0	60.3	81.9	91.6	95.5	97.5	98.4	98.4	98.7	98.1	99.2
Menstruation	Female	3.4	21.8	58.8	85.8	97.6	99.5	99.9	99.9	99.9	99.9	99.7	100.0	100.00
Sexual	Male	11.6	19.2	42.1	69.0	84.1	91.8	95.5	97.4	98.3	98.9	99.0	99.2	100.00
Interest	Female	5.6	9.9	24.8	44.3	59.9	72.3	81.1	85.3	89.6	92.1	94.4	96.0	97.7
Desire for	Male	9.6	14.4	32.1	54.1	71.0	82.2	89.0	92.3	94.5	95.8	96.6	97.3	98.4
Body Contact	Female	0.9	1.2	3.8	8.1	13.4	19.9	26.3	31.0	38.1	44.7	49.3	57.7	61.5
Sexual	Male	8.7	13.9	29.7	53.9	72.0	82.5	88.4	91.3	94.4	96.1	97.3	96.9	97.0
Excitement	Female	2.2	2.7	7.0	12.5	19.5	28.8	37.9	43.2	50.6	60.3	68.7	74.6	82.5
Desire	Male	5.2	7.6	17.5	32.5	46.5	61.4	70.2	74.8	80.8	84.4	88.0	89.8	89.5
to Kiss	Female	0.9	1.3	4.5	11.5	21.9	34.2	43.4	48.0	54.7	61.1	66.1	70.5	77.8
Masturbation	Male	4.7	9.3	25.1	51.6	73.4	85.5	91.5	95.2	96.1	96.7	97.7	97.8	97.0
	Female	3.4	4.4	8.6	12.7	17.4	21.2	25.5	27.9	31.9	34.6	41.3	41.0	39.5
Dating	Male	0.7	1.2	4.2	11.2	25.4	38.5	49.0	58.2	67.9	73.5	80.6	85.0	84.6
	Female	0.8	1.1	3.8	10.5	22.3	38.5	52.0	62.1	72.6	81.5	86.1	88.8	86.5
Have	Male	1.1	1.3	2.4	4.8	9.3	16.1	23.0	30.2	40.0	49.1	54.2	66.9	71.3
Kissed	Female	0.4	0.5	1.3	3.0	6.4	12.9	19.7	27.1	36.1	49.8	62.0	71.9	68.0
Petting	Male	0.0	0.2	0.4	1.1	3.6	7.9	12.7	17.4	26.6	36.4	47.7	56.1	66.2
	Female	0.0	0.1	0.3	0.8	2.3	6.3	11.2	15.9	20.1	30.9	41.9	50.9	58.0
Coitus	Male	0.0	0.0	0.1	0.5	1.4	3.9	6.8	9.8	17.6	26.0	37.4	46.8	56.1
	Female	0.0	0.1	0.1	0.2	0.7	2.4	5.3	7.6	10.4	17.1	28.0	36.5	37.7

Experience of Menstruation

To the question "Have you started menstruation?" 2,427 out of 2,432 definite answers were "yes." This is 99.8 percent, while it was 99.6 percent in the last survey. The age of girls who started menstruation ranges from eight or nine to 15, with most of them starting between the ages of eleven to 13. The cumulative percentage of those girls who have experienced menstruation is shown on Tables 28–1 and 28–2. It shows 50 percent of twelve-year-old girls and almost all 15-year-old girls have begun menstruation. This trend is exactly the same as that of the last survey in 1974. The trend of age decrease in the development of sexual maturity for girls is not the same as in the case of boys' ejaculation. Only 0.2 percent of the girls (5 out of 2,485) had not experienced menstruation by age 20. It is very rare or exceptional for them not to have had it by age 20. This differs from boys' ejaculation, for 107 out of 2,505 (4.3 percent) had not experienced it by age 20.

PSYCHOLOGICAL SEXUAL GROWTH

Interest in Sex

To the question "Have you ever had an interest in sexual matters?" 2,380 out of 2,474 definite answers by boys were "yes" (96.2 percent, compared with 96.9 percent in 1974) and 2,004 out of 2,356 definite answers by girls were "yes" (85.1 percent, compared with 90.3 percent in 1974). Most boys and girls start showing an interest in sexual matters around the age of twelve to 14. Studied from the percentages of cumulative experience of this survey, the result is almost unchanged among both boys and girls, and shows a similar trend compared to that of the last survey made in 1974.

Desire to Touch the Opposite Sex

To the question "Have you ever felt like touching the body of someone of the opposite sex?" 2,192 out of 2,446 definite answers by boys were "yes" (89.6 percent, compared with 91.8 percent in 1974) and 773 out of 2,345 definite answers by girls were "yes" (33.0 percent, compared with 40.0 percent in 1974). The ratio of the experienced has decreased compared to that of the last survey made in 1974. However, both in boys and girls the cumulative percentage of the experienced of this survey and that of the last one shows no difference. The largest age range for boys who begin to have a desire to touch the body of someone of the opposite sex is twelve to 14 and for girls is 13 to 21.

Sexual Excitement

To the question "Have you ever experienced sexual excitement?" 2,202 out of 2,437 definite answers by boys were "yes" (90.4 percent, compared with 91.2 percent in 1974) and 1,126 out of 2,233 definite answers by girls were "yes" (50.4 percent, compared with 54.6 percent in 1974). The ratio of the experienced boys is almost the same as that of the last survey made seven years ago. However, the ratio of experienced girls of this survey shows a decrease from the last one. Studied from the cumulative percentage of the experienced of this survey, the result shows not too much difference in both boys and girls from that of the last survey. As for the age of youths to start experiencing sexual excitement, boys of age twelve to 14 and girls of age 14 to 22 represent the largest ranges.

Desire to Kiss

To the question "Have you ever wanted to kiss in a sexual sense?" 1,841 out of 2,449 definite answers by boys were "yes" (75.2 percent, compared with 75.6 percent in 1974) and 1,258 out of 2,291 definite answers by girls (54.9 percent, compared with 55.0 percent in 1974). The ratio of experienced boys and also that of experienced girls are almost the same as those of the last survey made seven years ago. The cumulative percentage of the experienced indicates an increase among girls over 18 years old.

DEVELOPMENT OF SEXUAL ACTIVITY

Experience of Masturbation

To the question "Have you ever experienced masturbation?" 2,096 out of 2,270 definite answers by boys were "yes" (92.3 percent, compared with 90.6 percent in 1974) and 541 out of 1,955 definite answers by girls were "yes" (27.7 percent, compared with 24.4 percent in 1974). The cumulative percentage rates of experience shown on Tables 28–1 and 28–2 indicate an increasing trend of masturbation among both boys and girls; especially there is an increase among girls as they get older.

Experience of Dating

To the question "Have you ever dated?" 1,486 out of 2,486 definite answers by boys were "yes" (59.8 percent, compared with 61.5 percent in 1974) and 1,549 out of 2,461 definite answers by girls were "yes" (62.9 percent, compared with 62.4 percent in 1974). Comparing the boys with the girls, the percentage of experienced girls is higher than that of experienced boys in all ages. As the cumulative percentage of the experienced shown in the tables indicate, the percentage of experienced girls over 16 is higher than that of experienced boys.

Experience of Kissing
To the question "Have you ever kissed?" 907 out of 2,440 definite answers by boys were "yes" (37.2 percent, compared with 33.4 percent in 1974) and 876 out of 2,374 definite answers by girls were "yes" (36.9 percent, compared with 25.6 percent in 1974). The number of experienced boys and that of experienced girls has increased; especially there is a noticeable increase among girls. According to the cumulative percentage of the experienced shown in the tables, there is a noticeable increase among girls; the percentage of experienced girls of 20 to 21 surpasses that of boys. Almost 50 percent of both boys and girls of age 19 have experienced it.

Experience of Petting

To the question "Have you ever experienced petting?" 605 out of 2,314 definite answers by boys were "yes" (26.1 percent, compared with 20.8 percent in 1974) and 538 out of 2,244 definite answers by girls were "yes" (23.8 percent, compared with 11.5 percent in 1974). As for petting experience, there is a noticeable increase among girls. As the cumulative percentage of the experienced shows in the tables, an increase starts to be seen among girls of around 15 and a rapid increase is seen from around age 19. Fifty percent of both boys and girls have experienced it by age 21.

Experience of Sexual Intercourse

To the question "Have you ever had sexual intercourse?" 451 out of 2,414 definite answers by boys were "yes" (18.7

percent, compared with 15.1 percent in 1974) and 316 out of 2,365 definite answers by girls were "yes" (13.4 percent, compared with 6.6 percent in 1974). The number of both experienced boys and experienced girls has increased compared to that of the last survey. As the cumulative percentage of the experienced shows in the tables, a gradual increase starts to be seen among both boys and girls around age 15, showing a trend toward rapid increase with age. Comparing the results of this survey with those of the 1974 survey, the percentage of experienced boys and experienced girls has increased, but there is a noticeable increase among girls, as was also seen in the experiences of kissing and petting. This tendency attests to a more aggressive attitude in girls today toward sexual activity.

Items Relating to Coital Behavior

The percentage of those who had their first coital experience with a partner of the same age has increased from 39.4 percent to 48.6 percent in boys, but is almost unchanged in girls, from 37.3 percent to 36.3 percent. Among those who answered about the marital status of the partners, the rates of those who first had intercourse with unmarried partners increased from 91.5 percent to 98.4 percent in boys and from 89.0 percent to 96.5 percent in girls.

The place where a boy's first sexual intercourse takes place is their own house in 23.4 percent and their partner's in 23.2 percent, both showing an increase from 16.1 percent and 17.1 percent in 1974. For girls, the first coitus occurs in their own house in 10.2 percent and in the partner's in 28.6 percent. The rate in the girl's own house increased from 8.5 percent in seven years, but the rate in their partner's has not changed significantly from 29.1 percent. The number of those whose first coitus occurred in the partner's apartment or boardinghouse increased in girls from 9.4 percent to 24.0 percent. The rate in hotels or inns has decreased from 23.9 percent to 11.8 percent for boys and 22.3 percent to 18.1 percent for girls.

At the time of their first intercourse, 98.3 percent of boys and 93.0 percent of girls have some knowledge about contraception, but only 73.6 percent of boys and 67.0 percent of girls among those who insist they have knowledge practiced contraception, although the rates are significantly higher than those of 1974, which were 60.2 percent of boys and 46.1 percent of girls. Condoms are most commonly used in the first coitus. Their rate among contraceptives is 78.8 percent for boys and 71.4 percent for girls, which is almost the same as in 1974.

DISCUSSION

The survey on sexual behavior of Japanese students conducted in 1981 reveals a marked activation of Japanese adolescents, especially girls. This is recognizable in those aged 18 years and over, when the young people finish high school. Recently the number of people who enter colleges or universities increased, for girls especially. After rigorous preparation for the entrance examinations, entering college is a release not only from the severe competition, but also from parental control, partly because many of the schools are located away from the parents' houses.

Secondly, there was a youth rebellion in the late 1960s to early 1970s similar to other industrialized countries. Women's liberation movements also flourished. The old moral authority has lost its power and parents have no confidence in moral issues. In addition, Japan has recently become more affluent than ever and consumer commercial advertisements and vulgar magazines are prevalent in society. The number of the young who have their own rooms or cars is increasing these days. This is reflected in the fact that the first sexual intercourse occurs more and more in their own rooms or in their partners', and less and less in hotels or inns. Of course, these are only some of the causes for the increased sexual activity of today's youth. It is difficult to explain fully.

SUMMARY OF THIS SURVEY

A comparison of the results of this survey with those of the previous one conducted seven years ago in 1974 produces the following conclusions:

1. In the area of physiological sexual growth (ejaculation, menstruation) in boys and girls, almost no difference is seen between the two studies.
2. In psychological sexual growth (interest in sex, desire to touch the opposite sex, sexual excitement, desire to kiss), an apparent difference is found between boys and girls, as was also seen in the previous survey.
3. In the development of sexual activity (masturbation, dating, kissing, petting, sexual intercourse), an apparent increase among both boys and girls is no-

ticed. There especially is a noticeable increase among girls. As a result, two phenomena, called "convergence phenomenon" and "surpassing (cross-over) phenomenon" are observed. The former indicates that the difference between the percentage of girls and boys who have experienced such activities is getting smaller; the latter indicates that the percentage of experienced girls surpasses that of boys.

The following are noticeable points drawn from this study:

1. *A slowing of the decrease in age of physiological sexual maturity.* The percentage of boys who experienced ejaculation for the first time and of girls who began menstruation is almost the same as the percentages of the previous study. As was pointed out in the 1960s, the phenomenon of sexual maturity growth seems to be slowing down.
2. *An increase in the experience of masturbation among both boys and girls.* Though the percentage of experienced boys and that of experienced girls is apparently different, an increase is seen among boys over 13 and among girls of all ages, especially those over 18.
3. *Girls surpass boys in dating experience.* Girls over 16 surpassed boys of the same age in the 1974 survey; the same result was seen this time.
4. *The rate of girls is approaching that of boys in the experience of kissing.* The percentage of experience increased among both boys and girls; especially noticeable was the increase among girls. The percentage of both experienced boys and experienced girls at age 19 reaches 50 percent. The percentage of experienced girls surpasses that of experienced boys at the age of 20 to 21.
5. *More than 50 percent of both boys and girls age 21 have experienced petting.* The percentage of experience increased among both boys and girls; especially there was a noticeable increase among girls. The percentage of both experienced boys and experienced girls at 21 is over 50 percent.
6. *A rapid increase in the experience of sexual intercourse among girls.* The percentage of experience increase among both boys and girls. As was also observed in the experiences of kissing and petting, the difference in the percentages of boys and girls who have experienced intercourse is getting smaller.

The late Prof. Shinich Asayama, who was in charge of the last survey, had expected both the "convergence phenomenon," that is, the number of girls who have experienced sexual activities approaching that of experienced boys; and the "surpassing (cross-over) phenomena," that is, girls surpassing boys in these activities. This survey proved these hypotheses.

NOTES

1. The Japanese Association for Sex Education, *Sexual Activity of Youth*. Tokyo: Shogakukan, 1974.
2. The Japanese Association for Sex Education, *Sexual Activity of Youth, Second Survey*. Tokyo: Shogakukan, 1981.

29

Female Genital Mutilation in Egypt

A. A. Khattab

The World Health Organization estimated that about 65 million women were subjected to "female circumcision" in Africa. It is a sexual custom dating from before the time of the Pharaohs in Egypt. It is also practiced in other countries such as the Sudan, Ethiopia, Somali, Chad, Nigeria, Thailand, Kenya, and Indonesia. The operation entails the removal of the clitoris and labia minora. The person performing the operation is usually an old woman, a barber, or a non-medically trained person (a local Daya). The operation is rarely performed by medical personnel.

The surgery is done without anesthesia or analgesia under primitive conditions, usually in secrecy. Typically, the procedure is done to groups of girls together whose ages range between five and eleven years old. A razor blade or kitchen knife (the knife of honor) is used in the Sudan. In Chad, a piece of glass is used. Complications are numerous. Immediate complications include hemorrhage, shock, urinary retention, trauma to the urethra, vaginal introitus, sepsis, septicemia, tetanus, or bilateral salpingitis. Delayed complications include obstetrical delay of stage II of labor, perineal tears and post-partum hemorrhage, vesico-vaginal fistulae. Other medical complications include keloid formation, cysts, painful neuroma, tight introitus, dyspareunia, and vaginal adhesions. The psychological trauma is severe with the event being difficult to forget. Numerous sexological problems may result from the excision of important erogenous tissues and the resulting

293

scar tissue and damage. Pain, bleeding, and nonhealing of the area may interfere with sexual performance. Sexual aversion and anorgasmia are frequently encountered in such women.

It is of note that nothing in Islam or Christian religion advocates the performance of this ritual.

30

The Erotic Appeal
of the Female Breasts

A. Marlinata

THE EROTIC APPEAL OF THE FEMALE BREASTS

Mammary glands are the main characteristic of mammals.
They always serve as nutritive organs and nothing more.
For human beings this organ has also an erotic function,
not excepted in our South East Asian country, bordering
the Pacific. An analysis of what role the breasts play in
our sexual life and why they are so thrilling has been
made.

INTRODUCTION

One of the most important functions of life is reproduction.
To achieve this there must be a libido—a desire for sex
—of two opposite sexes. Hormones play an important role,
like the pheromones do in animals, to stimulate the libido.
The sense organs, too, add a lot to enhance the sexual
desire.

   The part of a woman's body which is capable of pro-
voking sexual arousal in men alters with time in history,
and differs from one country to another. Even within the
same population, the variation is significant.

   To get an idea of which part of the body is the most
attractive and why it is, hundreds of Indonesian males have
been studied; especially their erotic response to the young
adult female breasts, which in our language are euphemis-

tically called "treasures" of a woman, apples, coconuts, pomegranates, guavas and so on.

MATERIALS AND METHODS

Seven hundred and twenty-four male Indonesians, ages 18–25, were observed and studied by way of questionnaires. They were recruits of a police school and university students coming from all parts of Indonesia with different religions and customs—anthropologically, a melting pot of Malay, Mongol, Melanesia, and European origin. The research was done between 1976 and 1982.

Another study revealed that the conical breast is the most stimulating compared to the hemispheric, while the discoid form is regarded as infantile and the elongated breast considered as least appealing and even evil and demonic in Bali, where the appreciation of art and beauty is deep rooted.

TABLE 30-1. Which Organ Has the Strongest Erotic Appeal?

Anatomic Area	% Erotic Appeal	
	Recruits n = 513	Univ. Stud. n = 211
Breasts	81.7	97.2
Genitals	68.7	27.0
Thighs	56.2	33.6
Buttocks	35.1	4.7

TABLE 30-2. Which Sense Organ Stimulates Most?

Sense	% Most Exciting Stimulation	
	Recruits	Univ. Stud.
Visual	44.8	30.6
Tactile	51.4	58.2
Others	3.8	11.2

TABLE 30-3. Percent Breast Type of Indonesian Women

Discoid	14
Hemispheric	64
Conic	20
Elongated	2

DISCUSSION

The difference in perception among recruits and university students was due to educational and regional differences: police schoolmates have only finished nine years of elementary school while university students have passed high schools and a few years of university studies.

The first group came from villages and has a social level lower than the latter, who came mostly from big cities and well-to-do families.

The genitals are considered less attractive caused by the tropical heat and religious tabu. The thighs are mostly uncovered and not typically feminine. The buttocks are not so smooth in hot areas and are regarded as unclean because of their location near the anal opening and are not considered a gender symbol. Nevertheless, 35 percent of the recruits liked the steatopygeal posture of a female.

In our culture, the breast was not always covered. Pictures from ancient times show barebreasted women but still the breast was an erotic organ, adored and admired. Sculptures on the Borobudur temple reveal barebreasted beauties seducing men. In some areas where women do not cover their breasts, these organs have no visual erotic attractiveness, but are certainly libido-arousing by tactile contact.

After the arrival of the Moslem and Christian religion, the breasts were covered, loosely in villages where public baths and feeding infants are daily sceneries; and more tightly in cities where the mere showing of part of them is considered offensive. The contemporary government prohibits any visibility of the breasts in movies, posters, advertisements, visual press media, and all public shows.

The reason why the breasts are so tantalizing in this country can be attributed to several theories:

1. Psychoanalytic theory

    Indonesian babies get mother's milk for a long period of time—up to 2-3 years for economic, handy, and recently birth control reasons.

    This milk-producing organ gives also warmth, intimacy, satisfaction, and safety and impresses the child so deeply that subconsciously it is looked for during later periods of life, even after 60! When bottle-fed, the baby is still placed near the warm safety of the breasts.

2. Sociocultural theory

    The tight laws against obscenity and the scrupulous covering of the breasts tickle the curiosity of young men and adults while imported books, magazines, videotapes, and films show the passionate breast-adoring people of other countries. Prostitutes seduce their customers by showing the bustline as in other countries. Covered protruding organs trigger male fantasies and initiate curiosity.

3. Substitution theory

    According to Desmond Morris, since the *homo sapiens* stands erect and hides the genitals and buttocks, the breasts substitute for the primary erotic organs, which are covered in all human cultures. As our olfactory, auditory, and gustatory senses play a lesser role in sex appeal than in animals, our visual and tactile senses become more sensitive. So looking at, and touching, erotic organs like breasts arouse strong excitement for sex.

4. Phylogenetic theory

    Some scientists think that the appeal of the female breast is instinctive in men, like the urge to hunt.

The mammary glands of mammals are used for nutrition only and these glands develop only during the functional period of life. Human mammae reach the full size after puberty regardless of its nutritive function. After all, its size is larger than it should be to fit the baby's need. Compared to mammary glands of other mammals, humans' are relatively the biggest! And the areola (enhancing the beauty) is typically human.

Furthermore, the human breasts have a strong connection to the sexual organs: they swell during the menstrual periods; they form a secondary sex characteristic, and they respond sexually when stimulated as if there is a "hot line."

CONCLUSIONS

Mammary glands, nutritive organs since the early mammals, become erotic organs too in human beings. This appeal is enhanced by several psychoanalytic, sociocultural, evolutional, and phylogenetic factors.

Indonesian men, like most men from other parts of the world, consider these organs appealing. Big-bosomed stars from Hollywood and Italy are adored. Covering, scrupulous laws, mutilation, religious suppression, hiding, neglecting in decent conversation, are all preventive measures against sexual arousal and confirm the erotic appeal of the female breasts.

Booming practices of plastic surgeons and promotion by traditional medicine to beautify the breasts, are proofs of the erotic value of the "treasures of women."

Admiration of the breasts in men's magazines and in art, poetry and prose, sculptures and paintings, songs, and performances exaggerate the erotic appeal of the female breasts. Exploitation in advertisements, pornography, show-business and industry, confirm it. Will genetic selection create females with bigger mammae in the future? It is a probability.

In response to the "new ideal of beauty" (the sportsgirl) many men still are longing for the old-fashioned feminine image of lovely, beautiful, soft, warm, rounded, voluptuous, and tantalizing breasts.

NOTES

1. Morris, Desmond. *Intimate Behaviour.* New York: Bantam Books, 1977.

2. Morris, Desmond. *The Naked Ape.* New York: Dell Books, 1978.

3. Van Vloten-Elderinck, D.P.L. De sexueele Zeden in Woord en Beeld. Gebr.Graauw's Uitg My A'dam, 1978.

4. Weiss, E. *The Female Breast.* New York: Bantam Books, 1975.

5. Wilson, G., and D. Nias. *Liefdesgeheimen.* Amsterdam: Arbeiderspers, 1978.

6. Wilson, R. A. *The Book of the Breast.* Chicago: Playboy Press, 1976.

31

Rape in Germany

W. Kröhn and R. Wille

Worldwide discussion on social systems in East and West also incorporate the respective criminality which is clearly, and in places even dramatically, on the increase in almost all Western countries. Sexual offenses are an exception in the Federal Republic of Germany. According to both the absolute figures and the frequency figures, there is a remarkable constancy; in the case of nonviolent sexual offenses such as pedophilia and exhibitionism there is a decreasing tendency. Rape—that is, nonmarital coitus induced by force—has increased altogether over the last 20 years by only one percent per year in Germany, whereas there has been a slight, but still not dramatic increase in sexual assault, that is, sexual aggression without coital intention. Over the last ten years around 6,000 to 7,000 cases of rape per year and approximately 3,500 cases of sexual aggression have been reported. The 1980 frequency figures in the Federal Republic (that is rape offense charges per 100,000 inhabitants) have dropped to 10.8 compared with 11.5 in 1960, whereas over the same period in the United States they have tripled from 9.5 to 30.5. In spite of these obvious variations in criminal statistics, there has been a clear increase in West Germany in the sensitivity of the public, in particular of the women's movement, towards the violence of men against women. The number of rapes is regarded as an indicator of women's safety, just as the number of robberies is regarded as an indicator of public safety. Pertinent publications, however, and particularly those of the feminists, are rarely based on methodically secured investigation. Instead, they are based mostly on emotions and anger directed against the male-dominated structure of our social order, in particular the police and the judicial authorities. Nevertheless, a large number of publications issued since the beginning of the 1970s has brought home to the public the real repercussions of rape—the humiliation, the fears, and the androcentric reactions. The frequent ideological treatment of the subject has, however, led to extreme points of view and can contribute little to a realistic grasp of the complex problems. Prejudices and myths still reign, as well as the unreflected use of so-called legal rules-of-thumb in court.

In 1982, we conducted an empirical investigation and examined as thoroughly as possible all the cases of sexual aggression, that is, rape and sexual assault, reported in the county court district of Kiel. This investigation covered the person of the offender and the victim, as well as official reactions from the moment the court case was opened, right up until it was finally closed. We tried to combine the complete survey of a criminological field investigation with the individuality of a psychopathological-sexual-medical case investigation, so as to put ourselves in a position to provide representative evidence on the criminological features as well as on the motivation and personality structure of the offender and the reactions of the victim. Our methods of investigation included participatory observation of the victim from the moment the charge was reported to the police, as well as the recording of subsequent reactions one, three, six and twelve months after the offense. With this empirical approach we wanted to test the traditional stereotyped ideas against reality.

Our investigation material comprises

4	false charges	
114	cases of rape	with 119 offenders
	of which:	
	67 attempted	
	47 accomplished	

40	cases of sexual assault	with 28 offenders
	of which:	
	8 attempted	
	32 accomplished	

This adds up to a total of 154 sexual crimes of violence with 147 offenders.

Only those details of our preliminary results will be discussed which serve to refute or at least partially correct misconceptions.

MISCONCEPTION

Frequent False Charges because of Disappointment in Love or to Cover up Own Misdemeanors

False charges were rare. We found four cases in which women reporting rape admitted that the charges were false after proceedings had been initiated. In only one case, however, was it a false charge against a real person. In the other three cases the offender was fictitious. Rape is not, therefore, an offense with a disturbing quota of false charges. We found it not to be true that many men are sent to prison because of female vengefulness or insidiousness.

REALITY

False charges are rare—about 3 percent.

MISCONCEPTION

Rape Is a Perfect Crime—Risk of Punishment Is Low (≤ 1 Percent)

The risk of punishment is not 1 percent but approximately 25 percent. The "dark field," that is the number of unreported rapes, must, however, be left out of consideration here. If we convert our 114 cases into percent, we have 67 offenders traced out of 100 reported offenses. In 30 cases, the proceedings are not even usually begun because of actual or alleged evidential problems. This means that 37 offenders are charged. Of these, 28 are sentenced, 22 for rape and 6 for sexual assault. Six offenders were acquitted; in three cases proceedings were suspended or the defendant was committed to a psychiatric clinic. Rape is not, therefore, the perfect crime.

REALITY

> Risk of punishment for rape
> n = 114 = 100%

100%	charges
67%	offender known
	30% case not opened
37%	indictment lodged
28%	sentenced
	of which:
	22% (rape)
	6% (sexual assault)
6%	acquittal
3%	case suspended or
	committal to psychiatric hospital

MISCONCEPTION

All Women Want to Be Raped

None of the women wanted to be raped. All of the victims firmly condemned the act of violence committed against them. Twenty-two percent showed an initial liking for the subsequent offender; only 6 percent, however, expressed any sense of guilt in having aided and abetted the offense, and then in the form of over-encouragement before the offense. Approximately 30 percent of the victims reproached themselves afterwards with the thought that they might have perhaps been able to prevent the offense if they had been more careful.

REALITY

All the women rejected the use of violence—30 percent self-reproach

MISCONCEPTION

Delayed Charge—Offense Doubtful

Seventy-five percent of our women reported the incident within six hours, a total of 95 percent within 24 hours.

Only in five percent of the victims could a later charge justify a certain element of doubt. There was, however, no evidence of a connection between time of reporting charge, credibility of the report or indeed misrepresentation. The time at which the charge was preferred was essentially determined by the completely different psychical reactions and ways in which the trauma was overcome. A later reporting of the offense was, however, often declared in court as an apparently clear indication of a story which was either inconclusive or invented.

REALITY

No correlation between moment of charge and credibility.

MISCONCEPTION

Only Sobbing Women Have Really Been Raped

Thirty-eight percent of the victims were calm and collected when reporting the offense and had no problem communicating with the police. This does not mean that these women were emotionally undisturbed; their outer appearance and psychical attitude, however, gave the impression of definite control.

Thirty-three percent of the victims were still suffering from the effects of the incident, cried, sobbed and often inserted self-reproach in their statements. In spite of their immediate involvement, these women could not grasp, or simply just did not want to believe that anything like this could happen to them, of all people. On the whole, their attitudes and treatment of the matter were convincing and conclusive.

Another group of 29 percent, on the other hand, showed a definite and, to say the least, apparently paradoxical behavioral disorder. The leading symptom of affective and emotional strain manifested itself in various ways. Some were irritable, abrupt and unfriendly. Some—at least part of the time—lost in thought, torpid and hardly responsive. Others relieved the strain by inappropriate laughter or giggling; still others were restless or distracted themselves with mechanical actions. In a total of four cases the questioning had to be suspended as the victim was not capable of dealing with the police questions. In none of the cases, however, was there a complete breakdown or anything approaching psychotic behavior.

Most of the victims, without distinction in all three groups, spoke of the fears they had just suffered, or even of mortal fear, often at the same time registering relief that nothing worse had happened to them. They predominantly described the humiliation, the binding of their will and their degradation as far worse than the sexual act as such. On the whole, there was no indication of any definite connection between the various acute reactions which the victims showed when reporting the offense and other parameters such as age, attempted or accomplished rape, severity of the circumstances, use of violence, length or intensity of the rape itself.

REALITY

Victims' demeanor at time of charge:

- 40 percent outwardly calm and collected;
- 30 percent crying or sobbing;
- 30 percent torpid, giggling, irritable, restless.

MISCONCEPTION

A Rape is Merely Forced Coitus and Therefore Harmless

We were in contact with 70 percent of the victims after one month and with 60 percent again after three and six months. After six months, approximately 50 percent were more or less asymptomatic.

The reverse case, however, is that the sexual aggression still had a sometimes considerable affect on 50 to 60 percent of the victims of rape months later and that this was by no means being overcome asymptomatically.

The wide variety of psychical symptoms was striking at the examination after one month, when a breach in the victims' day-to-day routine occurred. Alongside this there was a preponderance of all around anxiety and timidity, loss of confidence and mistrust, perplexed inner dialogues, and depressions. Of rather less impact, but by no means to be ignored, is the impairment of sexual activity.

Three months after the incident, there was, on the whole, evidence of a general regression right through the above-listed symptoms, although not of any particular turning point. Many women try to forget what they had gone through and no longer wish to be reminded of it. They experience more and more problems with their own value as a woman, a person, with the control over their own lives and bodies, with confidence in their own capabilities.

These complaints continued after six months in 10 percent of the victims, with accompanying depression and vague feelings of anxiety. The remaining symptoms further abated and there was a clear indication of a reorganized life-style and new psychic equilibrium. Nevertheless, it must be emphasized that even after six months, only 50 percent of those examined were free of symptoms. In other words, at least one-third of the total sample had not overcome the experience and still showed symptoms.

In the first analysis, there was no definite connection between the victims' acute reaction and the appearance of subsequent symptoms. Above all, it cannot be deduced that a calm and collected reaction in the acute situation automatically indicates a positive outcome. This may perhaps be explained by the fact that, although a calm and controlled attitude was maintained when the offense was reported, the victims gave the impression of being psychically drained and exhausted, submitted to questioning rather than actively giving evidence.

REALITY

Repercussions

Symptoms	1 month	3 months	6 months
none	43%	42%	49%
feeling of guilt	29%	11%	6%
breach in daily routine	42%	40%	36%
fears, distrust	28%	26%	22%
reactive depression	22%	21%	19%
suppression	16%	29%	26%
feelings of worthlessness	19%	28%	25%

MISCONCEPTION

Coarse Police Methods—Secondary Victimization

Fifty-eight percent of the rape cases made positive comments about their dealings with the police, 39 percent were neutral and only 3 percent criticized the form of the questioning. On the whole, the sex of the official questioners was less important than their sensitivity and tactfulness.

In about 30 percent of the cases, however, details of the crime which appeared relevant to the researcher were either not inquired about or inadequately recorded. Ten percent of the defending counsel based their strategy on these inexactitudes to impair the victims' credibility.

REALITY

Fair method of questioning but inadequate recording (about 30 percent).

MISCONCEPTION

Offender = Conquering Ladies' Man
Victim = Morally Accused

In a further 18 percent of the court proceedings, the offenders were made out to be "ladies' men" who, perhaps in the heat of passion, succumbed to the woman's charms. Altogether in about 30 percent, there was a tendency of guilt reversal, that is blaming the victim. Inevitably, this was seen by the victims as secondary victimization.

REALITY

Confirmed in about 30 percent of cases.

MISCONCEPTION

Rapists Are Mentally Sick

About 20 percent of the offenders were inhibited youths and young men, usually still without coital experience and with fundamental problems in paving the way for hetero-sexual contact. These had, as a rule, mentally anticipated the act. Alcohol usually played no part here.

In 30 percent, it was a matter of men who were otherwise well-adjusted and inconspicuous, usually uninhibited by a certain amount of alcohol. These men either had coital experience but were transitorily without partner or had a permanent relationship with a partner, which was not fully satisfactory. The most apparent feature in those offenders whose masculine role was insufficient were conflicts of dominance. They tried to compensate for their problems by subjugating the woman in rape.

The largest group of about 40 percent consisted of inconsiderate, uncontrollably aggressive offenders, often with a considerable criminal record. They were of undiscriminating character and usually maintained impersonal relations, mostly showing little affection. The brief interaction with the victim before the offense was therefore crudely purposeful and egocentric.

A maximum of 10 percent of our delinquents were psychically abnormal. These were characterized by particular biographical peculiarities, were asocial outsiders, neurotically or mentally disturbed.

The typical rapist in our investigation was not, therefore, mentally sick, but "terribly normal."

REALITY

Maximum 10 percent mentally abnormal.

PART VIII

Other Topics

The range of topics included in the World Congress was extensive. This section includes representative papers from a wide range of subjects. Gilbert Tordjman's paper was included because of its interesting hypothesis that female orgasm which is experienced as deep and visceral, may be mediated over different spinal pathways than so-called clitoral orgasms. The other two papers include a philosophical paper by Dr. Herman Musaph on pedophilia, and a presentation by Dr. Bernard Apfelbaum on professional sex films.

32

Pedophilia in a Changing World

H. Musaph

Definition: We call pedophilia the sexual behavior pattern characterized by a compulsive desire to have sex with sexually immature children. Mostly, pedophiliacs are not able to build up a lasting satisfactory sexual relationship with adults. In modern sexology we call pedophilia a "paraphilia." The pathognomonic characteristic of all the paraphilias is that, for a given individual, erotic arousal is dependent on the imagery, or an erotic fantasy that differs from that pertaining strictly to a consenting erotic partner of the opposite sex (Money 1977).

The question: "Is pedophilia a psychopathological behavior" depends on the culture pattern in which the pedophilic lives. In some cultures, pedophilic behavior is accepted as a kind of sexual gratification in men. It is noteworthy to state that we in Western Europe live in a changing world, especially concerning sexual morals. We do not know how we shall judge pedophilia in the nineties and in the next century.

In our country, there is a pedophilia lobby, consisting of sexual reformers, pretending that pedophilia itself is not harmful to the child, when there is a loving relationship between the adult and the child. It is their belief that the psychological injuries are especially caused by the parents, the police, and society as a whole, who condemn this sexual behavior pattern as sinful. They find in their research many cases of children with pedophilic contacts who deliberately give the statement that they enjoyed these contacts

313

and that in their opinion no harm at all is done. This is perhaps true, but can we generalize this statement? And what kind of defense mechanism is there at work? And is this research not very much biased by the fact that the research workers are pedophiliacs themselves?

Every human being has the right to experience his own sexual attitude in his own way. We make the restriction that making love will never be noxious to oneself and the partner. Noxious also concerns psychological harm or psychological injury.

We never know if pedophilic contact will be harmful or harmless in the near and distant futures, so every pedophilic contact carries a risk for the child. The question is: How can the pedophilic, who has the right to be different, experience his sexual gratification without incurring these risks? I am not able to solve this problem. I think pedophilics themselves have to answer this question.

But what is our task? Pedophilia in psychiatric practice puts us in a conflict situation. We worship the attitude of tolerance, knowing that everybody has the right to reach happiness in his or her personal life through the roads he or she must choose. Tolerance is not the same as anarchy. Tolerance has its boundaries.

In sexual behavior patterns, this tolerance can be expressed in the slogan: Nobody has the right to condemn sexual activities in all its varieties, except when this activity does harm the individual or the partner. Tolerance has everything to do with freedom.

We have to stimulate people in experiencing their sexual activities, whatever they may be, in freedom. Every legal inhibition in this respect is unbearable, including the fundamental rule just mentioned. For freedom has the same limits as tolerance. Studying sexual behavior different from ours, it is necessary to change our frame of reference from person to person, from tribe to tribe, from nation to nation.

There is not such thing as an absolute standard of sexual behavior. We have to judge sexual behavior within the following frame:

· *The culture pattern.* In North Africa there are societies in which pedophilia between males and young boys is accepted.
· *The psychological age.* In our culture pattern many young people show an experimental phase in their psychosexual development before adulthood. In this phase, promiscuity is more rule than exception.

- *The intrapsychical emotional situation.* So: compulsive masturbation can be the only source of comfort in an overwhelming emotional conflict situation.
- *The personality structure.* For example, exhibitionism in an adult is mostly a regression to a period in emotional development, in which a normal sexual gratification was experienced, mostly in the third or fourth year of life.
- *The environmental situation, especially the mothering and fathering.* We know that the harm done by a pedophilic relationship is very much dependant upon the way in which the child is taken care of afterwards (Keilson 1978; Renshaw 1982).

Conclusion: Never transfer a situation from one period to another, from one person to another. Every sexual behavior in all its intervariability, has a meaning, has a function and is human.

Psychoanalysts corroborate this view, knowing that a person can alter after solving his unbearable emotional conflict situation. And not only psychoanalysts have this experience. Every skilled psychotherapist, whatever his technique of choice may be, will agree with this statement.

Pedophilics and many sexual reformers make out a good case for their own theories, biased or not. Sometimes the pedophilic image is counterphobic. It once was negatively stigmatized and has now been positively eroticized. The danger here is a running away, especially when harmless experiences are generalized.

In this judgment, a libidinization of anxiety, of guilt as a defense mechanism can be traced. But everybody uses this defense mechanism, also independent of pedophilia.

To sum up: In our culture pattern, in a changing world, pedophilia is still an unsolved problem in modern sexology. We need sexual reformers to improve the social status of pedophilics. And we need sexologists to improve the psychological status of children, who are suffering from a complicated situation, in which pedophilic contact is a source.

NOTES

Money, J. *Paraphilias.* In *Handbook of Sexology,* Chapter 72, 925–28. J. Money and H. Musaph, eds. Amsterdam/New York: Excerpta Medica, 1977.

Keilson, H. *Sequentielle Traumatisierung bei Kindern.* Stuttgart: Enke Verlag, 1978.

Renshaw, D. C. *Incest.* Boston: Little, Brown, 1982.

33

Similarities of the Sexual Responses of Men and Women

G. Tordjman

Investigators have, for a long time, been impressed by the similarity of the male and female genital organs. Gallien confirmed that the male copulatory organs were, in some ways, only an exteriorization of the female organs. Ambroise Paré expressed the same idea in other words: "What the man has outside the woman has inside."

Recent French and foreign studies on female sexuality have confirmed this structural similarity and have led us to propose an original conception of the female sexual response. We are going to try and demonstrate that in the woman as in the man there are circuits of sexual response which may be combined by medullary and pelvic associative fibers.

We shall support this concept in five ways:

- embryological arguments;
- histological arguments;
- chemical arguments based on studies of male and female ejaculates;
- arguments drawn from the study of paraplegic men and women;
- sexological observations.

THE EMBRYOLOGICAL ARGUMENTS

One cannot help but be amazed by the anatomical similarities of the male and female genital organs. They differ

only by the absence of the uterus in the man. The morphological differences of the external genitalia are more apparent than real. Embryological findings help explain this
similarity of structure.

The Urinary Tract

In both sexes, at the stage of differentiation, the Wolffian
ducts open into the wall of the uro-genital sinus.

In both sexes, the vesico-urethral part of this sinus
gives rise to the bladder and the prostatic urethra, given
that the whole of the female urethra corresponds to the
male prostatic urethra.

The uro-genital part of this sinus develops, in the male,
to form the membranous or perineal urethra.

In the female, the inferior part of the Wolffian ducts
atrophy to form Gartner's ducts, which extend from the
broad ligament to the vaginal vestibule, along the lateral
walls of the uterus and vagina, parallel to the urethra
which lies on the roof of the vagina. These embryological
remnants can give rise to cysts of variable size.

The Prostate and the Peri-Urethral Glands

They are derived from the prostatic utricle from remnants
of Muller's ducts which form the superior four-fifths of the
vagina in the female.

In the middle of the third month, in the region of the
anastomosis of the ejaculatory ducts, the posterior wall of
the urethra forms numerous glandular diverticula in the
surrounding mesenchyma. They constitute in the male, the
prostate which surrounds the ejaculatory ducts and the
inferior part of the seminal vesicles; in the female, the
peri-urethral glands whose ducts are interlinked like so
many branches around the trunk of a tree.

The best known of these glands are Skene's glands,
whose author said when he discovered them in 1880: "I do
not know anything about these glands; perhaps the future
will enlighten us as to their function" [1].

Moreover, ethnology (William Ashan) has demonstrated
that, in certain species like rats and rabbits, the female
has an undeniable prostate, although smaller than that of
the male.

The glandular homology between the two sexes can be
taken further: Cowper's glands in the male have their
equivalent in the female: Bartholin's glands which open
inside the vestibule.

The Erectile Organs

They are the primary erogenous zones. Do they have the same structural similarity between males and females? In appearance, the differences seem fundamental; as early as the eleventh week of embryological life, the genital tubercle becomes elongated to form the penis in the male and the clitoris in the female.

While the penis is formed by two corpora cavernosa which form a gutter for the corpus spongiosum which expands distally to form the glans, the clitoris is only formed by two corpora cavernosa. The corpus spongiosum is missing. How can we explain this difference when the penis and the clitoris have the same origin?

In the male, as the penile urethra extends along the uro-genital gutter, a mesenchymal lamina derived from the uro-rectal septum (Tourneaux's perineal spur) supports it like a floor and then surrounds it to form the corpus spongiosum (Hoang-Ncoc-Minh) [2,3]. In the female, as the membranous urethra does not become elongated, this perineal genital spur stops at the level of the bladder neck.

Subsequently, with the elongation of the vagina, this spur stays trapped between the bladder trigone and the neck of the urethra, anteriorly, and the anterior wall of the vagina, posteriorly. In other words, this mesenchymal lamina, which constitutes "Halban's fascia, represents, during embryogenesis, the equivalent or the homologue of the corpus spongiosum.

In summary, the copulatory organs of both sexes are formed from two fundamental structures: in the male, the two corpora cavernosa and the corpus spongiosum with its terminal expansion, the glans, are all erectile tissues which constitute the penis; in the female, the two corpora cavernosa form the clitoris, which is independent of Halban's fascia, the embryological homologue of the corpus spongiosum.

THE HISTOLOGICAL ARGUMENTS

Halban's fascia is therefore the homologue of the corpus spongiosum. It is not really an erectile body, but a fibro-elastic tissue rich in vascular lacunae.

If the corpus spongiosum was completely erectile, the urethral lumen in the male would be effaced and occluded at the moment of erection: ejaculation would be difficult to say the least.

The histology of Halban's fascia has been described in detail by Hoang-Ncoc-Minh and his team at the Research

Centre at Amiens. From an operative specimen, they describe it as follows [2]:

> The anterior vaginal wall is much thicker than the posterior wall due to the presence of a highly vascular muscular connective tissue: Halban's fascia. Within this musculo-connective lamina, we find numerous strong, muscular arteries and a rich network of arterioles and capillaries.
>
> The nervous system is particularly well developed: most of the nerve fibers lie close to the large arteries. Here and there, some fibers end in pseudo-corpuscular terminals which could have the same significance as the Krause bodies or pleasure corpuscles of the male copulatory organ.
>
> Halban's fascia is separated from the vaginal mucosa by a rather large connective tissue space which is poor in vessels and which allows a non-haemorrhagic cleavage of the fascia.
>
> Within Halban's fascia, there is a glandular system derived from the prostatic utricle. It can be compared to a tree, from which a large number of mucous glands and ducts branch out. These glands and ducts open into the distal female urethra into one or other of Skene's glands, via a very small orifice. These peri-urethral glands have been known for a long time to be the equivalent of the female prostate.
>
> Various studies, including those of Zwi Hoch [4], Perry, Whipple and our own, describe Halban's fascia as the primary vaginal erogenous zone.

As early as 1950, Grafenberg [5] stressed the specifically erogenous sensitivity of the female urethra, its congestion during the sexual act, especially in the orgasmic phase and its ability to secrete a fluid. This area has therefore been justly named after him. However, as we have described above, the G point is not a point, but a much more diffuse zone, rich in elastic fibers, vascular lacunae, pleasure nerve endings, and mucous glands, which make it the equivalent of the corpus spongiosum in the male. It is therefore a major erogenous zone on the same level as the clitoris. Its histological structures seem to be able to explain certain features of the female sexual response:

• because of the presence of pleasure nerve endings, it represents a primary erogenous sensory zone, as demonstrated by prolonged stimulation of the G point.

Its erogenous function is only comparable to that of the clitoris;

* because of the presence of vascular lacunae, it undoubtedly plays a role in the process of vaginal lubrication which we know to be due to vascular transudation and not to glandular secretion;
* by the process of congestion of the G point, the periurethral glandular system, the equivalent of the female prostate, is involved in the process of female ejaculation.

THE CHEMICAL ARGUMENTS IN FAVOR OF FEMALE EJACULATE

Several years ago, at the same time as Perry and after several older authors, we rediscovered the reality of the "female ejaculate" [6,7]. Since then, the evidence from numerous consultants, from couples who did not dare come forward before, and from explicit films, confirms this: An abundant fluid is secreted by certain women in certain circumstances during orgasm.

Where does this fluid come from and what is it exactly? The methylene blue test quickly excludes a vesical origin. The persistence of this "ejaculation" after hysterectomy allows us to exclude the participation of the uterine endocervical glands, whose secretion, if it exists, remains very small. The argument that the product of ejaculation is identical to the lubrication transudate cannot be supported. The features of the lubrication fluid are entirely different from those of the colorless, odorless, non-viscous orgasmic fluid.

In fact, the fluid secreted by some women at the moment of orgasm is similar to that of vasectomized men. It is an odorless, colorless or slightly opaline, fluid which we have been able to analyze. Of course, it does not contain any spermatozoa, but it is rich in acid phosphatase (the mean of ten samples is 100 units/ml, while the mean in urine is between 0.10 and 0.15 units). However, we have not been able to demonstrate an elevated glucose level in comparison with urine, as was shown by Belzer, Perry and Whipple. The mean magnesium level was 90 mg/l and the mean calcium level was 120 mg/l.

All of these samples were taken after three days of coital abstinence. The woman, in a dorsal position with the legs folded, was stimulated by her partner, using two fingers in the area of the G point. The fluid secreted was collected in a test-tube.

Conclusions on Female Ejaculation

Clinical experience has discredited the myth that ejaculation is a male privilege. Some women, even if they are a minority, ejaculate a fluid at the moment of orgasm which has a composition similar to that of the prostatic fraction of male ejaculate.

The trigger zone for this orgasmic emission, according to the majority of women who experience this phenomenon, is situated on the anterior wall of the vagina, in relation to the peri-urethral glandular system which has been appropriately called the "female prostate" [8].

In all of the women examined, this erogenous zone corresponds to Halban's fascia. In response to stimulation, it becomes congested, corrugated, and firm. Its stimulation can be compared to prostatic massage in the male by rectal examination.

In many men, and not only homosexuals, rectal examination and prostatic massage provoke a pleasure which culminates in the discharge of prostatic fluid. The individual variations in this peri-urethral glandular system in rodents could explain the inconstancy of the ejaculation process in women.

It is reasonable to suppose that the volume of the female prostate, like that of the male prostate, depends on the levels of circulating androgenic hormones. The fact that this ejaculation is more frequent in lesbians could be explained, perhaps, by a hormonal factor and also by the fact that the G point is more accessible to digital stimulation than to rubbing by the penis.

ARGUMENTS DRAWN FROM THE STUDY
OF PARAPLEGIC MEN AND WOMEN

Without going into the details of the clinical experimentation, which would weigh down this discussion, we can state that the study of paraplegic men and women has convinced us of the similarity of the sexual responses of the two sexes.

There are three types of erection in paraplegic men, depending on the level of the spinal lesion: (1) A psychogenic or voluntary erection which is usually of brief duration and often accompanied by premature ejaculation. This implies integrity of the spinal cord above T10. (2) A reflex mechanical erection which occurs involuntarily in response to a stimulus applied to a zone below the lesion. It lasts for as long as the stimulus which has provoked it.

This implies integrity of the S2–S4 terminal medullary cone. However, if the lower limit of the lesion involves T12–L2, there is only an isolated erection of the corpora cavernosa. The corpus spongiosum does not swell and the glans has the appearance of a faded flower on top of the shaft. (3) A mixed erection is possible, combining a psychogenic erection with a reflex erection, which demonstrates the existence of spinal associative fibers between T12–L2 and S2–S4. Destruction of these fibers leads to a desynchronization of the two types of orgasm.

Male ejaculation is a complex phenomenon with reflex arcs organized at two levels: the emission of seminal fluid is controlled at the lumbar level (T12–L2); the ejection is controlled at the sacral level (S2–S4) as was described by Déjerine in 1914.

The lumbar arc is essential and is subject to various inputs: certain inhibitory inputs from lower segments and other facilitatory inputs from higher structures. In fact, the seminal emission which is organized by the thoraco-lumbar segments via pelvic sympathetic nerves which cross the hypogastric plexus, always tends to be premature. In physiological conditions, it is the sacral level which prevents premature ejaculation.

Thus, in the male, the terminal phase of the sexual act and therefore the orgasm phase requires: (a) participation of the thoraco-lumbar spine to ensure pre-ejaculatory erection of corpus spongiosum (T10–T12) as well as imminent seminal emission (T12–L2) via the pelvic orthosympathetic system; (b) participation of the sacral spine (S2–S4) to ensure erection of the corpora cavernosa and the possibility of real spurting ejaculation. The integration between these two spinal levels is no longer possible in paraplegics with a lumbar lesion, but it remains intact in cases with mid-thoracic lesions.

The Study of Paraplegic Women

This revealed two levels of spinal organization of the sexual response [9]:

1. The thoraco-lumbar level T12–L1–L2 (a) conditions the whole of the response of Halban's fascia, which has the same embryological origin and the same consistency as the corpus spongiosum in the male, and (b) maintains uterine contractions.
   • A lesion of these segments causes the erogenous sensitivity of the G point to disappear, abolishes all

uterine contraction, making Caesarian section imperative in the pregnant woman and abolishes female ejaculation because of the secretory impossibility of the peri-urethral glandular system.

- The external clitoral and vulval orgasm, as described by Masters, remains possible, provided the sacral medullary cone is conserved in its entirety. Thus, the following functions remain possible: reflex clitoral erections, vaginal lubrication, the contractions of the orgasmic platform (the pubo-coccygeus muscle which is responsible for these contractions is innervated by the internal pudendal nerve derived from S2–S3–S4).

2. The sacral medullary cone level of organization—S2–S4 —conditions the reflex arc of what we have called the external or clitorido-vulval orgasm, including:
   - the primary sensory zone consisting of the clitoris and the external genital organs, which implies the erection of the clitoral corpora cavernosa; and
   - the periodic muscular contractions of the orgasmic platform (which grossly corresponds to the anterior portion of the pubo-coccygeus muscle).

However, a lesion of the sacral medullary cone which does not involve the T12–L1–L2 segments should not affect: the erogenous sensitivity of the G point; the swelling of Halban's fascia; nor the thin secretion of the peri-urethral glands which is not under pressure.

In fact, two difficulties interfere with the study of the sexual response of paraplegic women: (1) The frequency of the autonomic hyper-reflexive syndrome as the lower limit of the lesion rises. This syndrome consists of headaches, a feeling of tightness in the chest, sweats, vomiting, and contractures of the levator ani which close the vagina and prevent coitus. (2) The frequency of the transfer of erogenous zones to areas above the lesion (the lips, breasts and so on) which are often experienced as pleasurable.

The two levels of spinal organization, thoraco-lumbar and sacral, are connected by spinal, and no doubt, pelvic associative fibers, via sympathetic and para-sympathetic fibers of the hypogastric plexus. They are connected to the higher cortical centers of the diencephalon and neoencephalon which modulate the peripheral erogenous messages. These connections explain how the two orgasms, external and deep, can occur together or sequentially and they can be combined in various ways.

This also helps explain Masters' theory that all female orgasms reproduce the same basic physiological responses and are accompanied by both pelvic beating of the orgasmic platform and regular uterine contractions. These two spinal reflex arcs explain why some women can give preference to the external clitorido-vulval orgasm or the deep uterine orgasm, depending on their past experience.

In the male, for whom ejaculation represents an ontological imperative to ensure the perpetuation of the species, these two circuits are usually activated sequentially and harmoniously. Not only is female ejaculation not derived from the same necessity, it has also been repressed inasmuch as it has been interpreted as being a pathological sign of urinary incontinence or excessive lubrication.

SEXOLOGICAL OBSERVATIONS

Clinical observation confirms the findings of these studies. Let us examine the female first.

Women capable of two types of orgasm are precise in their descriptions. They distinguish between the external clitorido-vulval orgasm provoked by direct stimulation of the clitoris and the vulval area or adjacent perineal regions, and the deep coital orgasm which involves the personality of the partner and a relational dimension.

These women are not mistaken: there is a definite difference between the sensations obtained from stimulation of the clitoris and those obtained from the G point. One is immediate, intense and punctual. The clitoral sensation rapidly becomes unpleasant, irritating, and painful if it is renewed after a period of masturbation which has led to orgasm. The pleasurable sensitivity of the G point, however, only appears after several minutes of stimulation after the urgent desire to urinate has disappeared. This zone is able to be stimulated repeatedly.

The two orgasmic reflexes, external and deep, do not have the same expression. To achieve the external clitorido-vulval orgasm, the woman focuses all of her attention on the clitoral inducer and makes her body stiff and immobile. She knows that the least distraction will result in failure of the orgasm. Prolonged, persistent, punctual clitoral stimulation eventually leads to involuntary and regular contractions of the vaginal platform.

This type of orgasm, well described by Masters, depends on contractions of the levator ani, whose rhythmic beatings are separated by 0.8 seconds. It is accompanied by tenting and shortening of the lower one-third of the vagina and ballooning of the deeper part which loses contact. In contrast, the deep coital orgasm can only be achieved by active coital movements which repeatedly stimulate Halban's fascia. It requires lumbo-sacral flexibility and an adjustment of the partners until the preferential erogenous zone is discovered (the G point).

Two positions favor the pressure of the glans on the G point: (1) the woman lying on her back, on the edge of the bed, with the thighs flexed and the legs in the air, the partner on his knees; penetration at 90 degrees is not very deep, which is appropriate, as the G point is not situated deeply; and (2) Andromachus' position: the woman leans backwards between the thighs of her partner to approximate her G point to the penis. To a lesser degree, the woman in genu-pectoral position may be favorable.

The deep orgasm is characterized by: (1) regular and undulating uterine contractions, which are spaced one second apart, as Fox was able to record in the security of his bedroom and which Masters was never able to demonstrate under the usual laboratory conditions; and (2) the absence of contractions of the orgasmic platform.

On the contrary, in such an orgasm which is often accompanied by ejaculation, the reaction seems to be exactly the opposite of the phenomenon of ballooning provoked by contraction of the orgasmic platform. The women describe this phenomenon as a pushing downwards; the finger or the penis which stimulates the G point is pushed out of the vagina. This is not a tenting effect, but an A-shaped effect, as it was described by Perry and Whipple [10,11].

The same situation applies in the male. It is a common error that there is one sort of pleasure in men, while in women it takes on a variety of aspects. A more detailed analysis reveals that the man, like the woman, experiences two types of sensation and orgasm which are organized at the two spinal levels (thoraco-lumbar and sacral) which we have described above.

He experiences external, superficial, irritating sensations in the corpora cavernosa and the glans, comparable to clitoral sensations. They are drained towards the sacral medullary cone: this is the penile orgasm. He also experiences deeper sensations in the corpus spongiosum, the prostate, the prostatic urethra and the verumontanum: these sensations are drained towards T12–L2 and constitute the seminal orgasm.

The erotic message is therefore delivered in two phases. (1) The first is that of orgasmic imminence. This is the plateau phase of orgasm involving the corpus spongiosum and the prostate. (2) The second phase corresponds to the expulsive orgasmic contractions: this is the high point of the orgasm and involves all of the muscles of the pelvic floor.

The Practical Implications

Recent advances in female sexual physiology may explain the pathogenesis of certain anorgasmic conditions:

1. Secondary post-partum anorgasmia, which is very common, could be due to a cystocele which distends the elastic, musculo-connective tissue fibers of Halban's fascia during labor.
2. Anorgasmia can occur in cases of retroversion, just as in cases of hypertrophic elongation of the cervix. In both cases, the cervix fills the antero-superior one-third of the vagina and prevents any rubbing of this area. In these cases, the genu-pectoral position may cause the cervix to fall away from the antero-superior part of the vagina.
3. We can also understand the importance of preserving Halban's fascia in operations for cure of cystocele.
4. A contraceptive diaphragm may either stimulate or neutralize Halban's fascia during coitus.

The understanding of female ejaculation has allowed us to refute certain myths. This female ejaculate, present in many women, was readily confused with urinary incontinence or excessive vaginal lubrication, or even pathological lubrication. All sorts of drugs and even surgery were prescribed to modify this "physiological state." It is possible that a number of women, ashamed of this orgasmic emission which they confused with a loss of urine, learned to repress their orgasm and to contain this fluid or to present a retrograde ejaculation into the bladder.

The discovery of the erogenous nature of Halban's fascia corresponding to the G point described by Grafenberg in 1950, allows a remarkable approach to the treatment of deep anorgasmias, whether of intra-personal, conflictual or cultural origin without supplanting the other psychotherapeutic modalities which should always be combined. The treatment of both physical and psychological causes of anorgasmia can be accelerated by demonstration and stimulation of the G point. This revelation can lead to the discovery or the remodelling of the deep orgasm.

328 / G. Tordjman

How Can the G Point Be Located?

The zone of Halban's fascia or the G point is palpable and varies from 0.75 to 3 cm in diameter. It is located at the junction of the bladder and the urethra, at the level of the anterior wall of the vagina, half-way between the posterior border of the symphysis pubis and the cerivix.

It is easily located in the course of bimanual vaginal examination, when the external hand meets the vaginal finger just above the pubic bone. In response to digital or penile stimulation, the G point can swell from the size of a small bead to become the size of a 5-franc piece. Its size and its sensitivity are extremely variable from one woman to another, but just as for the breasts and the nipples, the size is not proportional to the sensitivity.

The woman may have some difficulty in finding the G point herself. It is easier if she is sitting or squatting: she can then locate it with her middle finger curved. She may prefer to stimulate the area externally by circular, retropubic, abdominal pressure. Direct circular pressure on the urethral orifice, which becomes congested and more prominent, is often effective. This type of masturbation has been known for a long time and can now be better understood as a result of recent anatomical and histological findings.

CONCLUSIONS

Thus, we can formulate three conclusions:

1. There are two orgasmic, spinal, reflex arcs in the female. One is external, clitorido-vulval, depending on the S2–S3–S4 segments and derived from the sensory zones of the clitoris and the adjacent areas rich in pleasurable nerve endings. The orgasmic contractions occur in the orgasmic platform. The other is deep, visceral, involving a total abandon and depending on thorasco-lumbar segments T12–L1– L2.

The sensory focus of this reflex arc is reported by the majority of women who experience this type of orgasm to be on the anterior wall of the vagina, in relation to the peri-urethral glandular system which has been called the "female prostate."

We have examined the specific histological features of Halban's fascia which can be considered to be the homologue of the corpus spongiosum in the male. The contractions of this type of orgasm occur, above all, in the uterus and the peri-urethral glands. These two reflex arcs are connected by spinal and pelvic associative fibers which pass by the hypogastric plexus. We can understand, therefore, all of the possible inter-relations of the two types of orgasm which are even further modified by interference of encephalo-limbic and cortical centers.

2. A certain number of women emit a fluid at the moment of orgasm. This fluid is emitted mostly by the peri-urethral glandular system. Its chemical composition, rich in acid phosphatase, is similar to that of prostatic fluid. It is possible that a transudate derived from the vascular lacunae of Halban's fascia during stimulation, is mixed with this glandular secretion.

3. The experience of deep orgasm and orgasmic ejaculation seem to be reinforced by appropriate exercises of the peri-vaginal and abdominal muscles. The peri-neometric study of Gragen's peri-vaginal muscles demonstrates a contractile force two or three times greater in women who have produced fluid during orgasm. This confirms Kegel's hypothesis which established a relationship between the strength of peri-vaginal muscles and sexual satisfaction.

NOTES

1. Skene, A. J. C.   The anatomy and pathology of two important glands of the female. *Am J Obst,* 1880, 13:265–70.

2. Hoang-Ncoc-Minh.   Similitude des organes copula-teurs mâles et femelles, une nouvelle conception embry-ologique. *Contraception, fertilité et sexualité,* 9, no. 4.

3. Hoang-Ncoc-Minh.   Rôle du Fascia de Halban dans la physiologie orgasmique féminine. *Cahiers de Sexologie clinique.*

4. Hoch, Zwi.   La zone sensorielle du´reflexe orgas-mique. *Les Cahiers de Sexologie clinique.*

5. Grafenberg E.   The role of urethra in female orgasm. *The International Journal of Sexology,* 1950, 3: 145–48.

6. Tordjman, G.   Nouvelles acquisitions dans´ l'etude des orgasmes féminins. *Contraception, fertilité et sexualité,* 1979, 7.

7. Tordjman, G.   Pour une meilleurs comprehension des orgasmes féminins. *Contraception, fertilité et sexu-*

alité, 1981, 9.

8. Sevely, J. L.. and J. W. Bennett. Concerning female ejaculation and female prostate. *J Sex Res,* 14/1/20.

9. Tordjman, G. New realities in the study of the female's orgasm. *Journal of Sex Education and Therapy,* 1980, 6:22–26.

10. Perry, J. D., and B. Whipple. "Multiple components of the female orgasm." In B. Graber, ed., *Circumvaginal musculature in sexual function.* S. Kreger, 1981, in press.

11. Perry, J. D. and B. Whipple. Pelvic muscle strength of female ejaculators: Evidence in support of a new theory of orgasm. *The Journal of Sex Research,* 17, no. 1:22–39.

34

Professional Sex Films Versus Sexual Reality

B. Apfelbaum

It has yet to be noted that all professional sex films share a common point of view. In fact, it is not at all clear that anyone has noticed that professional sex-film makers have a point of view.

I will first briefly suggest what distinguishes professional sex films from pornography. Then I will briefly say something about sexual reality. The body of this chapter will be devoted to descriptions from a revisionist film catalogue, a catalogue of sex films designed to remedy the deficiencies of the films presently available—a catalogue that expresses a contrasting point of view.

Although there may be a number of ways of differentiating sex films from pornography, what I find to be the essential distinguishing feature of the sex film is the casting of people who are already in established relationships. Perhaps what makes pornographic films most pornographic is the practice of having strangers engage in sexual contact.

The professional sex film aims to be a semi-documentary. It may be a free-form sexual encounter or it may be a couple doing a home assignment, but in either context the partners are not strangers to one another. The characters must be real and believable, because the professional sex-film maker wants to promote maximum identification of the audience with the figures in the film.

The goal of the pornographic film is to create sexual fantasies and the purpose is erotic arousal. The goal of the professional sex film is to create sexual reality and the purpose is reassurance. Seeing real people confirming and enhancing one another's sexuality is thought to be an effective way to liberate the viewer by showing how sex harms no one, is natural and easily available, and, above all, is not dirty. Professional sex films are thought to be an effective way to show people that their sexual fears and anxieties are groundless, irrational, and self-defeating.

What I want to argue is that the sexual reality found in professional sex films is a far cry from the sexual reality we all know, and that what it actually represents is a *denial* of sexual reality.

The people in sex films rarely have sex problems, and those they do have are easily solved. They always know what they want and they always ask for it with a smile, and they always get it with a smile. They are understanding and patient and never want more than their fair share. They also tend to have sex out-of-doors.

I remember a scene back in the early seventies in Berkeley. An especially zealous sex-missionary showed a series of professional sex films to a group of alienated and disaffected people from the Berkeley counter-culture. When it was over, one of the men, in commenting on one of the films, said that all he could identify with was "the pimples on the guy's back." In other words, he was oppressed by the film rather than liberated by it because he could not identify with the characters. The sexual reality they were trying to demonstrate had little of his own reality in it.

The best representation of sexual reality presently available in the professional literature is Masters and Johnson's (1979, 64–81) report of their observations of the sexual behavior of 307 committed heterosexual couples in the laboratory. Chosen for their freedom from sexual difficulties, these couples nonetheless revealed themselves to be just as constrained in sex as are the rest of us. For example, "there were many times when women were made physically uncomfortable by their husband's approaches to the breast." Although they admitted this to Masters and Johnson, on only three occasions did a woman ask her husband to be more gentle (out of thousands of observations) and no woman ever asked her husband to stop. The same problem arose over early and deep digital penetration of the vagina by their husbands, and the wives again endured their discomfort rather than puncture their husband's illusions. The most frequent complaint made to Masters and Johnson by the husbands was that their wives did not grasp the shaft of the penis tightly enough. Not one of the men had ever mentioned this to his wife.

Imagine a sex film based on these findings. Perhaps

titled *Endurance,* these normal (or better than normal) couples would be shown quietly suffering, afraid to say anything that might disturb their partner's concentration or might be taken as a slight.

Of course, all of us recoil from this side of sexual reality (with the possible exception of alienated literary minds), but it is this difficulty empathizing with our own and our partner's reality that creates all of our sexual difficulties. At least this is the ego-analytic formulation that forms the basis of my revisionist approach to sex films.

What would professional sex films look like that did represent reality? To answer this question I have produced a revisionist film catalogue, with the titles and descriptions of 11 films offered by Didjacome Films, Inc.

1. *The Latin Lover.* This film is based on a play that was popular in Rio de Janeiro in 1979. A married man has a sexual encounter while on a business trip. He contracts gonorrhea. When he returns his wife passionately demands sex. This puts him in a terrible dilemma. He cannot reveal his extramarital contact and he cannot reveal the fact that he has gonorrhea. On the other hand, what other good reason could he have for refusing sex with his wife? He has no alternative but to go ahead and infect her.

    In our modification of this plot, the wife does not want sex either, having contracted gonorrhea from *her* lover, but she thinks her husband wants her to act as though she is passionately desirous and so she feels she has no choice.

    We have also added a short film on to the end of *The Latin Lover* which shows how this man could easily have avoided sex with his wife. It is titled: *Pretending to be Drunk.* It also includes a section for those needing to refuse sex for extended periods; this section is called *Pretending to be an Alcoholic.*

2. *The Inquiring Finger.* This short film is based on a prototypic scene described by Van de Velde in his classic *Ideal Marriage* (1930, 167). He says that if in response to the inquiring hand, the female partner keeps her thighs together, the male partner should back off and retrace his steps. If, when he returns, he gains "access," he should use the inquiring finger to determine whether she is aroused. If she is dry, he should do clitoral stimulation until the inquiring finger comes up moist. The woman is simulated by a

lifelike rubber doll since this best illustrates the nature of the interaction.

3. *Conscientiousness.* This film is in two parts. Part I shows a couple in which the woman is doing manual stimulation of her partner's genitals. It requires over an hour for him to reach orgasm. In Part II we see a man performing oral sex continuously for over an hour, although he fails to induce the desired result. He is shown telling his partner that he enjoyed doing it anyway, and also trying to straighten out his neck. This is one of our least popular films.

4. *Getting There.* This film is designed for the teenage boy and is in three parts: (1) Getting to first base, (2) Getting to home plate, and (3) Popping out to the infield. This film is ideal for the teenage boy since he has to know how to get to home plate. This information is not relevant to the teenage girl since she *is* home plate.

5. *More Getting There.* This film was inspired by Alex Comfort's *Joy of Sex* (1972, 56). In it he advises that "each partner, moreover, should practice removing the clothes of the other sex without clumsiness or holdups, and preferably with one hand." In this film we see two partners removing each other's clothes with one hand, blindfolded, and under water.

6. *Honey, It Will Just Take a Minute.* This is another one of our most unpopular films. At bedtime a husband pleads with his wife for a quickie but she refuses. He argues that he has a big business deal the next day and if he is not up for it they will not be able to make their mortgage payments and may lose the old homestead.

   His wife argues that it has been only four days since the last time, and that he has always let her go for five. He then scales his demand down to 30 seconds of manual stimulation. She agrees on the condition that she can do it with her back turned.

   As it happens, 30 seconds is just short of the time he needs and he does not make it.

7. *Beyond Linda Lovelace.* As is well known, Linda Lovelace, in her recent book, *Inside Linda Lovelace* (1981), reveals that she did not want to make *Deep Throat* and, in fact, hated doing it, but only realized this two years later. In this fictionalized version, one that many women can identify with, she never realizes it.

8. *Afterglow, the New Climax.* This film shows how to prolong afterglow. A couple is shown enjoying afterglow

for six hours following intercourse and orgasm. This film was made by Andy Warhol.

9. *Sex is Communication.* This is one of our most practical films. It shows how sex is the best form of communication. A couple is shown communicating in sex, demonstrating the use of popular sex communications, such as "This feels good"; "This feels fantastic"; "This never felt so good"; "I love it"; "Oh, stop it's too much"; "Oh God, I'm coming"; and "Didja come?" This last example is, of course, the name of our film company.

10. *How to Ask for Sex.* In *The Sensuous Man* (1971, 124), "M" advises the man (he is the one who asks for sex) not to ask for sex directly since women are not ready yet. He suggests using a signal, like "turning off a light or two," or, "You might take off your shoes, sigh, and lie back on the couch." In this film, the husband follows this advice, but his wife appears not to notice. He then sneaks his shoes back on, once again taking them off, sighing, and lying back on the couch. After he repeats this several times, his wife makes a mental note to find an intimate moment in which to tell him that he should buy a new pair of shoes.

11. *The Advantages of Orgasm.* This true-to-life film exposes the way that a couple can have sex when neither of them desires it, although each thinks that the other wants it. She first touches him and he feels obliged to touch her back, which makes her feel the need to reassure him with a hug, which makes him feel compelled to reciprocate. As we follow this couple through foreplay and coitus, we see the advantage of orgasm, that is, male orgasm. It puts an end to the sex act.

Now, I am sure that the professional sex-film makers are well aware of these sexual realities, but they think that these are *distortions* of sex. They think that if people would only let go and be natural that all these distortions of sex would be eliminated. They are not alone in this belief. Few people think that what actually goes on in sex is the reality of sex. As I like to put it: "Sex is beautiful, it's just people that ruin it."

So with the intent of liberation, sex-film makers discredit the reality of the audience. Those who *are* able to make the hoped-for identification may enjoy the films. They are likely to be the same people who enjoy pornography.

However, it is the people who feel upstaged by the sex-film figures and who are oppressed by both pornographic films and professional sex films who are the ones we need to reach, and they may be in the majority.

I might add that these people are not likely to find fault with the films, only with themselves for not being able to be like the people in them.

NOTES

1. Comfort, A. *The Joy of Sex*. New York: Crown, 1972.
2. Lovelace, Linda. *Inside Linda Lovelace*. New York: Grove Press, 1981.
3. "M." *The Sensuous Man*. New York: Dell, 1971.
4. Van de Velde, T. H. *Ideal Marriage: Its Physiology and Technique*. New York: Random House, (1926) 1930.

35

Training Programs in Human Sexuality

B. Goldstein, D. Calderwood, K. D. George, J. J. Levy, P. Nijs, W. B. Pomeroy, and J. M. Reinisch

Overview: Training Programs in Human Sexuality
B. Goldstein

What constitutes a quality university education in the emerging field of sexology? The answer to this question will be complex and will reflect various meanings and perceptions of the terms quality, education, and sexology. It will also depend upon the goals of sexological education. A systematic survey and typology of sexology programs which may provide a quality education at the university and college level is not currently available. Several abstracts describing a sample of successful sexology programs, both national and international, are included in this chapter. The abstracts are distillations of the presentations given at the Sixth World Congress of Sexology by a panel entitled, *Sexology at the University Level.*

Each panelist was invited to give a 15 to 20 minute presentation describing the goals, priorities, and outcomes of his or her program in the academic and political context of the university or institutional environment. It was suggested that panelists provide data and information on the following additional areas of program development and maintenance: (1) student demand and the characteristics and numbers of students enrolled in each program, (2) methods of career planning and placement for students who complete their studies, (3) recommendations for a possible *core* or *basic* curriculum to be required of all students in sexology, (4) methods of bringing interdisciplinary faculty together for support and to discuss the development of goals and priorities, (5) minimum levels of audio-visual aids, library resources, and student and technical assistance necessary for efficient operation of a sexology program, (6) political ramifications of the program's establishment and maintenance including the pitfalls, difficulties, and successful routes through administrative review processes, and (7) methods of program evaluation and quality control.

The Human Sexuality Program at New York University
Deryck Calderwood

The educational model used at New York University provides the framework for our experiential methodology, our courses in specialization and internships, and international aspects of the program. The program provides attention to each of the four components of the SURE model: Self-evaluation, Unlearning, Relearning, and Exercise. The outcome for graduates is that, ideally, they will:

- Have a solid basic knowledge of the content in the field of sexuality, a system of access to specialized knowledge, ability to apply knowledge to professional practice and to make evaluative judgments as to the efficacy and utility of this knowledge.
- Have analyzed their attitudes and values so they may successfully integrate or separate personal concerns from professional functions, in order to effectively compartmentalize different aspects of personal and professional life and to be capable of selectively combining areas where constructive outcomes are possible.
- Have mastered leadership and facilitation skills, and to have demonstrated their ability to accept, understand, and empathize with those with whom they work and, in appropriate situations, to express assertively their position on sexual issues.

The Human Sexuality Program at
The University of Pennsylvania
Kenneth D. George

The Graduate School of Education at the University of Pennsylvania approved an M.S. and Ph.D. program in human sexuality in 1977. The major purpose of the program is to prepare educational professionals and researchers in the field of human sexuality to serve colleges, universities, graduate professional schools, social agencies, state Boards of Education, and school systems. The focus of the program is scholarship. Experiential education is used to support the learning that has occurred through readings, lectures, discussions, and research.

Ph.D. students begin the program in our introductory courses where they learn the basic concepts and become more comfortable with sensitive topics. Then the students move into the foundational courses where they acquire knowledge in the biological, psychological, historical, and anthropological areas that compose the core of this field.

The second phase of the program is centered around preparing the students to become effective educators through acquisition of a strong foundation in teaching models and curriculum theory. They then test these theories by planning, implementing, and evaluating an in-depth teaching situation at different levels with students of all ages in diverse, motivating, and appropriate modalities.

The final phase of the program begins with students examining the recent research literature in order to identify researchable areas of interest. After identification, students review the literature in that area and develop a dissertation proposal.

During 1982–83, approximately 300 undergraduate students took the introductory courses in human sexuality. At the same time, there were 30 Ph.D. students in the program. The program is in the fortunate position of growing, and the undergraduate tuition income is able to financially support the program and provide scholarship aid for the graduate students who come from a variety of disciplines. They are teachers, nurses, clergy, social workers, and counselors who have expressed a desire to be teachers and researchers in the field of human sexuality.

Sexology at San Francisco State University
Bernard Goldstein

A Human Sexuality Studies Program including an undergraduate minor of 23–26 semester units, a monthly faculty staff meeting, and a developing certificate program for professionals has been in operation for two years at San Francisco State University. The interdisciplinary minor provides an educational foundation for those students interested in going on to advanced levels of education in sex counseling, research, and teaching as well as for those who want only a better understanding of sexuality. The minor may be coupled with any major but is particularly useful in those fields where human services are provided. The general objectives of the minor are to provide basic knowledge of sexology and to help students develop an appreciation for the importance of different approaches and perspectives to a fuller understanding of human sexuality. Students are encouraged to examine the ways in which professionals investigate and collect data and how they go about generating new ideas. Ultimately, it is hoped that students will be more capable of critically analyzing reports in the scientific and popular media.

The minor curriculum is essentially interdisciplinary with a core requirement including courses dealing with the biological, psychological, social-cultural, and interpersonal aspects of sexuality. Students have some flexibility as to which specific courses in each area they may take, but all must have exposure to the fundamental perspectives of sexology. An introductory course provides an opportunity for students to meet most faculty in the program, and a colloquium presents recent advances in the field and allows for some integration of the perspectives. Electives may be chosen from ten emphases ranging from biology and behavior to variations in sexual expression. A special seminar on research methodology, data collection and analysis is available as an elective.

The teaching faculty of the program come from eleven departments and four schools within the University and is augmented by an adjunct professor from the Institute for Advanced Study of Human Sexuality. The program also maintains close ties with a student organization on campus that provides education and referral services in sexuality for peers.

Over the past four years, approximately 7,000 students were enrolled in 15 courses dealing with human sexuality. A survey conducted in 1979 indicated that 38 percent of the 457 students polled felt that a minor in human sexuality would be relevant to their career plans. As of Spring 1983, only 28 students are enrolled in the minor program, and 7 more are contemplating joining the program. Although sex courses continue to fill up, fewer students actually joined the minor than was indicated from the preliminary data on student demand. There are many possible reasons for this discrepancy among which we can cite the current political climate, the vagaries of the job market, and the newness of the program. Students in the minor are mostly women (69 percent), somewhat older than the average student at SFSU (27 years old), psychology majors, and more experienced in terms of marriage, divorce, cohab- itation, and bisexual relationships compared to students taking a sex class but not enrolled in the minor.

The Program of Sexology at
Université du Québec à Montréal
Joseph Josy Levy

The Université du Québec à Montréal (UQAM) is the young- est French university in Montréal and is affiliated with a network of universities scattered in the main cities of the province of Quebec. Its enrollment is around 20,000 part- time and full-time students, and it offers programs in many fields.

Sexology at UQAM started in 1969 as a minor (30 cred- its) for the B.S. in Education. In 1972, the minor was expanded and became a 60-credit major in sexology, and in 1978, a full three-year B.A. program (90 credits) was established. In 1980, a M.A. program (45 credits) was added, and a Ph.D. program is actually in preparation.

The three-year B.A. program offers two specializa- tions—one in sex education and the other in the field of sexology within the framework of social and health services. No emphasis in therapy is given at the B.A. level. Both programs deliver a B.A. in Sexology plus a teaching permit for those specializing in the sex education program. The program consists of 18 obligatory courses dealing with the fundamentals of sexology. The rest of the courses deal with the chosen field of intervention and probationary periods.

The two-year M.A. program also offers two specializa- tions—one in sex education and one in sex therapy and counseling. To be admitted into the sex counseling pro- gram, the students must have worked in therapy for at least one year and must also attend a few courses in psy- chology or sexology for a year.

Around 500 students are actually enrolled in the B.A. program and 80 in the M.A. program. Eighty percent of the students are women and 70 percent are full-time students. The students entering the program are chosen according to a set of criteria: results in previous studies, motivation for entering the field, and marks obtained in a three-hour examination where they must analyze a paper in sexology and answer a set of questions. For the M.A., a lengthy questionnaire is used to evaluate the students.

The fully autonomous Department of Sexology is interdis- ciplinary and involves 18 full-time professors (four women and 14 men) whose specialities cover the whole register of the field of sexology from philosophy to biology. They also do research in their different fields of interest. Furthermore, a group of professor researchers in clinical sexology is in charge of a program of research and a university clinic dealing with problems of sexual dysfunctions and gender identity.

As for the services, the University possesses a library and an audiovisual service dealing with sexological topics. They give an annual budget to the department to buy the material evaluated as being of teaching value.

The department and its program constitute an example of an original approach in sexology and show the possibility of developing an interdisciplinary endeavor in this field.

Training of Specialists in Family Sciences as Sexologists
Piet Nijs

Since 1961, the interacting "Institute of Familial and Sexological Sciences" of the University of Leuven (KUL) has been offering a postgraduate specialization in sexology. This program is only offered to people with a university diploma.

The more than 20 years of experience with this program indicates that the important clinical segment is strengthened by a two-year basic training in sexological sciences. The basic training program includes courses in cultural anthropology, familial sociology, psychology, sexual pedagogics, physiology of fertility, and bioethics. The clinical training includes education in sexual psychopathology, psychiatry, methods of psychotherapy, marriage counseling and therapy, nondirective psychotherapy, communication and sex therapy, and family planning and fertility control.

A one-year full-time training program in marriage counseling and therapy and communication therapy may be undertaken only after the above-mentioned basic theoretical studies have been completed. Training is under the auspices of the Department of Marriage and Family and the Communication Center and Clinic for Sexual Dysfunctions.

The experience of this program supports the following conclusions:

- Every sexologist needs basic studies on family sciences, since the family system remains a key system of sexuality.
- Every specialist in family sciences needs basic studies on sexological sciences, since the family system is also founded upon sexuality.

- Sex Therapy and Family Therapy are both specialization *after* basic psych-therapeutical training (on an individual and group-therapeutical level)
- Efficient modern family therapy and efficient new sex therapy both need a foundation in traditional psychotherapy.
- Modern infatuation with the new sex therapies, the abundance of family theapies, and the confabulation on sexology need interacting teaching and interdisciplinary research on a university level.

Since 1982, there is a one-year M.D. program, "Human Fertility and Sexology," offered for medical doctors.

The Institute for Advanced Study of Human Sexuality
Wardell B. Pomeroy

The Institute for Advanced Study of Human Sexuality opened formally in 1976. It is approved by the State of California to grant four degrees (Master of Human Sexuality, Doctor of Human Sexuality, Doctor of Education in Human Sexuality, Doctor of Philosophy in Human Sexuality). Similar to other graduate schools, it takes about two to four years to earn a doctorate and one to two years for a Master's degree. The Institute is accredited by The National Association of Private, Non-Traditional Schools and Colleges. In addition to the degree programs, the Institute offers a variety of programs leading to a certificate as sex therapist, sex counselor, or instructor/advisor of human sexuality. These courses take about 700 classroom hours and 700 hours of preparation.

A residency of two to three weeks every trimester is required except for our clinical programs where residence of five continuous months is necessary. Students in the clinical program spend a minimum of 100 client hours and 100 supervision hours to fulfill their course requirements. Five different supervisors are available. Every trimester, our Basic Lecture Series presents ten lectures by well-known experts in sexology and related fields. The series plus eight other courses are required for all students. A host of courses ranging from anatomy and physiology to massage to geriatrics and disability to sex therapy are available.

Currently, we have about 85 students with a wide variety of backgrounds. Most of them are mid-career professionals, mainly with Master's degrees and some with M.D. or Ph.D. degrees. Graduates find jobs in sex therapy, sex education, and sex research. Trained individuals are so scarce (our Institute is unique in the world) that, for the most part, our graduates have an easy time finding work in the sex field.

The Institute has a faculty well trained in sexology including specialists in history, sex therapy, childhood sexuality, and sexual minorities, women's issues, and sex research. It includes ten as resident faculty, 15 as consulting faculty and 13 as adjunct faculty.

The Kinsey Institute for Research in Sex, Gender, and Reproduction
June Machover Reinisch

This has been an exceptional year in the Institute's history. I was appointed Director of the Institute on August 1, 1982, the third person to hold the directorship since the Institute's founding in 1947. My work in the area of behavioral endocrinology and child development and my commitment to broadening the research interests of the Institute match well with the recommendations made by the University's review of the Institute in 1980 and its recommended goals for the Institute.

A number of other specific changes were made:

• The official name of the Institute was changed to "The Kinsey Institute for Research in Sex, Gender, and Reproduction" to reflect the Institute's expansion of research into biological, medical, and other scientific areas.
• A Scientific Advisory Board consisting of seven distinguished sex researchers was appointed and held its first meeting December 1982. The Board is charged with assisting the Institute in strengthening its research function.

The Institute conducts several types of activities simultaneously. These activities include research, grant and contract development, and maintenance of library facilities and collections of flat art, objects, films, and photographs dealing with human sexuality. The Institute also provides information, lectures, and sponsorships for appropriate programs both nationally and internationally.

The Institute's interdisciplinary minor program in Human Sexuality was first formally listed in the Graduate School Bulletin for the 1982 Fall Semester. Administered by Dr. Paul H. Gebhard, the minor has already attracted eight graduate level students. Dr. Gebhard also taught a required core course in the minor, "Basics of Human Sexuality."

Students at all levels of higher education may apply to use the collections for their academic work. This requires only a letter of sponsorship from a faculty member. The Information Service also assists students. Additionally, the staff conducts slide lectures and tours for academic and professional groups. In the preceding fiscal year, such events were offered to university classes in history, forensics, French literature, and library science, to list a few.

Index

About the Editors

Robert Taylor Segraves, M.D., Ph.D., is Associate Professor of Psychiatry at the University of Chicago, Director of Adult Psychiatry outpatient services, and Director of the Sexual Disorders and Behavioral Medicine subclinics. He is also the author of *Marital Therapy: A Combined Behavioral Psychodynamic Approach.*

Erwin J. Haeberle, Ph.D., Ed.D., is Director of Historical Research at the Institute for Advanced Study of Human Sexuality in San Francisco, California, and Adjunct Professor at San Francisco State University. He is also a Research Associate at The Kinsey Institute for Research in Sex, Gender and Reproduction, Indiana University, Bloomington, Indiana, and, in the fall and winter of 1983–84, he will be a visiting professor at the University of Kiel Medical School, Kiel, West Germany. Haeberle is also the author of a sexological textbook, *The Sex Atlas,* and of an illustrated booklet, *The Birth of Sexology,* which was distributed to the Congress participants as a gift from the city of Berlin and the West German government.